Complementary and Integrative Treatments
in Psychiatric Practice

Complementary and Integrative Treatments
in Psychiatric Practice

edited by

Patricia L. Gerbarg, M.D.
Philip R. Muskin, M.D., M.A.
Richard P. Brown, M.D.

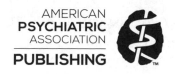

AMERICAN
PSYCHIATRIC
ASSOCIATION
PUBLISHING

If you wish to buy 50 or more copies of the same title, please go to www.appi.org/specialdiscounts for more information.

Copyright © 2017 American Psychiatric Association Publishing

ALL RIGHTS RESERVED

First Edition

Manufactured in the United States of America on acid-free paper
23   4

American Psychiatric Association Publishing
1000 Wilson Boulevard
Arlington, VA 22209-3901
www.appi.org

Library of Congress Cataloging-in-Publication Data
Names: Gerbarg, Patricia L., editor. | Muskin, Philip R., editor. | Brown, Richard P., editor | American Psychiatric Association, issuing body.
Title: Complementary and integrative treatments in psychiatric practice / edited by Patricia L. Gerbarg, Philip R. Muskin, Richard P. Brown.
Description: First edition. | Arlington, VA : American Psychiatric Association Publishing, [2017] | Includes bibliographical references and index.
Identifiers: LCCN 2017010071 (print) | LCCN 2017011850 (ebook) | ISBN 9781615371358 (eb) | ISBN 9781615370313 (pb : alk. paper)
Subjects: | MESH: Mental Disorders—therapy | Complementary Therapies | Integrative Medicine—methods
Classification: LCC RC480 (ebook) | LCC RC480 (print) | NLM WM 400 | DDC 616.89/1—dc23
LC record available at https://lccn.loc.gov/2017010071

British Library Cataloguing in Publication Data
A CIP record is available from the British Library.

Contents

I

Defining CAIM: Diagnoses, Target Symptoms, and Treatment Strategies

II
Nutrients in Psychiatric Care

III
Plant-Based Medicines

IV
Neurohormones

V
Mind-Body Practices

VI
Technologies

Contributors

Ryan Abbott, M.D., J.D., MTOM
Professor of Law and Health Sciences, University of Surrey School of Law, Guildford, United Kingdom; Adjunct Assistant Professor, Division of General Internal Medicine and Health Services Research, Department of Medicine, David Geffen School of Medicine at University of California, Los Angeles, Los Angeles, California

Shahin Akhondzadeh, Ph.D., F.B.Ph.S.
Professor of Clinical Neuroscience, Psychiatric Research Center, Roozbeh Hospital, Tehran University of Medical Sciences, Tehran, Iran

Jay D. Amsterdam, M.D.
Professor of Psychiatry and Director, Depression Research Unit, Department of Psychiatry, Perelman School of Medicine, University of Pennsylvania, Philadelphia, Pennsylvania

Acharya Balkrishna
Chairman, Patanjali Research Foundation, Haridwar, India

Timothy Barclay, Ph.D.
Associate Professor, Department of Psychology, Liberty University, Lynchburg, Virginia

Benjamin Barone, M.A.
Associate, Brain Wellness and Biofeedback Center of Washington, Bethesda, Maryland

Mark Blumenthal, Ph.D. (Honoris Causa)
Founder and Executive Director, American Botanical Council; Editor-in-Chief, *HerbalGram*; Director, ABC-AHP-NCNPR Botanical Adulterants Program, Austin, Texas

Teodoro Bottiglieri, Ph.D.
Program Director, Center of Metabolomics, Institute of Metabolic Disease, Baylor Research Institute, Dallas, Texas

Richard P. Brown, M.D.
Associate Clinical Professor of Psychiatry, Columbia University College of Physicians and Surgeons, New York, New York

Carlo Calabrese, N.D., M.P.H.
Affiliate Associate Professor, Department of Neurology, Oregon Health and Science University, and Visiting Research Professor, National College of Natural Medicine, Portland, Oregon

C. Sue Carter, Ph.D.
Director and Rudy Professor of Biology, Kinsey Institute, Indiana University, Bloomington, Indiana

Donald D. Chang, Ph.D.
M.D. candidate, School of Medicine, University of Queensland–Ochsner Clinical School, Brisbane, Queensland, Australia

Ka-Fai Chung, M.B.B.S., M.R.C.Psych.
Clinical Associate Professor, Department of Psychiatry, University of Hong Kong, Hong Kong SAR, China

Bruce J. Diamond, Ph.D., M.Ed.
Professor, Department of Psychology, and Director of the Neuropsychology, Cognitive and Clinical Neuroscience Lab, William Paterson University, Wayne, New Jersey

Mary Lee Esty, Ph.D.
President, Brain Wellness and Biofeedback Center of Washington, Bethesda, Maryland

Harris Eyre, Ph.D., M.B.B.S.
Honorary Research Fellow, Department of Psychiatry, University of Melbourne, Melbourne, Victoria, Australia

Lester G. Fehmi, Ph.D.
Director, Princeton Biofeedback Centre, Princeton, New Jersey

Patricia L. Gerbarg, M.D.
Assistant Clinical Professor of Psychiatry, New York Medical College, Valhalla, New York

Nigel Gericke, B.Sc. (Hons), M.B.B.Ch.
Director of Science, Nektium Pharma SL, Las Palmas de Gran Canaria, Spain

Olga Gericke, M.D., F.C.Psych.
Psychiatrist, Private Practice, Cape Town, South Africa

Bonnie J. Kaplan, Ph.D.
Professor Emeritus of Paediatrics, Cumming School of Medicine, University of Calgary, Calgary, Alberta, Canada

Melvin Kaplan, O.D.
Director, The Center for Visual Management, Tarrytown, New York

Ladan Kashani, M.D.
Associate Professor of Gynecology and Obstetrics, Infertility Ward, Arash Hospital, Tehran University of Medical Sciences, Tehran, Iran

Edward T. Kenny, M.D.
Faculty, The Columbia University Center for Psychoanalytic Training and Research, New York, New York

Daniel L. Kirsch, Ph.D.
President, American Institute of Stress, Fort Worth, Texas

Danusha Selva Kumar, B.A.
Research Coordinator, CASPIR, Northwell Health, Great Neck, and Feinstein Institute for Medical Research, Manhasset, New York

Helen Lavretsky, M.D., M.S.
Professor of Psychiatry and Director of Late-Life Mood, Stress and Wellness Research Program, Semel Institute for Neuroscience and Human Behavior, University of California, Los Angeles, Los Angeles, California

Kirk D. Little, Psy.D.
President, International Society for Neurofeedback and Research, Miami, Florida, and Little Psychological Services, PLLC, Florence, Kentucky

Joel F. Lubar, Ph.D., BCIA-EEG Senior Fellow, QEEG Diplomate
Professor Emeritus, University of Tennessee, Knoxville, Tennessee, and Past President of International Society for Neurofeedback and Research, Southeastern Neurofeedback Institute, Inc., Pompano Beach, Florida

William R. Marchand, M.D.
Chief of Psychiatry and Associate Chief of Mental Health, George E. Wahlen Veterans Affairs Medical Center, and Clinical Associate Professor, Department of Psychiatry, University of Utah School of Medicine, Salt Lake City, Utah

Jeff Marksberry, M.D.
Vice-President of Science and Education, Electromedical Products, Inc., Mineral Wells, Texas

Lila Massoumi, M.D., ABIHM
Assistant Clinical Professor of Psychiatry, Michigan State University, Detroit, Michigan

Amirhossein Modabbernia, M.D.
Postdoctoral Research Fellow, Department of Psychiatry, Icahn School of Medicine at Mount Sinai, New York, New York

Ashley Mondragon, B.A.
Lab Coordinator, Neuropsychology, Cognitive and Clinical Neuroscience Lab, Department of Psychology, William Paterson University, Wayne, New Jersey

Frederick Muench, Ph.D.
Director of Digital Health Interventions, Northwell Health, Great Neck, New York, and Associate Professor, Feinstein Institute for Medical Research, Manhasset, New York

Philip R. Muskin, M.D., M.A.
Professor of Psychiatry, Columbia University Medical Center, New York, New York

David V. Nelson, Ph.D.
Associate Professor of Psychology, Department of Psychology and Philosophy, Sam Houston State University, Huntsville, Texas

Chi-Un Pae, M.D., Ph.D.
Professor, Department of Psychiatry, Catholic University of Korea College of Medicine, Seoul, Republic of Korea, and Adjunct Professor, Department of Psychiatry and Behavioral Sciences, Duke University Medical Center, Durham, North Carolina

Alexander Panossian, Ph.D., D.Sci.
Science and Research Director, EuroPharma USA Inc., Green Bay, Wisconsin

Judith E. Pentz, M.D.
Assistant Professor, Department of Psychiatry, University of New Mexico, Albuquerque, New Mexico

Charles Popper, M.D.
Clinical Associate in Psychiatry, McLean Hospital, Belmont, Massachusetts, and Instructor in Psychiatry, Harvard Medical School, Boston, Massachusetts

Stephen W. Porges, Ph.D.
Distinguished University Scientist, Kinsey Institute, Indiana University, Bloomington, Indiana

Julia J. Rucklidge, Ph.D., C.Psych.
Professor of Clinical Psychology, Department of Psychology, University of Canterbury, Christchurch, New Zealand

Jerome Sarris, N.D., M.H.Sc., Ph.D.
Professor of Integrative Mental Health and Deputy Director, NICM, Western Sydney University, Sydney, New South Wales, Australia, and Honorary Principal Research Fellow, Department of Psychiatry, Melbourne University, Melbourne, Victoria, Australia

Jenna Saul, M.D., DFAACAP
Co-chair, AACAP Committee on Integrative Medicine; Clinical Assistant Professor, Medical College of Wisconsin, Wausau, Wisconsin; Child and Adolescent Psychiatry Consulting, Marshfield, Wisconsin

Susan B. Shor, L.C.S.W.
Executive Director, Princeton Biofeedback Centre, Princeton, New Jersey

Deborah R. Simkin, M.D., DFAACAP, Diplomat ABIHM, BCN
Co-chair, AACAP Committee on Integrative Medicine; Clinical Assistant Professor, Department of Psychiatry, Emory School of Medicine, Atlanta, Georgia; President, Attention, Memory and Cognition Center, Destin, Florida

Nilkamal Singh, M.Sc.
Scientist 'C', Patanjali Research Foundation, Haridwar, India

Dan J. Stein, Ph.D., FRCPC
Professor and Chair, Department of Psychiatry, University of Cape Town, Cape Town, South Africa

Shirley Telles, Ph.D.
Director, Patanjali Research Foundation, Haridwar, India

Robert W. Thatcher, Ph.D.
President, Applied Neuroscience, Neuroimaging Lab, Applied Neuroscience Research Institute, Seminole, Florida

Sheng-Min Wang, M.D., Ph.D.
Clinical Assistant Professor, International Health Care Center, Seoul St. Mary's Hospital, Catholic University of Korea, and Professor, Department of Psychiatry, Catholic University of Korea College of Medicine, Seoul, Republic of Korea

Michel Woodbury-Farina, M.D.
Associate Professor, University of Puerto Rico, San Juan, Puerto Rico

Wing-Fai Yeung, Ph.D., B.C.M.
Assistant Professor, School of Nursing, Hong Kong Polytechnic University, Hong Kong SAR, China

Disclosures

The following contributors to this book have indicated a financial interest in or other affiliation with a commercial supporter, a manufacturer of a commercial product, a provider of a commercial service, a nongovernmental organization, and/or a government agency, as listed below.

Mark Blumenthal, Ph.D. (Honoris Causa), is founder and executive director of the American Botanical Council (ABC) and editor-in-chief of *HerbalGram*, ABC's peer-reviewed journal (www.herbalgram.org).

Teodoro Bottiglieri, Ph.D., reports having been a member of the advisory board for Methylation Sciences Inc.; holding stock options on Methylation Sciences Inc.; serving as scientific advisor to Gnosis S.p.A. and Nestle Health Sciences, Pamlab Inc.; and having received research funding from Nestle Health Sciences, Pamlab Inc., distributor of B vitamins as a medical food.

Richard P. Brown, M.D., received grant support from NCCAM and is a research consultant for Humanetics, with future royalties on a patent for use of 7-Keto DHEA treatment for posttraumatic stress disorder; faculty member and speaker for Breath-Body-Mind at the Kripalu Center for Yoga & Health; and coauthor receiving royalties for various books, CDs, and DVDs on complementary and integrative medicine.

Patricia L. Gerbarg, M.D., received grant support from NCCAM and is a faculty member and speaker for Breath-Body-Mind at the Kripalu Center for Yoga & Health and coauthor receiving royalties for various books, CDs, and DVDs on complementary and integrative medicine.

Nigel Gericke, B.Sc. (Hons), M.B.B.Ch., is the Director, Medical and Scientific, of HG&H Pharmaceuticals, which has developed a standardized and clinically studied extract of *Sceletium tortuosum*.

Helen Lavretsky, M.D., M.S., reports research grants from Forest Research Institute, the Alzheimer's Research and Prevention Foundation, NCCIH/NIH, and NIMH/NIH.

Jeff Marksberry, M.D., reports having been a speaker for Pfizer and a clinical consultant with Electro-Medical Products International, Inc.

Alexander Panossian, Ph.D., D.Sci., is an independent contractor with the title Science and Research Director at EuroPharma USA, a company that markets herbal products, including *Rhodiola rosea*, ashwaganda, and other adaptogens. He conducts research on adaptogens but does not benefit from marketing of these products

Charles Popper, M.D., reports having been on the scientific advisory board for Hardy Nutritionals and a consultant for Truehope Nutritionals.

Jerome Sarris, N.D., M.H.Sc., Ph.D., is supported by a CR Roper Fellowship at the University of Melbourne.

Robert W. Thatcher, Ph.D., works for Applied Neuroscience, Inc.

The following contributors have indicated that they have no financial interests or other affiliations that represent or could appear to represent a competing interest with their contributions to this book:

Shahin Akhondzadeh, Ph.D., F.B.Ph.S.; Benjamin Barone, M.A.; Carlos Calabrese, N.D., M.P.H.; C. Sue Carter, Ph.D.; Ka-Fai Chung, M.B.B.S., M.R.C.Psych.; Bruce J. Diamond, Ph.D., M.Ed.; Mary Lee Esty, Ph.D.; Harris Eyre, Ph.D., M.B.B.S.; Olga Gericke, M.D., F.C.Psych.; Bonnie J. Kaplan, Ph.D.; Melvin Kaplan, O.D.; Danusha Selva Kumar, B.A.; Kirk D. Little, Psy.D.; Joel F. Lubar, Ph.D., BCIA-EEG Senior Fellow, QEEG Diplomate; William R. Marchand, M.D.; Lila Massoumi, M.D., ABIHM; Amirhossein Modabbernia, M.D.; Frederick Muench, Ph.D.; Philip R. Muskin, M.D., M.A.; David V. Nelson, Ph.D.; Chi-Un Pae, M.D., Ph.D.; Judith E. Pentz, M.D.; Stephen W. Porges, Ph.D.; Julia J. Rucklidge, Ph.D., C. Psych.; Jenna Saul, M.D., DFAACAP; Deborah R. Simkin, M.D., DFAACP, Diplomat ABIHM, BCN; Nilkamal Singh, M.Sc.; Shirley Telles, Ph.D.; Wing-Fai Yeung, Ph.D., B.C.M.

Preface

For this book, we invited an international group of experts, researchers, and clinicians to discuss their perspectives on scientific studies, treatment considerations, and future directions in complementary, alternative, and integrative medicine (CAIM). From an enormous and burgeoning body of preclinical and clinical research, various topics were chosen on the basis of therapeutic potential, strength of evidence, safety, clinical experience, geographical and cultural diversity, and public interest. We hope to provide enough information for clinicians to become interested in discovering more, developing confidence in prescribing, and learning how to make appropriate referrals for patients interested in a wider selection of treatment options. This includes knowing the evidence base, risks and benefits, guidelines for treatment, and informative resources.

In Chapter 1, the evolution of the concept of CAIM is recounted. In Chapter 2, flowcharts outline a decision-making process for prioritizing and combining CAIM treatments in five diagnostic categories: depressive disorders, anxiety disorders, trauma- and stressor-related disorders, bipolar disorders, and schizophrenia spectrum and other psychotic disorders. The chapter on CAIM in child and adolescent psychiatry showcases nutrition, equine therapy, art therapy, and neurotherapy, providing a glimpse into the diversity of approaches being used.

A broad range of therapies is represented in this volume. Lesser-known ancient herbs, including saffron from Persia, *Rhodiola* from Eurasia, *Bacopa* from South Asia, *Kava* from Polynesia, and *Sceletium* from Africa, are promising treatments for disorders of mood and cognitive function. Some have an extensive evidence base (e.g., S-adenosyl-L-methionine, St. John's wort, ginkgo, omega-3 fatty acids, acetyl-L-carnitine, and melatonin). Some that were once rejected by the medical establishment (e.g., neurotherapy and cranial electrotherapy stimulation) are now being studied and developed at medical centers. Mind-body practices, including yoga, qigong, and tai chi, that were on the fringe of health care for decades are now being embraced by clinics, hospitals, schools, and even the military.

Polyvagal theory, based on the evolution of the autonomic nervous system, sharpens the framework for understanding the vicissitudes of the social engagement network and defense systems. Through the polyvagal lens, we are better able to understand and study the effects of mind-body treatments, particularly therapeutic breathing practices, on stress response, trauma resolution, cognitive function, empathy, and connectedness.

We introduce two systems of treatment that are virtually unknown in psychiatric circles. Visual management therapy, by correcting disorders of visual processing, can improve symptoms of attention-deficit/hyperactivity disorder. Open Focus attention training, derived from neurofeedback and Zen and first developed for pain management, also offers relief from emotional pain and somatic symptoms. Chapter 29 presents digital health technologies.

There are clear data indicating that most clinicians are treating patients who are already using some form of CAIM. Data also indicate that many patients do not volunteer such information to their physicians. The onus is on the clinician to ask about CAIM use, preferably in a nonjudgmental manner that invites patients to fully share their experience and concerns. If the treatment has been helping the patient and is not causing adverse effects, then it can become part of an ongoing treatment plan. The clinician should try to verify that the products being used are reliable and free of toxic contaminants and check for potential interactions with prescribed medications. Simply consulting formularies is insufficient, particularly when they contain indiscriminate collections of in vitro cytochrome P450 testing (rarely validated by in vivo or human trials), poorly documented case reports, and extensive lists of "potential adverse interactions," most of which have never occurred and are highly unlikely to occur. The chapters in this volume provide a more clinically balanced perspective on interactions with drugs.

Patients who exhaust all conventional treatments and remain symptomatic may seek out CAIM approaches but may have difficulty deciding which are likely to be beneficial and safe. Most patients would prefer to consult their personal physician for advice. Others, who distrust prescription medications or who cannot afford them, may be open to trying supplements, nutrients, herbs, or mind-body practices. The clinician who becomes knowledgeable about complementary treatments will be better able to meet the patient's need for guidance, monitor CAIM trials, and integrate complementary treatments with conventional therapies.

Concerns about malpractice prevent many clinicians from recommending CAIM. Such risks can be mitigated by careful documentation of the reasons for the CAIM recommendation and disclosure to the patient of potential risks, benefits, and comparisons with conventional treatment options. It helps to keep in mind that most CAIM treatments are far less likely to cause adverse reactions than most of the medications we prescribe every day.

CAIM treatments have been viewed as an optional part of psychiatric care, but given the fact that more than 50% of psychiatric patients use them, they have become an unavoidable part of clinical practice. Disavowing CAIM because it was not taught during medical training or because one is not satisfied with the evidence base may not serve the patient's best interests. Professionals are obligated to become knowledgeable about all psychoactive substances their patients are taking, not only to prevent adverse interactions but, more importantly, to optimize and integrate all treatments that may enhance mental health outcomes and quality of life.

Patricia L. Gerbarg. M.D.
Richard P. Brown, M.D.
Philip R. Muskin, M.D., M.A.

SECTION I

Defining CAIM

Diagnoses, Target Symptoms, and Treatment Strategies

CHAPTER 1

The Growth of Complementary and Integrative Medicine

Lila Massoumi, M.D., ABIHM

Definitions and Historical Contexts

This chapter traces the evolution of the concepts of *complementary* and *integrative medicine* and their relationship to conventional medicine. *Conventional medicine* encompasses those healing philosophies and practices taught extensively at medical schools and/or that meet the requirements of the generally accepted standard of care within a specific country. It is the practice of medicine by the dominant culture at the present time. One could argue that the standard of care in psychiatry involves a careful evaluation and treatment with medication, psychotherapies, behavioral and cognitive therapies, and/or certain electrotherapies.

The practice of medicine that falls outside the mainstream has been described by an evolving nomenclature, as evidenced by the name changes of the National Institutes of Health's (NIH's) center on nonpharmacological therapies. The NIH center, established in 1991, was initially named the Office of Alternative Medicine, whereby "alternative medicine" meant nonmainstream practices *in place of* conventional medicine. In 1998, the center changed its name to the National Center for Complementary and Alternative Medicine (NCCAM), whereby "complementary" meant nonmainstream practices used *in addition to* conventional medicine. In 2014, NCCAM became the National Center for Complementary and Integrative Health (NCCIH). *Integrative health* or *integrative medicine* denotes nonmainstream practices integrated with conventional medicine practices, with the physician as provider or coordinator. The following terms are currently in use: *complementary and alternative medicine* (CAM), *integrative medicine* (IM), and *complementary, alternative, and integrative medicine* (CAIM). Integrative medicine should not be confused with integrated medicine. *Integrated medicine/care* is the integration of primary care and behavioral health care at the time of the patient's appointment with the primary care doctor, whereby the patient perceives the behavioral health component to be a routine part of general medical care. In contrast, with the collaborative care model, the patient perceives behavioral health care as a separate service by a mental health specialist who collaborates with the primary care doctor. Psychiatrists who use CAIM sometimes refer to their field as *integrative psychiatry* or *integrative medicine in psychiatry*.

CAIM Treatments

Whether a given treatment or conceptual paradigm falls under conventional medicine or CAIM is not always clear-cut. As the evidence supporting a nonmainstream practice mounts, that practice can transition into the mainstream. The time course for a given therapy to acquire substantial evidence and become widely utilized has been estimated to be 15–20 years, per the science of "dissemination and implementation" (Green et al. 2009). CAIM treatments are diverse and lack a formalized taxonomy. The NCCAM classification system divides CAIM into five broad categories, although a given treatment may fall into more than one (Table 1–1).

TABLE 1–1. NCCAM categorization of CAIM modalities

Category	Examples of modalities
Whole medical systems	Traditional Chinese medicine, Ayurveda, homeopathy, naturopathy
Dietary supplements	Herbs, nutrients (e.g., vitamins, minerals, fish oil), probiotics
Mind-body medicine	Meditation, yoga, prayer, tai chi, qigong
Manipulative body-based practices	Massage, spinal manipulation (e.g., chiropractic, osteopathic)
Energy therapies	Reiki, therapeutic touch

Note. CAIM=complementary, alternative, and integrative medicine; NCCAM=National Center for Complementary and Alternative Medicine.

Clinically, it may be more useful to use the following three categories when educating patients about nonmedication treatments: supplements, lifestyle factors, and electromagnetic treatments (Table 1–2).

TABLE 1–2. Simplified categorization of CAIM modalities

Treatment	Description	Examples
Supplements	Substances available over the counter	Herbs, vitamins, minerals, fish oil, probiotics, nutraceuticals
Lifestyle factors	Behaviors under the patient's control that require a time commitment	Diet, exercise, mind-body practices, counseling, love and companionship, life purpose (including religion/spirituality)
Electromagnetic treatments	Use of electricity or magnetic fields to effect biological change	Cranial electrotherapy stimulation, neurofeedback, transcranial magnetic stimulation

Note. CAIM=complementary, alternative, and integrative medicine.

CAIM Practitioners

Clinicians who practice IM are characterized not only by their incorporation of non-mainstream therapies but also by philosophical tenets or values that guide treatment. These tenets include an emphasis on the long-term safety of treatments; the importance of the doctor-patient relationship; education and empowerment of the patient; defining health as "optimal wellness" as opposed to "absence of disease"; and prevention of chronic diseases by addressing lifestyle factors such as diet, exercise, and stress management. Although most of these tenets are fundamental to all fields of medical practice, the proponents of IM feel that in light of certain trends in modern medicine, we need to refocus on humanistic values.

CAIM Use Among Patients

One reliable source of data on CAIM usage in the United States is the National Health Interview Survey (NHIS) administered by the U.S. Census Bureau. The NHIS is given to approximately 35,000 adults annually, with interview questions about their personal and family members' health practices, representing approximately 100,000 persons. Findings from the last three data sets with questions about CAIM (2002, 2007, and 2012) consistently indicate that CAIM is used by approximately 33% of Americans (Clarke et al. 2015). As of 2012, supplements other than vitamins or minerals (e.g., fish oil) were used by 17% of the population (https://nccih.nih.gov/research/statistics/NHIS/2012/natural-products). The CAIM modality showing the most growth was yoga, increasing from 5% in 2002 to 9.5% in 2012 (Purohit et al. 2013).

Analysis of NHIS data from 2007 revealed that the presence of a neuropsychiatric symptom (e.g., anxiety, depression, insomnia/hypersomnia, headaches, memory, attention problems) increased the likelihood of CAIM use from 33% to 44% (Purohit et al. 2013). Similarly, a representative U.S. sample survey of 2,500 respondents noted that those with self-reported depression or anxiety had more than a 50% chance of using CAIM (Kessler et al. 2001). Among hospitalized psychiatric patients, 63% reported using CAIM (Elkins et al. 2005). Of particular significance to clinicians is the consistent finding across studies that most patients who use CAIM do not disclose such use to their psychiatrist.

Why Learn About CAIM?

The high prevalence of CAIM use in psychiatric populations (44%–63%) is one reason why psychiatrists who become educated about CAIM are better equipped to advise their patients. Knowledge of evidence-based CAIM treatments can benefit particular psychiatric populations, including patients with treatment-resistant disorders, medication-sensitive patients, patients taking conventional medications who require augmentation, geriatric patients, minority groups with unique pharmacogenetic profiles who may have been underrepresented in drug trials, children and adolescents, pregnant women, military special forces who might have biochemical differences, and depressed patients at risk for suicide attempts via drug overdose.

CAIM Controversies

CAIM has been criticized historically for lack of evidence for efficacy, safety, and supplement-drug interactions. The relatively smaller body of research is due in part to the high cost of clinical trials, which cannot be recovered in sales because most natural substances cannot be patented. Nonetheless, research into CAIM has grown exponentially in the past decade, most notably in the field of mind-body practices. Additionally, the NCCIH made the study of supplement-drug interactions one of its priorities and in 2015 established a Center of Excellence for Natural Product Drug Interaction Research at the University of Washington.

The Future of CAIM

The Academic Consortium for Integrative Medicine and Health—comprising universities and academic institutions that have integrative medicine centers—has increased in membership from 11 U.S. centers in 2002 to 56 in 2012. In 2013, board certification in integrative medicine was established through the American Board of Physician Specialties (ABPS). The ABPS is one of three national board certifying organizations for doctors of medicine (M.D.) and doctors of osteopathic medicine (D.O.). Although the ABPS is not as well known as the American Board of Medical Specialties or the American Osteopathic Association Bureau of Osteopathic Specialists, ABPS certification is a step toward establishing standards for the practice of integrative medicine.

KEY POINTS

- For nonmainstream therapies, the following terms are in current use: integrative medicine (IM), complementary and alternative medicine (CAM), and complementary, alternative, and integrative medicine (CAIM).

- IM, which combines mainstream and less conventional therapies, is guided by principles that include long-term safety of prescription medications, lifestyle factors, and prevention.

- The National Health Interview Survey data from 2002, 2007, and 2012 consistently show that CAM is used by 33% of the population. Estimates of use in psychiatric populations are higher.

- The number of CAM educational programs and treatment centers is growing in the United States, and board certification is available for physicians.

References

Clarke TC, Black LI, Stussman BJ, et al: Trends in the use of complementary health approaches among adults: United States, 2002–2012. Natl Health Stat Report Feb 10(79):1–16, 2015 25671660

Elkins G, Rajab MH, Marcus J: Complementary and alternative medicine use by psychiatric inpatients. Psychol Rep 96(1):163–166, 2005 15825920

Green LW, Ottoson JM, García C, Hiatt RA: Diffusion theory and knowledge dissemination, utilization, and integration in public health. Annu Rev Public Health 30:151–174, 2009 19705558

Kessler RC, Soukup J, Davis RB, et al: The use of complementary and alternative therapies to treat anxiety and depression in the United States. Am J Psychiatry 158(2):289–294, 2001 11156813

Purohit MP, Wells RE, Zafonte RD, et al: Neuropsychiatric symptoms and the use of complementary and alternative medicine. PM R 5(1):24–31, 2013 23098832

CHAPTER 2

Complementary and Integrative Medicine, DSM-5, and Clinical Decision Making

Patricia L. Gerbarg, M.D.

Richard P. Brown, M.D.

Philip R. Muskin, M.D., M.A.

Leave no stone unturned.

The Oracle of Delphi, Euripides, Heracleidae

Psychiatrists and consumers face a proliferation of complementary, alternative, and integrative medicine (CAIM) treatments. Assessing which of these approaches may be beneficial and safe is one challenge; deciding which CAIM treatments should be tried first and how to integrate them with conventional psychotropics is another. In this chapter, we take up these challenges by providing decision-making flowcharts for clinicians interested in offering patients a wider range of therapeutic options. Developing skills in CAIM is essential in treating patients who do not respond well to conventional treatments and in minimizing short- and long-term adverse effects of medication (Gerbarg and Brown 2016; Sarris et al. 2015).

The evidence base for many CAIM treatments is robust, but for others it is moderate or minimal. How far to expand one's repertoire of treatments to get patients well depends in part on each clinician's level of confidence in his or her ability to select and administer potentially efficacious treatments safely. In this book, we aim to equip clinicians with the information necessary for providing CAIM treatments or for referring patients to practitioners who have that expertise. CAIM strategies for five of the major DSM-5 (American Psychiatric Association 2013) categories of disorders will be proposed: depressive disorders, anxiety disorders, trauma- and stressor-related disorders, bipolar disorders, and schizophrenia spectrum and other psychotic disorders. Detailed information on each treatment is provided in the CAIM-specific chapters that follow. The proposed decision-making flowcharts offer guidelines for clinical decision making based on research evidence, traditional use, and the clinical experience of the authors in treating complex cases for more than 30 years. In general, treatments that should be tried first appear at the top of each list toward the left, with further augmentations moving down in order and to the right, depending on likelihood of response. A layering approach, wherein addition of each CAIM treatment incrementally increases response, can cumulatively yield better outcomes. These flowcharts are not the only approach; rather, they are a starting point from which clinicians can develop CAIM treatments on the basis of their professional experience and the needs of patients in their practices.

Depressive Disorders

Clinical trials of antidepressant medications indicate that less than 30% of depressed patients achieve full remission within 8 weeks (Thase 2003), about 30% are partial responders, and 30% are nonresponders (Baghai et al. 2006). Many discontinue antidepressants because of side effects. Three-year nonadherence rates as high as 75% have been documented among patients taking antidepressants (Bambauer et al. 2006). In comparison, CAIM treatments have fewer side effects and can be used to reduce side effects from prescription psychotropics (Brown et al. 2009). Because residual symptoms are associated with increased risk of relapse (Fava 2006), CAIM approaches are indicated for patients whose depression does not remit after optimal antidepressant trials, switching, combining treatments, and addressing comorbid psychiatric or medical disorders. Antidepressants alone do not necessarily counteract the multiple dysfunctions in neural circuits and neuroendocrine systems affecting depressive symptomatology (Culpepper et al. 2015). CAIM treatments bring different mechanisms of action to bear on complex dysfunctions that are not corrected by antidepressant drugs designed to target one or two neurotransmitters.

As with any treatment decision, the choice of CAIM for patients with depressive disorders takes into account target symptoms, responses and adverse reactions to previous treatments, comorbid conditions, current medications, patient preferences, cultural issues, and cost. The following decision-making flowchart outlines a clinical decision-making process (see Figure 2–1).

When a patient reports partial response to any treatment, it is important to assess the degree of improvement and the nature of the residual symptoms. Rather than administering a standardized test during each office visit, a simple method is to ask the patient the percentage improvement in depression. Patients can learn to estimate mild (10%–25%), moderate (26%–69%), or substantial (70%–95%) improvement and remission (96%–100%). This provides a means to assess target symptoms and re-

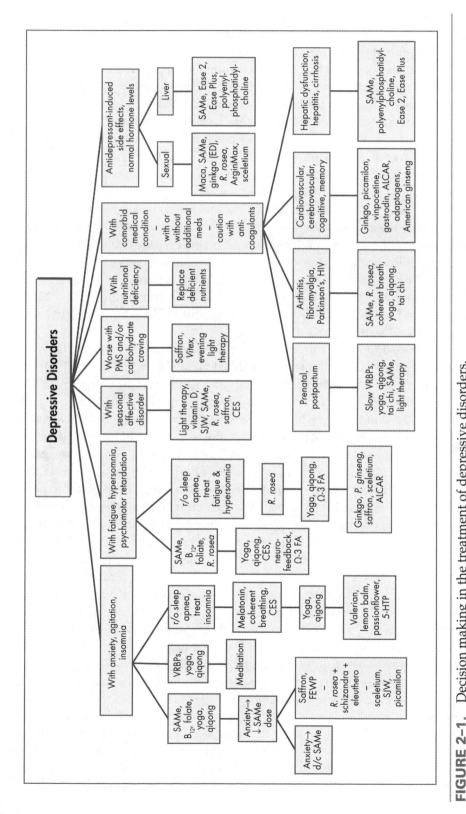

FIGURE 2–1. Decision making in the treatment of depressive disorders.

ALCAR=Acetyl-L-carnitine; CES=cranial electrotherapy stimulation; ED=erectile dysfunction; FA=fatty acid; FEWP=Free and Easy Wanderer Plus; 5-HTP=5-hydroxytryptophan; PMS=premenstrual syndrome; r/o=rule out; SAMe=S-adenosylmethionine; SJW=St. John's wort; VRBPs=voluntarily regulated breathing practices.

sponses to subsequent trials. If the patient believes that the current antidepressant is providing even mild benefits and if the maximum tolerable dose has been reached, then it can be continued with an augmentation strategy.

Controlled studies document that significant numbers of patients who have partial response to antidepressants or whose antidepressants have lost their effectiveness can benefit from augmentation with S-adenosylmethionine (SAMe), and a subset improve with B vitamins and folate (Bottiglieri 2013) (see Chapter 4, "S-Adenosylmethionine"). These supplements safely combine with every class of antidepressant and have few side effects (Brown et al. 2009; Torta et al. 1988). SAMe can be a first-line antidepressant, monotherapy, or augmentation, with the following caveats: As is the case with other antidepressants, SAMe can trigger symptoms of mania in patients with bipolar disorder. In depressed patients with anxiety or insomnia, activation by SAMe may temporarily exacerbate these symptoms, necessitating the use of an anxiolytic or sedative hypnotic during the first 2 weeks until antidepressant effects are established. If anxiety persists, even after lowering the dose of SAMe, other treatment options would include saffron, Free and Easy Wanderer Plus, and ADAPT-232 (combination of *Rhodiola rosea*, *Schisandra chinensis*, and *Eleutherococcus senticosus*) (Ravindran and da Silva 2013). CAIM treatments for anxiety disorders can be helpful in depressed patients who manifest anxiety and insomnia (See Figure 2–2).

A heterogeneous literature supports multicomponent mind-body practices, including yoga, qigong, tai chi, voluntarily regulated breathing practices (VRBPs), and mindfulness, for alleviating depression, anxiety, and insomnia (see Chapters 21–25). The evidence base, mechanisms of action, and clinical applications for mind-body approaches are discussed in Chapters 20–25. Recent trends toward higher-quality studies and identification of specific components that are most effective will facilitate development of programs that have more impact, are less time-consuming, and are more easily integrated into conventional treatment settings. For example, a meta-analysis of randomized controlled trials of yoga for prenatal depression distinguished between physical exercise–based yoga and integrated yoga, which includes physical exercises, VRBPs (pranayama), meditation, or deep relaxation (Gong et al. 2015). Depression significantly decreased with integrated yoga (standardized mean difference [SMD], –0.79; confidence interval [CI], –1.07 to –0.51; $P<0.00001$) compared to physical exercise–based yoga (SMD, –0.41; CI, –1.01 to –0.18; $P=0.17$). Many studies of mind-body practices are carried out with elderly patients and those with medical illnesses such as cancer, multiple sclerosis, cardiovascular disease, or neurocognitive symptoms. Although these subjects may not carry a primary diagnosis of major depressive disorder, their symptoms of depression and anxiety can be improved by participation in mind-body programs. Therefore, such programs should be considered adjunctive treatments for patients with any depressive disorder. One challenge in prescribing mind-body treatments to depressed patients is their lack of motivation. Participation requires attending a regular class or using training DVDs at home. The patient must practice between 3 and 7 days per week to obtain benefits. Clinicians must educate and motivate patients and monitor compliance with mind-body practices.

Neurofeedback and brain stimulation technologies are useful in treating depression, anxiety, and sleep disorders. (See Chapter 26 on neurotherapy, Chapter 27 on

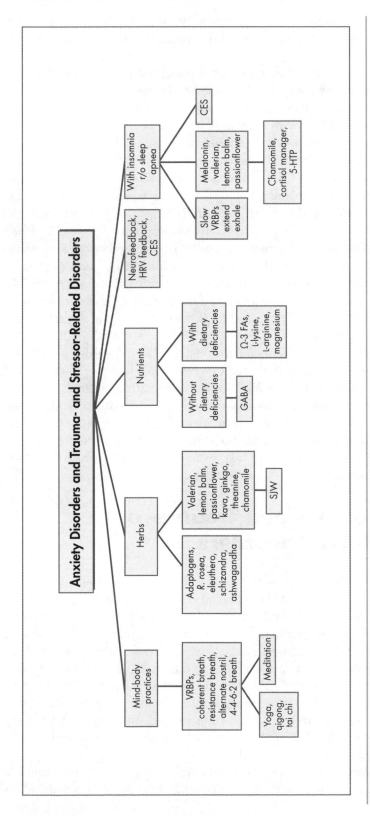

FIGURE 2–2. Decision making in the treatment of anxiety disorders.

CES=cranial electrotherapy stimulation; FA=fatty acid; GABA=γ-aminobutyric acid; 5-HTP=5-hydroxytryptophan; HRV=heart rate variability; r/o=rule out; SJW=St. John's wort; VRBP=voluntarily regulated breathing practice.

cranial electrotherapy stimulation, and Chapter 29 on technologies.) These approaches can be combined with pharmacotherapy, phytomedicines, nutrients, and mind-body practices.

In contrast to the anxious or agitated depressed patient, those with psychomotor retardation, hypersomnia, low energy, and fatigue need more activating treatments. SAMe, B vitamins, and folate constitute a reasonable first trial. If there are improvements on maximal doses of SAMe with vitamin B_{12} and folate but residual symptoms persist, then the adaptogenic herb *R. rosea* should be considered to increase mental and physical energy (see Chapter 8, "Adaptogens in Psychiatric Practice," and Chapter 9, "Integrating *Rhodiola rosea* in Clinical Practice"). *R. rosea* works well with SAMe and other antidepressants. Ginkgo and ginseng (*Panax ginseng* or Asian ginseng) can provide additional activation, and they are particularly helpful in patients with mild cognitive or memory decline (see Chapter 11, "*Ginkgo biloba*," and Chapter 13, "*Panax Ginseng* and American Ginseng in Psychiatric Practice"). Mind-body practices, particularly slow VRBPs, can rapidly reduce anxiety and insomnia (see Chapter 21, "Breathing Techniques in Psychiatric Treatments"). A careful history may reveal a seasonal component to the depression. If a trial of light therapy does not fully resolve the seasonal component, St. John's wort, SAMe, *R. rosea*, saffron, or cranial electrotherapy stimulation can be beneficial.

Although studies of antidepressants for major depressive disorder usually exclude patients with significant comorbid medical conditions, in the real world most psychiatrists find that patients with medical illnesses constitute a large portion of their practices. The stress of medical illness and medical treatments can cause or exacerbate depression. CAIM is particularly useful in such patients because they are at greater risk for adverse reactions to medications and medication interactions. Furthermore, many CAIM treatments used to treat psychiatric disorders also have therapeutic effects on medical conditions (see Chapter 4).

Anxiety Disorders and Trauma- or Stressor-Related Disorders

Multicomponent mind-body practices can be potentially beneficial in patients with any anxiety or stress-related disorder and should be an essential part of integrative treatments (see Figure 2–2 and Chapters 20–25). It is well worth the time and effort needed to convince patients to learn and maintain these practices. For mild anxiety or insomnia, herbs can be combined for additive effects: valerian, lemon balm, passionflower, theanine, and lavender. EGb 761, a special extract of ginkgo with anxiolytic effects in controlled trials, is particularly beneficial in elderly patients (Kasper 2015). Some patients benefit from less potent treatments, such as 5-hydroxytryptamine (5-HTP) and chamomile. For more severe anxiety and trauma-related disorders, adaptogenic herbs, particularly the ADAPT-232 combination of *R. rosea*, *S. chinensis*, and *E. senticosus*, are recommended (see Chapters 8 and 9).

In patients without dietary deficiencies, γ-aminobutyric acid (GABA) may be calming. Tests for dietary deficiencies will indicate if supplemental nutrients are needed. Neurofeedback and other technologies are useful additions to CAIM regiments for anxiety and insomnia (see Chapters 26, 27, and 29). Patients whose insomnia is not caused by physical problems, such as obstructive sleep apnea, often do well with melatonin (in doses up to 10 mg hs) and slow VRBPs with prolonged exhalation and resistance breathing (see Chapter 19, "Melatonin and Melatonin Analogues for Psychiatric Disorders," and Chapter 21).

Bipolar Disorders

CAIM can be used for treating bipolar disorders to augment mood stabilizers, reduce comorbid symptoms, and counteract medication side effects (see Figure 2–3). Using milder anxiolytic herbs, such as ashwagandha, lemon balm, and passionflower, reduces the risk of exacerbating hypomanic or manic symptoms. For persistent depression, trials of saffron, *S. chinensis*, *E. senticosus*, and traditional Chinese medicine, such as Free and Easy Wanderer Plus, can be of benefit (see Chapters 8, 15, and 16). Antipsychotic-induced side effects, such as extrapyramidal symptoms, can improve with *N*-acetylcysteine, vitamin B_6, and omega-3 fatty acids (Brown et al. 2009). Melatonin and other supplements listed in Figure 2–3 are worthwhile. Valproate-induced hepatotoxicity may respond to carnitine-pantothenic acid (Felker et al. 2014).

Schizophrenia Spectrum and Other Psychotic Disorders

Antipsychotic medication can be augmented with VRBPs, *N*-acetylcysteine, and ginkgo. Preliminary evidence suggests that slow VRBPs (e.g., coherent breathing) may improve social engagement and the ability to recognize facial emotional expressions (see Figure 2–4 and Chapter 21). Furthermore, *N*-acetylcysteine, vitamin B_6, omega-3 fatty acids, melatonin, dehydroepiandrosterone (DHEA), ginkgo, and *R. rosea* can reduce extrapyramidal symptoms. *R. rosea* and walking (while listening to music and doing slow VRBPs) can reduce fatigue and sedation.

Acupuncture

Clinical research supports the use of acupuncture for pain management, but evidence in psychiatric disorders is limited by methodological problems (Pilkington 2010, 2013). One systematic review concluded that acupuncture may be an effective add-on treatment for depression and, to a lesser degree, in schizophrenia (Bosch et al. 2015). Another systematic review and meta-analysis suggested that acupuncture combined with antidepressant medication may be more effective than selective serotonin reuptake inhibitor therapy alone and that it is safe and well tolerated over the first 6-week treatment period (Chan et al. 2015). A systematic review noted positive reports on acupuncture for generalized anxiety disorder and anxiety neurosis and limited evidence for auricular acupuncture in perioperative anxiety but overall found insufficient evidence for firm conclusions (Pilkington 2010). A review and meta-analysis could not

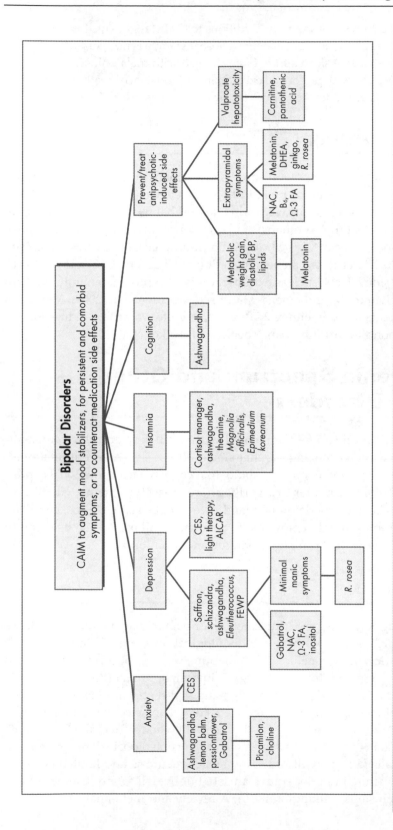

FIGURE 2–3.   Decision making in the treatment of bipolar disorders.

ALCAR=acetyl-L-carnitine; BP= blood pressure; CAIM=complementary, alternative, and integrative medicine; CES=cranial electrotherapy stimulation; DHEA=dehydroepiandrosterone; FA=fatty acid; FEWP=Free and Easy Wanderer Plus; NAC=N-acetylcysteine.

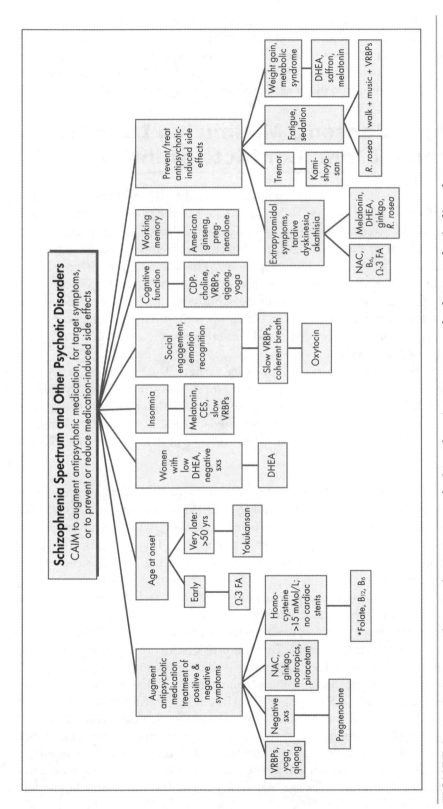

FIGURE 2–4. Decision making in the treatment of schizophrenia spectrum and other psychotic disorders.

CAIM=complementary, alternative, and integrative medicine; CES=cranial electrotherapy stimulation; DHEA=dehydroepiandrosterone; FA=fatty acid; mMol/L=micromoles per liter; NAC=*N*-acetylcysteine; sxs=symptoms; VRBPs=voluntarily regulated breathing practices.

*Folate, B12, and B6 should be given only to patients with no cardiac stents.

confirm that acupuncture was an effective treatment for psychological symptoms associated with opioid addiction (Boyuan et al. 2014). However, one randomized controlled trial (RCT) of laser acupuncture for neonatal abstinence syndrome found a significantly reduced duration of morphine therapy (Raith et al. 2015). All reviews called for more high-quality RCTs to evaluate the benefits and long-term effectiveness of acupuncture.

Informed Consent, Minimizing Liability, Malpractice, and Conflicts of Interest

Physician education includes learning how to empathically inform a patient and be confident that the individual has fully participated in the process of informed consent. This process is crucial to the patient-physician relationship and will minimize the liability risks of practicing medicine. As is true with conventional medical practice, developing a caring, consistent, responsive professional relationship with each patient and including the patient in decision making through informed consent are necessary to provide good care and minimize liability. No different from conventional medical practice, malpractice categories that apply to CAIM are misdiagnosis, failure to treat, failure of informed consent, fraud and misrepresentation, abandonment, vicarious liability, and breach of confidentiality.

Rules and regulations governing CAIM vary by state. The Federation of State Medical Boards (FSMB) provides model guidelines for CAIM (https://www.fsmb.org/Media/Default/PDF/FSMB/Advocacy/2002_grpol_Complementary_Alternative_Therapies.pdf). All that we know about informed consent in conventional medicine applies to CAIM with the following guidelines (Brown et al. 2009; Cohen 2002; Cohen et al. 2013).

1. *Prescribe CAIM treatments for which there is some published evidence of safety and efficacy.* Before you consider recommending a CAIM treatment, you should obtain knowledge about the CAIM treatment being prescribed, whether you are prescribing them yourself or referring to another practitioner. If you are referring the patient, it should be clear that your colleague is following a similar procedure of informed consent.
2. *Follow the customary procedures for diagnostic evaluation, including obtaining the relevant history, examination, testing, and medical records.*
3. *Provide the information necessary for informed consent and fully document this discussion in the patient's medical record.* This requires disclosure to the patient or legal guardian of all known risks and benefits, full *discussion and comparison with the risks and benefits of conventional treatment options*, and discussion of the impact of no treatment. The rationale for using CAIM should be carefully discussed with the patient and family and should be documented in the medical record. Reasons for administering CAIM could include failure to achieve remission with conventional treatments, adverse reactions or contraindications to conventional treatments, patient preference and the reasons why the patient prefers CAIM or refuses conventional treatment, and lack of access or inability to pay for conventional treatments.

4. *Do not recommend CAIM when patients have acute severe or life-threatening illnesses, including acute suicidality, such that delaying conventional treatment could result in harm.* Discussing the risks and benefits of treatment or no treatment, either traditional or CAIM, is one of the most important interactions with patients.
5. *Determine the extent to which CAIM treatment could interfere with other ongoing treatments.*
6. *If you decide the patient would benefit from referral to a more experienced CAIM practitioner, carefully determine that the CAIM provider is competent, to ensure that the patient is best served.*
7. *Monitor the patient and document treatment response, adverse reactions, and ongoing discussions with the patient about treatment decisions* regardless of whether you are prescribing or delivering the CAIM therapy.
8. *Avoid actual or the appearance of a conflict of interest.* For example, selling CAIM products such as supplements to patients is a conflict of interest. However, selling CAIM products at cost (with no profit to the clinician) to provide treatments that are not readily available is not a conflict of interest.

KEY POINTS

- Decision-making flowcharts can help clinicians decide the order of complementary, alternative, and integrative medicine (CAIM) treatment trials for patients whose response to prescription psychotropics is insufficient.

- The proposed CAIM flowcharts have heuristic value and provide a framework for future evaluation and optimization of integrative treatments.

- Keys to minimizing liability are learning about safe and effective CAIM, establishing and maintaining a positive doctor-patient relationship, obtaining full informed consent, and monitoring treatments.

References

American Psychiatric Association: Diagnostic and Statistical Manual of Mental Disorders, 5th Edition. Arlington, VA, American Psychiatric Association, 2013

Baghai TC, Möller HJ, Rupprecht R: Recent progress in pharmacological and non-pharmacological treatment options of major depression. Curr Pharm Des 12(4):503–515, 2006 16472142

Bambauer KZ, Adams AS, Zhang F, et al: Physician alerts to increase antidepressant adherence: fax or fiction? Arch Intern Med 166(5):498–504, 2006 16534035

Bosch P, van den Noort M, Staudte H, Lim S: Schizophrenia and depression: a systematic review of the effectiveness and the working mechanisms behind acupuncture. Explore (NY) 11(4):281–291, 2015 26007331

Bottiglieri T: Folate, vitamin B12, and S-adenosylmethionine. Psychiatr Clin North Am 36(1):1–13, 2013 23538072

Boyuan Z, Yang C, Ke C, et al: Efficacy of acupuncture for psychological symptoms associated with opioid addiction: a systematic review and meta-analysis. Evid Based Complement Alternat Med 2014:313549, 2014 25530779

Brown RP, Gerbarg PL, Muskin RP: How to Use Herbs, Nutrients and Yoga in Mental Health Care. New York, WW Norton, 2009

Chan YY, Lo WY, Yang SN, et al: The benefit of combined acupuncture and antidepressant medication for depression: a systematic review and meta-analysis. J Affect Disord 176:106–117, 2015 25704563

Cohen MH: Legal issues in complementary and integrative medicine: a guide for the clinician. Med Clin North Am 86(1):185–196, 2002 1179969

Cohen MH, Natbony SR, Abbott RB: Complementary and alternative medicine in child and adolescent psychiatry: legal considerations. Child Adolesc Psychiatr Clin N Am 22(3):493–507, 2013 23806316

Culpepper L, Muskin PR, Stahl SM: Major depressive disorder: understanding the significance of residual symptoms and balancing efficacy with tolerability. Am J Med 128(9 suppl):S1–S15, 2015 26337210

Fava M: Pharmacological approaches to the treatment of residual symptoms. J Psychopharmacol 20(3 suppl):29–34, 2006 16644769

Felker D, Lynn A, Wang S, et al: Evidence for a potential protective effect of carnitine-pantothenic acid co-treatment on valproic acid-induced hepatotoxicity. Expert Rev Clin Pharmacol 7(2):211–218, 2014 24450420

Gerbarg PL, Brown RP: Therapeutic nutrients and herbs, in Psychiatric Care of the Medical Patient, 4th Edition. Edited by D'Addona D, Fogel B, Greenberg D. New York, Oxford University Press, 2016, pp 545–610

Gong H, Ni C, Shen X, et al: Yoga for prenatal depression: a systematic review and meta-analysis. BMC Psychiatry 15:14, 2015 25652267

Kasper S: Phytopharmaceutical treatment of anxiety, depression, and dementia in the elderly: evidence from randomized, controlled clinical trials. Wien Med Wochenschr 165(11–12):217–228, 2015 26092515

Pilkington K: Anxiety, depression and acupuncture: a review of the clinical research. Auton Neurosci 157(1–2):91–95, 2010 20451469

Pilkington K: Acupuncture therapy for psychiatric illness. Int Rev Neurobiol 111:197–216, 2013 24215924

Raith W, Schmölzer GM, Resch B, et al: Laser acupuncture for neonatal abstinence syndrome: a randomized controlled trial. Pediatrics 136(5):876–884, 2015 26504123

Ravindran AV, da Silva TL: Complementary and alternative therapies as add-on to pharmacotherapy for mood and anxiety disorders: a systematic review. J Affect Disord 150(3):707–719, 2013

Sarris J, Gerbarg PL, Brown RP, Muskin PR: Integrative and complementary medicine in psychiatry, in Psychiatry, 4th Edition, Edited by Tasman AJ, Lieberman JA, First MB, Riba M. London, Wiley, 2015, pp 2261–2290

Thase ME: Achieving remission and managing relapse in depression. J Clin Psychiatry 64 (suppl 18):3–7, 2003 14700448

Torta R, Zanalda F, Rocca P, et al: Inhibitory activity of S-adenosyl-L-methionine on serum gamma-glutamyl-transpeptidase increase induced by psychodrugs and anticonvulsants. Curr Ther Res 44:144–159, 1988

CHAPTER 3

Complementary and Integrative Medicine in Child and Adolescent Psychiatric Disorders

Nutrition, Equine-Assisted Therapy, Art Therapy, and Neurofeedback

Deborah R. Simkin, M.D., DFAACAP, Diplomat ABIHM, BCN

Jenna Saul, M.D., DFAACAP

Judith E. Pentz, M.D.

Joel F. Lubar, Ph.D., BCIA-EEG Senior Fellow, QEEG Diplomate

Kirk D. Little, Psy.D.

Robert W. Thatcher, Ph.D.

A healthy PFC [prefontal cortex] means a healthy cognitive grip over the world with very little elements of prejudice.

Abhijit Naskar, Principia Humanitas

From the many contemporary developments in the complementary and integrative treatment of children and adolescents, we selected four areas for review: nutrition, equine-assisted therapy, art therapy, and neurofeedback. These modalities have the potential to benefit a broad range of children seen in psychiatric practice. The reader is referred to Simkin et al. (2014) for a review of movement and dance therapy and to

Yinger and Gooding (2014) for a review of music therapy. The weight of evidence varies among complementary, alternative, and integrative medicine (CAIM) treatments; however, as low-risk approaches, they warrant consideration and further research. Keeping in mind that children—particularly those with trauma histories, learning disabilities, and impaired social engagement—commonly have difficulty verbalizing thoughts and feelings, nonverbal CAIM modalities provide much needed pathways for expression and communication.

Nutrition in Child and Adolescent Psychiatry

The standard American diet may lack sufficient nutrients to support optimal physical and mental development in children. In addition, an optimal diet may not be sufficient, for example, in children with high pesticide levels, polymorphisms, or slow metabolisms.

Food Additives, Preservatives, and Pesticides

Evidence suggests that food sensitivities or allergies can shift mood, cause irritability, reduce focus, and exacerbate hyperactivity. In an open-label study of 76 children with attention-deficit/hyperactivity disorder (ADHD) placed on an oligoantigenic diet of foods with the least risk of allergic reaction, 68 had reduction in ADHD symptoms (Egger et al. 1985). This group (n=68) entered a double-blind randomized placebo-controlled trial (DBRPCT). One group was offered an allergen-free drink; the other, a drink with an allergen containing artificial colors or flavors, wheat, dairy, and soy. Only children given the allergen drink had a return of ADHD symptoms. This study was repeated in 1992, with similar results (Egger et al. 1992). A randomized controlled trial (RCT) of preschoolers showed a significantly greater increase in hyperactivity symptoms on active challenge with dye (20 mg/day) or sodium benzoate (45 mg/day) versus placebo, by parent ratings, with a small to medium effect (Bateman et al. 2004). McCann et al. (2007) repeated the Bateman study in preschoolers, with similar effects. A higher level of dye given to 8- to 9-year-olds resulted in a small but significant effect (Stevenson et al. 2010). Gene polymorphism moderated the dye effects on hyperactivity by histamine gene *HNMT Thr105Ile*. However, in the 8- to 9-year-olds, hyperactivity was also significantly decreased with histamine gene *HNMT T939C* and dopamine gene *DAT1*. A C allele in the *HNMT T939C* genotype in 40% of subjects protected against the dye effect (Stevenson et al. 2010). In an open-label study of the few foods diet (rice, meat, vegetables, pears, and water) complemented with specific foods such as potatoes, fruits, and wheat given to 78 children diagnosed with ADHD, 59 improved. After 2 weeks, if no changes occurred, other foods were eliminated; when the children were reexposed to the foods, 47 (60%) relapsed. There was no correlation between dietary changes and food sensitivity laboratory results (Pelser et al. 2001). In a DBRPCT of the food elimination diet in 26 children with ADHD, 19 (73%) responded with reduced symptoms (Boris and Mandel 1994). Children with a family history of allergies reacted most strongly.

High levels of organophosphate pesticides were found in 94% of 1,139 youths with ADHD; those with higher levels had a tenfold increase in risk of ADHD (Bouchard et al. 2010). Slow metabolism of pesticides by cytochrome P450 (CYP) 2D6 enzyme may increase the risk associated with high environmental exposure. Slow CYP2D6 metabolizers are at higher risk for developing Parkinson's disease, a risk that increases with exposure to pesticides (Mann and Tyndale 2010). Pesticides can deplete glutathione (a major antioxidant). *N*-acetylcysteine (NAC) is a safe, well-tolerated antidote for cysteine/glutathione deficiency (Atkuri et al. 2007). In a 12-week DBRPCT in children with autism ($n=33$), 14 children were randomly assigned to NAC (initiated at 900 mg/day for 4 weeks, followed by 900 mg bid for 4 weeks and 900 mg tid for 4 weeks). Compared with placebo, NAC resulted in significant improvements on the Aberrant Behavior Checklist (ABC) Irritability subscale ($F=6.80$; $P<0.001$; $d=0.96$) and was well tolerated (Hardan et al. 2012). On the basis of available research, it is important to consider sensitivities to foods, artificial coloring, and preservatives in the diagnosis and treatment of youths with mental health issues. Genetic testing of CYP2D6 may help identify children at greater risk for adverse effects of pesticides. Laboratory tests for food sensitivities may not correlate with reactions to foods.

Determining if youths have food sensitivities associated with hyperactivity entails elimination of foods commonly known to cause sensitivities for 3 weeks and then reexposure to these foods (one at a time) every 3–4 days to see if a reaction (e.g., bloating, worse hyperactivity, fatigue, poor concentration, rash) occurs. Common foods sensitivities include wheat, gluten, caffeine, dairy, eggs, gluten grains (e.g., barley, rye, spelt, wheat), white sugar, cane syrup, beet sugar, shellfish, soy, beef, pork, peanuts, processed meats, and chocolate.

Omega-3 Fatty Acids

Omega-3 fatty acid (FA) research for brain health was reviewed by Gow and Hibbeln (2014). Omega-3 FAs are marine- and plant-based lipids essential for cell membrane fluidity and for eye development (Chalon 2006). Because of changes in food production (e.g., large-scale fish farming) and dietary habits, omega-6 and omega-9 FAs are consumed in larger quantities than omega-3 FAs, an imbalance that is associated with increased inflammatory markers. In a 16-week DBRPCT, 40 boys ages 8–14 years with ADHD and 39 matched (according to age, handedness, and body mass index) typically developing boys were randomly assigned to receive 10 g/day of either nonfortified margarine or margarine fortified with 650 mg eicosapentaenoic acid (EPA) and 650 mg docosahexaenoic acid (DHA; Bos et al. 2015). Phospholipid DHA level at follow-up was higher for all children receiving EPA/DHA supplements than placebo. There was no effect of EPA/DHA supplementation on cognitive control or functional magnetic resonance imaging (fMRI) measures of brain activity. After supplementation with EPA and DHA, scores on the Child Behavior Checklist for attention problems improved in comparison with placebo ($F(1,67)=14.99$; $P<0.001$). In subjects with ADHD, higher levels of DHA were associated with less severe attention problems at baseline and follow-up.

In an open-label study of 18 children and adolescents with juvenile bipolar disorder, supplementation with 360 mg/day EPA and 1,560 mg/day DHA for 6 weeks resulted in significantly higher red blood cell EPA and DHA and significant improvements on the Young Mania Rating Scale ($P=0.004$) and Hamilton Depression Rating Scale ($P=0.002$); 40% of participants had "much improved" or "very much improved" symptoms on the Clinical Global Improvement Scale; and parent ratings of internalizing and externalizing behaviors were significantly improved ($P=0.046$) (Clayton et al. 2009).

In an Austrian RCT, 13- to 25-year-olds ($N=81$) with "subthreshold psychosis" were given 1.2 g/day of omega-3 FA or placebo for 12 weeks and were followed for 40 weeks. After 52 weeks, among the 76 completers (93.8%), 2 of the 41 (4.9%) in the omega-3 FA group transitioned to psychosis compared with 11 of the 40 (27.5%) in the placebo group. Positive and negative symptoms, general symptoms, and functioning improved in the omega-3 FA group compared with placebo. At follow-up 6.7 years later, most of the omega-3 FA group did not show severe functional impairment. Omega-3 FAs may reduce the risk of progression to psychotic disorder and psychiatric morbidity (Amminger et al. 2015).

Omega-3 FA supplementation is a promising adjunctive treatment for ADHD, major depressive disorder, bipolar disorder, and possibly first-episode psychotic disorder in youths. A prescription food, Vayarin, contains omega-3 FAs plus phosphatidylserine, which is thought to enable omega-3 FAs to pass through the blood-brain barrier. The phosphatidylserine dose is 100 mg/day. The recommended proportion of EPA/DHA is 2:1 at 1,000 mg/day or more for latency-age children. A reliable resource for high-quality omega-3 FAs is Nordic Naturals.

Three Important Minerals: Zinc, Iron, and Magnesium

Low levels of zinc, magnesium, and iron have been found in children with ADHD, and low levels of zinc have been found in children with inattentive ADHD (Arnold et al. 2013a; Mahmoud et al. 2011). The severity of ADHD symptoms has been correlated with low levels of ferritin (Konofal et al. 2008). Ferritin levels should be between 40 and 60 ng/mL. Serum ferritin must be monitored during supplementation because excess iron can cause hemochromatosis. Evidence suggests that in patients whose serum levels of magnesium, zinc, or iron are low, supplementation with the deficient mineral can improve symptoms. The pediatric dose of zinc picolinate is 15 mg/day with a gradual increase to 30 mg/day. Iron is best administered in chelated form 30 mg/day or as ferrous sulfate 325 mg/day. Magnesium (chelated as citrate or glycerate) is dosed by body weight at 2–3 mg/lb. These mineral formulations are more completely absorbed by the body and cause less nausea, cramping, or constipation. Symptom improvement may require weeks to months of daily supplementation.

Probiotics, Attention-Deficit/Hyperactivity Disorder, and Autism

The term *microbiome* refers to bacteria cohabiting the gastrointestinal tract. Microbes contain more than 150 times the number of genes in the human body, and 90% of our DNA is microbial in origin. Research suggests that gut microbiota, through bottom-up effects, can influence brain development; brain function; and behavior via immune, endocrine, and neural pathways. This could lend credibility to the "leaky gut" hypothesis that deficits in gut permeability may underlie chronic low-grade inflammation in disorders such as depression (Kelly et al. 2015). It is now thought that corticotropin-releasing factor (CRF) and its receptors (CRFR1 and CRFR2) are important in stress-induced gut permeability dysfunction (Rodiño-Janeiro et al. 2015), whereby larger-than-usual molecules from the gut enter the bloodstream, where they are seen as foreign, thus setting the stage for inflammatory response.

During early development, disruptions of the intestinal barrier by food can predispose immature infants to autoimmune diseases (Groschwitz and Hogan 2009). In addition, the gut microbiota is necessary for normal development of the hypothalamic-pituitary axis (Moloney et al. 2014), which can influence psychiatric illnesses. In an RCT, 75 infants who were randomly assigned to receive *Lactobacillus rhamnosus* or placebo during the first 6 months of life were followed for 13 years (Pärtty et al. 2015). Gut microbiota was assessed at ages 3 weeks; 3, 6, 12, 18, and 24 months; and 13 years. At age 13 years, ADHD or autism spectrum disorder was diagnosed in 6 of 35 children (17.1%) in the placebo group and was not diagnosed in any children in the probiotic group ($P=0.008$). The mean numbers of *Bifidobacterium* species in feces during the first 6 months of life were lower in affected children (8.26 ± 1.24 standard deviation [SD] log cells per gram), than in healthy children (9.12 ± 0.64 SD log cells per gram), $P=0.03$, suggesting a possible link between the use of probiotics and decreased risk for ADHD and autism. Larger studies are needed to determine whether probiotics given early in life may reduce the risk of later neuropsychiatric disorders.

Imbalance of flora in the gut can also lead to nutritional deficiencies. Furthermore, gut microbes participate in synthesis of key nutrients such as B_{12} and other B vitamins. Prebiotics, food sources for healthy bacteria, include foods containing inulin and other forms of fiber (e.g., almonds and bananas). Although more research is needed, supplementation with probiotics is a low-risk approach that may be beneficial, especially early in life.

Most probiotics require refrigeration and are not suitable for travel. Among those probiotics that do not need refrigeration, Klaire Labs has good choices for children.

Equine-Facilitated Therapies

As parents and providers seek novel therapeutic interventions for children with treatment-refractory illness, equine-facilitated therapy (EFT) programs have proliferated. Studies show that EFT can facilitate prosocial behavior, modulate stress response, and improve self-esteem in children with autistic, learning, and behavioral problems and histories of abuse.

Therapeutic Horseback Riding

Therapeutic riding (TR) entails riding in small groups led by a certified instructor who teaches horsemanship skills while targeting therapeutic goals, which include improving communication, social skills, adaptive skills, and/or behaviors. When only horsemanship skills are used, the intervention may be called therapeutic horse-manship.

Equine-Assisted Psychotherapy

Equine-assisted psychotherapy (EAP) incorporates horses experientially for mental and behavioral therapy and personal development. This requires a licensed psychotherapist with expertise as an equine specialist or a therapist who works with an equine specialist who facilitates experiences with horses. EAP can facilitate cognitive-behavioral therapy, acceptance and commitment therapy, metaphor therapy, dialectical behavior therapy, and other types of therapy.

Equine-Assisted Learning

Equine-assisted learning focuses on personal or group learning or educational goals such as improved teamwork for members of a company or agency, leadership skills for a school group, resiliency training for military troops, social skills, or assertiveness training.

Research Review of Equine-Facilitated Therapies

EQUINE-FACILITATED THERAPIES IN TREATMENT OF AUTISM SPECTRUM DISORDER

Children with autism spectrum disorder need interventions to reduce stress-related maladaptive behaviors and improve social communication (Gabriels et al. 2015). The majority of animal-assisted interventions for autism spectrum disorder involve TR and therapeutic horsemanship. A comprehensive review by O'Haire (2013) of animal-assisted interventions targeting individuals with autism spectrum disorder identified 14 empirical studies from 1840 to 2011 that included a live animal and identified improvements in social interaction, communication skills, behaviors, and stress level. The studies were methodologically weak but supported animal-assisted intervention as a "probably efficacious treatment."

In a large-scale RCT, 127 youths with autism spectrum disorder were randomly assigned to either TR or barn activity groups (Gabriels et al. 2015). The barn activity group had no contact with horses, but a life-sized stuffed horse was present for teaching horsemanship skills. Participants in the TR group showed significantly more improvements in irritability ($P=0.02$) and hyperactivity ($P=0.01$) on the Autism Behavioral Checklist, Social Cognition and Communication subscales of the Social Responsiveness Scale, the number of words spoken, and the number of new words. Such findings support EFTs for children and adolescents with autism spectrum disorder.

REVIEW OF EQUINE-ASSISTED PSYCHOTHERAPY RESEARCH IN YOUTHS

A 2007 review of literature on EAP with children and adolescents indicated that at-risk youths and children with histories of neglect, abuse, and eating disorders may benefit from EAP and noted the need for more robust research (Lentini and Knox 2009). A 2014 systematic review concluded that equine-related treatments for mental disorders lack empirical support (Anestis et al. 2014). Since then, several studies suggesting efficacy of EAP have been published (e.g., Hauge et al. 2014; Kemp et al. 2014).

Lentini and Knox (2015) identified eight case series of at-risk youths wherein EAP resulted in mild to moderate improvements in self-esteem, social development, self-control, and transferable skills, as well as reduced adjudications and maladaptive behavior. In an open-label study, 30 youths ages 8–17 referred for treatment of sexual abuse responded (regardless of age, gender, or ethnicity) to the Equine-Assisted Growth and Learning Association (EAGALA) program with significant reductions in symptoms of traumatic stress, depression, anxiety, and undesirable behaviors (Kemp et al. 2014).

Evidence suggests that EAP may improve engagement in therapy for children and youths who reject or who are unlikely to benefit from traditional office-based therapies. In an RCT, "at-risk" 11- to 17-year-olds (Texas Education Association criteria) assigned to a 5-week EAGALA EAP group ($n=14$) showed significantly more improvement on Hope scores (Adolescent Domain-Specific Hope Scale; $P=0.037$; effect size=2.536) and on the Beck Depression Inventory ($P=1.08$) compared with a group given treatment as usual ($n=12$) (Frederick et al. 2015; Waite and Bourke 2013). Lentini and Knox (2015) reviewed 34 studies of EAP in a total of 672 children and adolescents. In eight studies including children or youths with suicidal ideation, ADHD, anxiety, history of sexual abuse, posttraumatic stress disorder (PTSD), history of bereavement, or other social and behavioral problems, improvements were noted in "warm emotion," quality of life, empowerment, anxiety, depression, enthusiasm, and happiness. Two studies (Drinkhouse et al. 2012; Yorke et al. 2013) documented correlations of cortisol and heart rate between human and horse pairs. Most studies showed mild to moderate benefits of EAP for children and adolescents.

HOW HUMAN-EQUINE INTERACTIONS FACILITATE PROSOCIAL BEHAVIORS AND EMOTION REGULATION

Several hypotheses have been proposed to explain how human-equine interactions facilitate prosocial behaviors (Hauge et al. 2014). Kersten and Thomas (2004) posit that self-esteem, confidence, communication skills, trust, and boundaries are improved when a person succeeds with the challenge of controlling the movement of a 1,000-pound creature. Horses are prey animals who exhibit a flight response prior to a fight response (Skipper 2005). Horses also readily habituate to situations with behavioral flexibility and, like humans, may respond in both unique and common ways to certain stimuli (McGreevy and McLean 2010). This shared tendency between horses and humans provides a point of connection. Horses are herd animals who live in a social hierarchy with a repertoire of social behaviors. During ground-based interactions between humans and tamed horses, the horses demonstrate the same behavior repertoires as when they are in the herd. The implication is that humans receive direct and immediate nonjudgmental nonverbal feedback regarding their actions. Persons in EAP sessions are physically and mentally engaged. If the horse does not act as intended, then the person may change his or her approach to get a different response. This provides opportunities for both children and therapists to assess the child's emotional and behavioral responses, which can then be explored therapeutically. Thus, EAP enables distancing and self-reflection. Finally, observing the horse and exploring observations objectively facilitate the generation of metaphors that can be explored with the patient. Campbell (2012) proposed that within the human mind-body system all significant thoughts, feelings, beliefs, and experiences are initially conceived in the brain as images, and thereafter words are applied. She referred to these images as "internalized metaphors," the majority of which lie hidden in the unconscious. The exploration of metaphors allows deep-seated needs, conflicts, or knowledge to be brought into consciousness, facilitating self-discovery and unique personal solutions.

From another viewpoint, animal-human interactions provide opportunities for coregulation, balancing of stress response systems, and activation of parasympathetic pathways involved in relatedness, connection, bonding, and love (see Chapter 20, "Polyvagal Theory and the Social Engagement System," and Chapter 21, "Breathing Techniques in Psychiatric Treatment"). Calm animals can moderate stress response and reduce cardiovascular reactivity in children. This calming may be related to the size, warmth, and rhythmic movements of the horse. Horses respond to the child's body language and mirror his or her movements. The sense of connectedness with the animal, enhanced by physical contact, particularly petting, grooming, hugging, and riding, provides an experience of intimacy, closeness, safety, and social support. Children may experience therapy animals as more predictable and approachable than humans. Grooming and feeding a horse gives the child a chance to nurture and care for the animal, as well as to gain competence and mastery of skills. These aspects could account for observations that children who have difficulty relating to humans may first bond with an animal, and later, having experienced and "learned" connectedness, they may subsequently transfer this capacity to relationships with humans.

Art Therapy

Review of Art Therapy

Art therapy has a long tradition of helping people of all ages engage in creative activities that facilitate expression of their experiences and enhance well-being (Malchiodi 2011). For children and adolescents, art therapy offers a sensory-rich, emotionally rewarding experience that can match their developmental, cultural, and relational needs. Children often have difficulty verbalizing thoughts and feelings. In trauma cases, when the abuser has frightened the victim into silence or when trauma is encoded subsymbolically (without language), art therapy can circumvent the inability to verbalize by providing a nonverbal means for communication.

Art Therapy Research in Youths

Several studies have suggested that art therapy can ameliorate psychosocial problems in children and adolescents, including reducing anxious attachment (Ball 2002), managing mood disorders (Henley 2007), improving relatedness to parents (Hosea 2006), and coping with emotional distress and adjustment difficulties (Lee 2013).

Many empirical studies of art therapy have focused on youths with a history of trauma, disruptive behaviors, and impaired coping. An open-label study ($N=41$) of cognitive-behavioral art therapy found significant reduction ($P<0.05$) on 9 of 10 Briere's Trauma Symptom Checklist for Children subscales (Pifalo 2006). An RCT of inpatient adolescents ($N=29$) with PTSD found that youths receiving trauma-focused group art therapy had significant reduction in trauma symptoms on the UCLA Posttraumatic Stress Disorder Reaction Index compared with a control group receiving treatment-as-usual art activities ($P<0.01$) (Lyshak-Stelzer et al. 2007).

In an open trial of individual art therapy, 94 emotionally and behaviorally disturbed youths ages 2–16 years showed significant improvement in measures of 24 symptomatic behaviors ($P=0.001$) and significantly decreased frequency of disturbed behaviors ($P=0.006$) (Saunders and Saunders 2000). Participation in a 12-week art therapy program for children ages 4–21 years ($N=67$) affected by familial substance abuse was associated with improved competencies and reduced behavior problems (Springer et al. 1992). A nonrandomized study of children with leukemia ages 2–14 years ($N=32$) showed that prehospitalization group art therapy promoted cooperative behavior during painful medical interventions compared with a control group of youths hospitalized before art therapy (Favara-Scacco et al. 2001).

Neurofeedback in Child and Adolescent Psychiatric Disorders

Neurofeedback, a form of electroencephalographic biofeedback derived from operant conditioning, supported by more than 40 years of research, is used to treat children with ADHD, autism spectrum disorder, and learning disorders by changing brain wave patterns in malfunctioning circuitry (Simkin et al. 2014). Howe and Sterman (1972) noticed that a cat waiting for a tone to stop (before getting food) learned to produce a 12-Hz to 15-Hz brain frequency rhythm he called sensorimotor rhythm (SMR). Howe and Sterman (1972) used SMR training over sensory motor cortex to decrease seizures in animals, as did Lubar and Shouse (1976) in humans. Using SMR training with a hyperactive child, placing electrodes at the C3 and C4 positions on the scalp to train up 12-Hz to 15-Hz beta rhythm until theta rhythm (4–8 Hz) was no longer seen, Shouse and Lubar (1979) found increased attention and reduced hyperactivity. Some ADHD patients did not respond to SMR or theta/beta ratio (TBR) training. Lubar (1991) incorporated quantitative electroencephalograms (qEEGs) to target symptoms associated with specific brain wave abnormalities using the TBR protocol in ADHD patients who had high theta/low beta ratio. Today abnormal brain wave patterns are compared with a normative database so that neurofeedback protocols can be tailored to the baseline qEEG, clinical status, and history of the patient. qEEG has been cross-correlated with diffuse tensor imaging, fMRI, single-photon emission computed tomography, and positron emission tomography, supporting its validity. On the basis of 10 "gold standards," six qEEG reliable normative databases have been identified (Johnstone et al. 2005; Simkin and Black 2014; Thatcher and Lubar 2009).

Types of Neurofeedback

Hammond (2011) described seven types of neurofeedback, summarized in Table 3–1, that have been used for ADHD (Hurt et al. 2014). Surface qEEG neurofeedback targets amplitudes, frequencies, or rhythms. In z-score neurofeedback (ZNF), training targets are the calculated real-time qEEG z-scores identified as abnormal by comparison with a normative database that has been integrated into neurofeedback software (Krigbaum and Wigton 2014). The focus is on shifting excessive live (real-time) z-score metrics (standard deviations) toward mean ($z=0$) normalization. Low-resolution electromagnetic tomographic analysis (LORETA) allows the clinician to translate qEEG data into a three-dimensional image that corresponds to an fMRI image. During neurofeedback treatment, as brain waveforms adjust toward normal, three-dimensional LORETA images become more consistent with a normal fMRI (Simkin and Black 2014; http://uzh.ch/keyinst/loreta.htm).

TABLE 3–1. Description of neurofeedback therapies

Type	Date	How it works
Traditional frequency/power (surface neurofeedback)	1960s	Changes amplitude or speed of specific brain wave in specific brain area with two to four electrodes
Slow cortical potential neurofeedback (SCP-NF)	1993	Modifies direction (positive or negative) of slow cortical potentials
Low Energy Neurofeedback System (LENS)	1992	Changes brain waves through passive delivery of very weak electromagnetic signal
Hemoencephalographic (HEG) neurofeedback	1994	Provides neurofeedback based on blood flow
Live z-score neurofeedback	1998	Compares multiple variables (e.g., phase lag, coherence) to normative database using moment-to-moment feedback
Low-Resolution Electromagnetic Tomographic Analysis (LORETA) neurofeedback	1994	Monitors phase, power, and coherence with 19 electrodes
Functional magnetic resonance imaging (fMRI) neurofeedback	2003	Allows patient to regulate feedback in deep cortical structures

Comparing Surface Neurofeedback, z-Score Neurofeedback, and LORETA z-Score Neurofeedback

Two similar types of ZNF, surface 1–19 channel ZNF and LORETA ZNF (LZNF), have one fundamental difference (Krigbaum and Wigton 2014; Simkin et al. 2014; Thatcher 2012). Surface neurofeedback measures the amplitude of neurons directly beneath an electrode, where 95% of the neurons arise from a distance of 6 cm and all frequencies are mixed together at each electrode. In contrast, LORETA unscrambles frequencies beneath each electrode and links to three-dimensional sources deeper inside the brain with accuracies of approximately 1 cm in many locations. Surface ZNF calculates the z-score at 10–20 surface sites, whereas with LZNF, z-score is calculated for voxels in deeper structures (e.g., Brodmann areas, cingulate gyrus). Clinical reports of ZNF and LZNF indicate positive outcomes after 10–20 sessions for traumatic brain injury, PTSD, anxiety, ADHD, postneurosurgery depression, and mood disorders. Other types of neurofeedback may require 40–80 sessions. With LZNF, brain networks and hubs are targeted for training with specificity and localization similar to that of fMRI. This facilitates linkage of clinical symptoms with brain regions (with deviant z-scores) whose scores can be moved toward the mean ($z=0$) to stabilize brain functioning (Simkin and Black 2014).

Slow Cortical Potential, Theta/Beta Ratio, Sensory Motor Rhythm, Quantitative EEG, z-Score Neurofeedback, and Low-Resolution Electromagnetic Tomography

NEUROTHERAPY STUDIES IN ATTENTION-DEFICIT/HYPERACTIVITY DISORDER

Although numerous double-blind, randomized, placebo-controlled trials (DBRPCTs) of neurofeedback have targeted ADHD, many of these studies used research methods that are not recognized as valid techniques (Arns and Strehl 2013; Pigott and Cannon 2014). Five such DBRPCTs did not find a difference between sham and neurofeedback (Arnold et al. 2013b; DeBeus and Kaiser 2011; Landsbergen et al. 2011; Perreau-Linck et al. 2010; van Dongen-Boomsma et al. 2013). However, a closer look at these studies can account for the negative conclusions. Four of the five studies used unconventional neurofeedback protocols. Two studies used auto thresholding, whereby a child is always rewarded whether or not active learning is taking place. Furthermore, in two studies, reinforcement was set at 80%, which was so high that learning may not have occurred because it was too easy to obtain reinforcement. Three studies used overly complex feedback such as exciting Sony PlayStations or movies instead of simple auditory or visual feedback. Such methods make it difficult to differentiate between feedback reinforcement due to entertainment versus reinforcement from the neurofeedback treatment. In one study ($n=9$), the authors could not evaluate specific neurofeedback results because of the small sample size. In a meta-analysis by Sonuga-Barke et al. (2013) and a recent meta-analysis by Cortese et al. (2016), many of the included studies had methodological flaws. Moreover, none of the included studies used qEEG. Clinical trials with better methodologies, including those using pretreatment qEEGs have shown positive benefits of neurofeedback for ADHD as a solo treatment or as augmentation with stimulant medications.

In an RCT of 81 children with ADHD, neurofeedback TBR at Cz (a centrally located position on the vertex for electrode placement) for 19–30 sessions compared with methylphenidate led to comparable reductions in theta power that were greater than physical exercise ($P=0.08$ and $P=0.12$, respectively) (Janssen et al. 2016). Using qEEG with neurofeedback substantially increases the effect sizes. Arns et al. (2012), testing five neurofeedback protocols based on baseline qEEG data, reported effect sizes for attention of 1.78 and for hyperactivity of 1.22. Meta-analysis of stimulant medication in ADHD found effect size=0.84 for inattention and 1.01 for hyperactivity/impulsivity (Faraone and Buitelaar 2010). Highlighting the need for pretreatment qEEG, Kerson and Collaborative Neurofeedback Group (2013) received the first 5-year National Institutes of Health grant to study neurofeedback for ADHD. Long-term studies (Gevensleben et al. 2010; Leins et al. 2007) showed that neurofeedback effects persisted after 6 months and continued to improve, especially with respect to impulsivity and hyperactivity. In an RCT by Steiner et al. (2011), neurofeedback students maintained their medication dosage at 6 months; students getting cognitive training and control subjects needed significant medication increases (9 mg, $P \le 0.002$ vs. 13 mg, $P \le 0.001$). In a study of qEEG-based neurofeedback (Monastra et al. 2002), all subjects were taking medication. When medication was discontinued at the end of the study, only neurofeedback participants sustained improvements.

NEUROTHERAPY STUDIES IN LEARNING DISORDERS

In an RCT, 21 children with dyslexia (1.5–2 years delayed), excluding confounding neurological or psychiatric diagnoses, received sessions of two-channel connectivity-guided EEG coherence neurofeedback twice a week for 20 weeks (Coben et al. 2015). On the basis of qEEG, areas with prominent hypocoherence (low coherence) were targeted for training. The control group ($n=21$) received resource room assistance but no neurofeedback. Mean reading scores increased by 1.243 years in the treatment group, whereas the control group reading scores decreased by 0.2 years. Small studies indicated TBR neurofeedback and slow cortical potential neurofeedback may improve symptoms in learning disorders. In a study of 5 children with learning disorders (Becerra et al. 2006), enduring effects—positive behavioral changes and a spurt of EEG maturation—were shown from theta/alpha neurofeedback training 2 years earlier.

NEUROTHERAPY STUDIES IN AUTISM SPECTRUM DISORDER

The first study of surface neurofeedback in youths with autism spectrum disorder assigned 14 children ages 8–12 to treatment or wait-list groups according to the order of applying (Kouijzer et al. 2009). After 40 sessions, 70% of neurofeedback participants had reduced theta ($P<0.05$), increased low beta ($P<0.05$), and significant improvements in neuropsychological indices: attention, $P<0.05$; set-shifting, $P<0.05$; inhibition, $P<0.05$; verbal inhibition, $P<0.0$; and motor inhibition and planning, $P<0.05$. Significant gains were made in nonverbal communication, stereotypic behaviors, and social interaction communication skills, which would be expected to improve before communication skills. Follow-up tests 1 year later found lasting improvements. In a surface neurofeedback study of autism using qEEG, 60% of 20 neurofeedback participants had reduced theta and significant improvements in cognitive flexibility, social interactions, and communication compared with control participants. Improvements endured at 6-month follow-up (Kouijzer et al. 2010).

In a third surface neurofeedback RCT of 20 children with autism spectrum disorder, 60% of surface neurofeedback participants in the neurofeedback group showed decreased theta (Coben et al. 2011) after 40 or more (average 64.5) sessions. After neurofeedback, significant improvements were found on the Autism Treatment Evaluation Checklist (ATEC; two-sample t test, $t=11.302$; degrees of freedom [df] 19; $P<0.000$), Gilliam Asperger's Disorder Scale (GADS; two-sample t test, $t=8.332$; df 19; $P<0.000$), Behavior Rating Inventory of Executive Function (BRIEF; two-sample t test, $t=5.370$; df 19; $P<0.000$), and Personality Inventory for Children (PIC-2; two-sample t test, $t=6.320$; df 19; $P<0.000$). No significant changes were found on parent rating scales. Retesting after a mean of 10.1 months during which no other treatments were administered indicated that the effects lasted up to 2 years after neurofeedback. Coben (2015) used multivariate coherence neurofeedback to target hypercoherences (too much activity shared between brain areas) and hypocoherences in 42 subjects receiving 40 sessions of neurofeedback. At 10-month follow-up, improvements in attention/executive function, visual-motor skills, language, and parent rating scales were maintained.

Larsen and Sherlin (2013) graded neurofeedback evidence on a 1 to 5 efficacy scale, wherein 1 means not empirically supported (case studies or anecdotal reports) and 5 indicates superiority to placebo in RCTs at a minimum of two independent sites. Neurofeedback was deemed efficacious (level 4) or efficacious and specific (level 5) for epilepsy, ADHD, and anxiety disorders; probably efficacious (level 3) for traumatic brain injury, alcoholism/substance abuse, insomnia, and optimal/peak performance; and insufficient (level 2) for depressive disorders, autism spectrum disorder, PTSD, and tinnitus. Subsequent RCTs by Coben et al. (2015) raised dyslexia from level 3 to level 4 and autism to level 3.

KEY POINTS

- Neurofeedback shows promise in treating attention-deficit/hyperactivity disorder (ADHD), autism spectrum disorder, and learning disorders, with evidence of enduring effects.

- Food sensitivities and nutrient deficiencies can impact mental health.

- Omega-3 fatty acids show promise as an adjunct in the treatment of ADHD, mood disorders, bipolar disorder, and first-time psychotic episodes.

- Probiotics may modulate brain function and behavior via immune, endocrine, and neural pathways. Studies may validate probiotics as preventive treatments, especially early in life.

- Equine-assisted psychotherapy may reduce maladaptive behaviors, anxiety, and depression in youths.

- Art therapy can facilitate treatment of posttraumatic stress disorder, mood disorders, and disruptive disorders.

References

Amminger GP, Schäfer MR, Schlögelhofer M, et al: Longer-term outcome in the prevention of psychotic disorders by the Vienna omega-3 study. Nat Commun 6(6):7934, 2015 26263244

Anestis MD, Anestis JC, Zawilinski LL, et al: Equine-related treatments for mental disorders lack empirical support: a systematic review of empirical investigations. J Clin Psychol 70(12):1115–1132, 2014 24953870

Arnold LE, Hurt E, Lofthouse N: Attention-deficit hyperactivity disorder: dietary and nutritional treatments. Child Adolesc Psychiatr Clin N Am 22(3):381–402, 2013a 23806311

Arnold LE, Lofthouse N, Hersch S, et al: EEG neurofeedback for ADHD: double-blind sham-controlled randomized pilot feasibility trial. J Atten Disord 17(5):410–419, 2013b 22617866

Arns M, Strehl U: Evidence for efficacy of neurofeedback in ADHD? Am J Psychiatry 170(7):799–800, 2013 23820843

Arns M, Drinkenburg W, Leon Kenemans J: The effects of QEEG-informed neurofeedback in ADHD: an open-label pilot study. Appl Psychophysiol Biofeedback 37(3):171–180, 2012 22446998

Atkuri KR, Mantovani JJ, Herzenberg LA, et al: N-Acetylcysteine—a safe antidote for cysteine/glutathione deficiency. Curr Opin Pharmacol 7(4):355–359, 2007 17602868

Ball B: Moments of change in the art therapy process. Arts Psychother 29(2):79–92, 2002

Bateman B, Warner JO, Hutchinson E, et al: The effects of a double blind, placebo controlled, artificial food colourings and benzoate preservative challenge on hyperactivity in a general population sample of preschool children. Arch Dis Child 89(6):506–511, 2004 15155391

Becerra J, Fernández T, Harmony T, et al: Follow-up study of learning-disabled children treated with neurofeedback or placebo. Clin EEG Neurosci 37(3):198–203, 2006 16929704

Boris M, Mandel FS: Foods and additives are common causes of the attention deficit hyperactive disorder in children. Ann Allergy 72(5):462–468, 1994 8179235

Bos DJ, Oranje B, Veerhoek ES, et al: Reduced symptoms of inattention after dietary omega-3 fatty acid supplementation in boys with and without attention deficit/hyperactivity disorder. Neuropsychopharmacology 40(10):2298–2306, 2015 25790022

Bouchard MF, Bellinger DC, Wright RO, et al: Attention-deficit/hyperactivity disorder and urinary metabolites of organophosphate pesticides. Pediatrics 125(6):e1270–e1277, 2010 20478945

Campbell G: Mining Your Client's Metaphors: A How-To Workbook on Clean Language and Symbolic Meaning. Bloomington, IN, Balboa Press, 2012

Chalon S: Omega-3 fatty acids and monoamine neurotransmission. Prostaglandins Leukot Essent Fatty Acids 75(4–5):259–269, 2006 16963244

Clayton EH, Hanstock TL, Hirneth SJ, et al: Reduced mania and depression in juvenile bipolar disorder associated with long-chain omega-3 polyunsaturated fatty acid supplementation. Eur J Clin Nutr 63(8):1037–1040, 2009 19156158

Coben R: Four Channel Multivariate Coherence Training: Rationale and Findings (plenary session). Presented at the ISNR 22nd Annual Conference, San Diego, CA, October 2015

Coben R, Arns M, Kouijzer M: Enduring effects of neurofeedback in children, in Neurofeedback and Neuromodulation Techniques and Applications. Edited by Coben R, Evans JR. San Diego, CA, Academic Press, 2011, pp 403–422

Coben R, Wright E, Decker S, et al: The impact of coherence neurofeedback on reading delays in learning disabled children: a randomized controlled study. NeuroRegulation 2(4):168–178, 2015

Cortese S, Ferrin M, Brandeis D, et al: Neurofeedback for attention-deficit/hyperactivity disorder: meta-analysis of clinical and neuropsychological outcomes from randomized controlled trials. J Am Acad Child Adolesc Psychiatry 55(6):444–455, 2016 27238063

DeBeus R, Kaiser D: Neurofeedback with children with attention deficit hyperactivity disorder: a randomized double-blind placebo-controlled study, in Neurofeedback and Neuromodulation: Techniques and Applications, Vol 1. Edited by Coben R, Evans J. San Diego, CA, Elsevier. 2011, pp 127–152

Drinkhouse M, Birmingham SS, Fillman R, et al: Correlation of human and horse heart rates during equine-assisted therapy sessions with at-risk youths: a pilot study. Journal of Student Research 1(3):22–25, 2012

Egger J, Carter CM, Graham PJ, et al: Controlled trial of oligoantigenic treatment in the hyperkinetic syndrome. Lancet 1(8428):540–545, 1985 2857900

Egger J, Carter CH, Soothill JF, et al: Effect of diet treatment on enuresis in children with migraine or hyperkinetic behavior. Clin Pediatr (Phila) 31(5):302–307, 1992 1582098

Faraone SV, Buitelaar J: Comparing the efficacy of stimulants for ADHD in children and adolescents using meta-analysis. Eur Child Adolesc Psychiatry 19(4):353–364, 2010 19763664

Favara-Scacco C, Smirne G, Schilirò G, et al: Art therapy as support for children with leukemia during painful procedures. Med Pediatr Oncol 36(4):474–480, 2001 11260571

Frederick KE, Ivey Hatz J, Lanning B: Not just horsing around: the impact of equine-assisted learning on levels of hope and depression in at-risk adolescents. Community Ment Health J 51(7):809–817, 2015 25698076

Gabriels RL, Pan Z, Dechant B, et al: Randomized controlled trial of therapeutic horseback riding in children and adolescents with autism spectrum disorder. J Am Acad Child Adolesc Psychiatry 54(7):541–549, 2015 26088658

Gevensleben H, Holl B, Albrecht B, et al: Neurofeedback training in children with ADHD: 6-month follow-up of a randomised controlled trial. Eur Child Adolesc Psychiatry 19(9):715–724, 2010 20499120

Gow RV, Hibbeln JR: Omega-3 fatty acid and nutrient deficits in adverse neurodevelopment and childhood behaviors. Child Adolesc Psychiatr Clin N Am 23(3):555–590, 2014 24975625

Groschwitz KR, Hogan SP: Intestinal barrier function: molecular regulation and disease pathogenesis. J Allergy Clin Immunol 124(1):3–20, quiz 21–22, 2009 19560575

Hammond DC: What is neurofeedback: an update. J Neurother 15(4):305–336, 2011

Hardan AY, Fung LK, Libove RA, et al: A randomized controlled pilot trial of oral N-acetylcysteine in children with autism. Biol Psychiatry 71(11):956–961, 2012 22342106

Hauge H, Kvalem IL, Berget B, et al: Equine-assisted activities and the impact on perceived social support, self-esteem and self-efficacy among adolescents—an intervention study. Int J Adolesc Youth 19(1):1–21, 2014 24833811

Henley D: Naming the enemy: an art therapy intervention for children with bipolar and comorbid disorders. Art Ther 24(3):104–111, 2007

Hosea H: "The brush's footmarks": parents and infants paint together in a small community art therapy group. International Journal of Art Therapy 11(2):69–78, 2006

Howe RC, Sterman MB: Cortical-subcortical EEG correlates of suppressed motor behavior during sleep and waking in the cat. Electroencephalogr Clin Neurophysiol 32(6):681–695, 1972 4121518

Hurt E, Arnold LE, Lofthouse N: Quantitative EEG neurofeedback for the treatment of pediatric attention-deficit/hyperactivity disorder, autism spectrum disorders, learning disorders, and epilepsy. Child Adolesc Psychiatr Clin N Am 23(3):465–486, 2014 24975622

Janssen TW, Bink M, Geladé K, et al: A randomized controlled trial into the effects of neurofeedback, methylphenidate, and physical activity on EEG power spectra in children with ADHD. J Child Psychol Psychiatry 57(5):633–644, 2016 26748531

Johnstone J, Gunkelman J, Lunt J: Clinical database development: characterization of EEG phenotypes. Clin EEG Neurosci 36(2):99–107, 2005 15999905

Kelly JR, Kennedy PJ, Cryan JF, et al: Breaking down the barriers: the gut microbiome, intestinal permeability and stress-related psychiatric disorders. Front Cell Neurosci 9:392, 2015 26528128

Kemp K, Signal T, Botros H, et al: Equine facilitated therapy with children and adolescents who have been sexually abused: a program evaluation study. J Child Fam Stud 23(3):558–566, 2014

Kerson C; Collaborative Neurofeedback Group: A proposed multisite double-blind randomized clinical trial of neurofeedback for ADHD: need, rationale, and strategy. J Atten Disord 17(5):420–436, 2013 23590978

Kersten G, Thomas L: Equine Assisted Psychotherapy and Learning Training Manual. Santaquin, UT, EAGALA, 2004

Konofal E, Lecendreux M, Deron J, et al: Effects of iron supplementation on attention deficit hyperactivity disorder in children. Pediatr Neurol 38(1):20–26, 2008 18054688

Kouijzer M, de Moor J, Gerrits B: Long-term effects of neurofeedback treatment in autism. Res Autism Spectr Disord 3(2):496–501, 2009

Kouijzer ME, van Schie HT, de Moor JM: Neurofeedback treatment in autism: preliminary findings in behavioral, cognitive, and neurophysiological functioning. Res Autism Spectr Disord 4(3):386–399, 2010

Krigbaum G, Wigton NL: When discussing neurofeedback, does modality matter? NeuroRegulation 1(1):48–60, 2014

Lansbergen MM, van Dongen-Boomsma M, Buitelaar JK, et al: ADHD and EEG-neurofeedback: a double-blind randomized placebo-controlled feasibility study. J Neural Transm (Vienna) 118(2):275–284, 2011 21165661

Larsen S, Sherlin L: Neurofeedback: an emerging technology for treating central nervous system dysregulation. Psychiatr Clin North Am 36(1):163–168, 2013 23538085

Lee SY: "Flow" in art therapy: empowering immigrant Korean children with adjustment disorders. Art Ther 30(2):56–63, 2013

Leins U, Goth G, Hinterberger T, et al: Neurofeedback for children with ADHD: a comparison of SCP and Theta/Beta protocols. Appl Psychophysiol Biofeedback 32(2):73–88, 2007 17356905

Lentini JA, Knox MS: A qualitative and quantitative review of equine-facilitated psychotherapy (EFP) with children and adolescents. Open Complement Med J 1(1):51–57, 2009

Lentini JA, Knox MS: Equine-facilitated psychotherapy with children and adolescents: an update and literature review. Journal of Creativity in Mental Health 10(3):278–305, 2015

Lubar JF: Discourse on the development of EEG diagnostics and biofeedback for attention-deficit/hyperactivity disorders. Biofeedback Self Regul 16(3):201–225, 1991 1932259

Lubar JF, Shouse MN: EEG and behavioral changes in a hyperkinetic child concurrent with training of the sensorimotor rhythm (SMR): a preliminary report. Biofeedback Self Regul 1(3):293–306, 1976 990366

Lyshak-Stelzer F, Singer P, St. John P, et al: Art therapy for adolescents with posttraumatic stress disorder symptoms: a pilot study. Art Ther 24(4):163–169, 2007

Mahmoud MM, El-Mazary AA, Maher RM, et al: Zinc, ferritin, magnesium and copper in a group of Egyptian children with attention deficit hyperactivity disorder. Ital J Pediatr 37:60, 2011 22206662

Malchiodi CA: Handbook of Art Therapy, 2nd Edition. New York, Guilford, 2011

Mann A, Tyndale RF: Cytochrome P450 2D6 enzyme neuroprotects against 1-methyl-4-phenylpyridinium toxicity in SH-SY5Y neuronal cells. Eur J Neurosci 31(7):1185–1193, 2010 20345925

McCann D, Barrett A, Cooper A, et al: Food additives and hyperactive behaviour in 3-year-old and 8/9-year-old children in the community: a randomised, double-blinded, placebo-controlled trial. Lancet 370(9598):1560–1567, 2007 17825405

McGreevy P, McLean A: Equitation Science. Oxford, UK, Wiley-Blackwell, 2010

Moloney RD, Desbonnet L, Clarke G, et al: The microbiome: stress, health and disease. Mamm Genome 25(1–2):49–74, 2014 24281320

Monastra VJ, Monastra DM, George S: The effects of stimulant therapy, EEG biofeedback, and parenting style on the primary symptoms of attention-deficit/hyperactivity disorder. Appl Psychophysiol Biofeedback 27(4):231–249, 2002 12557451

O'Haire ME: Animal-assisted intervention for autism spectrum disorder: a systematic literature review. J Autism Dev Disord 43(7):1606–1622, 2013 23124442

Pärtty A, Kalliomäki M, Wacklin P, et al: A possible link between early probiotic intervention and the risk of neuropsychiatric disorders later in childhood: a randomized trial. Pediatr Res 77(6):823–828, 2015 25760553

Pelser L, Frankena K, Toorman J, et al: Effects of a restricted elimination diet on the behaviour of children with attention-deficit hyperactivity disorder (INCA study): a randomized controlled trial. Lancet 377(9764):494–503, 2001

Perreau-Linck E, Lessard N, Levesque J, Beauregard M: Effects of neurofeedback training on inhibitory capacities in ADHD children: a single-blind, randomized, placebo-controlled study. J Neurother 14(3):229–242, 2010

Pifalo T: Art therapy with sexually abused children and adolescents: extended research study. Art Ther 23(4):181–185, 200e

Pigott H, Cannon R: Neurofeedback requires better Evidence of efficacy before it should be considered a legitimate treatment for ADHD: what is the evidence for this claim? NeuroRegulation 1(1):25–45, 2014

Rodiño-Janeiro BK, Alonso-Cotoner C, Pigrau M, et al: Role of corticotropin-releasing factor in gastrointestinal permeability. J Neurogastroenterol Motil 21(1):33–50, 2015 25537677

Saunders E, Saunders J: Evaluating the effectiveness of art therapy through a quantitative, outcomes-focused study. Arts Psychother 27(2):99–106, 2000

Shouse MN, Lubar JF: Operant conditioning of EEG rhythms and Ritalin in the treatment of hyperkinesis. Biofeedback Self Regul 4(4):299–312, 1979 526475

Simkin DR, Black NB: Meditation and mindfulness in clinical practice. Child Adolesc Psychiatr Clin N Am 23(3):487–534, 2014 24975623

Simkin D, Thatcher RW, Lubar J: Quantitative EEG and neurofeedback in children and adolescents: anxiety disorders, depressive disorders, comorbid addiction and attention-deficit/hyperactivity disorder, and brain injury. Child Adolesc Psychiatr Clin N Am 23(3):427–464, 2014 24975621

Skipper L: Let Horses Be Horses: The Horse Owners' Guide to Ethical Training and Management. London, JA Allen, 2005

Sonuga-Barke EJ, Brandeis D, Cortese S, et al; European ADHD Guidelines Group: Nonpharmacological interventions for ADHD: systematic review and meta-analyses of randomized controlled trials of dietary and psychological treatments. Am J Psychiatry 170(3):275–289, 2013 23360949

Springer J, Phillips J, Phillips L, et al: CODA: a creative therapy program for children in families affected by alcohol or other drugs. J Community Psychol 1(1):55–74, 1992

Steiner NJ, Sheldrick RC, Gotthelf D, et al: Computer-based attention training in the schools for children with attention deficit/hyperactivity disorder: a preliminary trial. Clin Pediatr (Phila) 50(7):615–622, 2011 21561933

Stevenson J, Sonuga-Barke E, McCann D, et al: The role of histamine degradation gene polymorphisms in moderating the effects of food additives on children's ADHD symptoms. Am J Psychiatry 167(9):1108–1115, 2010 20551163

Thatcher RW: Introduction, in Handbook on Quantitative Electroencephalography and EEG Biofeedback. Edited by Thatcher R. St Petersburg, FL, Anipublishing, 2012, pp 10–145

Thatcher RW, Lubar J: History of the scientific standards of QEEG normative databases, in Introduction to Quantitative EEG and Neurofeedback: Advanced Theory and Applications, 2nd Edition. Edited by Budzynski, T, Budzynski H, Evans J, et al. Philadelphia, PA, Elsevier, 2009, pp 29–59

van Dongen-Boomsma M, Vollebreqt MA, Slaats-Willemse D, Buitelaar JK: A randomized placebo-controlled trial of electroencephalographic (EEG) neurofeedback in children with attention-deficit/hyperactivity disorder. J Clin Psychiatry 74(8):821–827, 2013 24021501

Waite C, Bourke L: "It's different with a horse": horses as a tool for engagement in a horse therapy program for marginalised young people. Youth Studies Australia 32(4):15–24, 2013

Yinger OS, Gooding L: Music therapy and music medicine for children and adolescents. Child Adolesc Psychiatr Clin N Am 23(3):535–553, 2014 24975624

Yorke J, Nugent W, Strand E, et al: Equine-assisted therapy and its impact on cortisol levels of children and horses: a pilot study and meta-analysis. Early Child Development and Care 183(7):874–894, 2013

SECTION II

Nutrients in Psychiatric Care

CHAPTER 4

S-Adenosylmethionine

Teodoro Bottiglieri, Ph.D.

Patricia L. Gerbarg, M.D.

Richard P. Brown, M.D.

Give sorrow words; the grief that does not speak knits up the o'er wrought heart and bids it break.

William Shakespeare, Macbeth, *act 4, scene 3*

S-Adenosylmethionine (SAMe; also referred to as *S*-adenosyl-L-methionine or ademetionine) was discovered in 1950 by Giulio Cantoni, former director of biochemistry at the National Institute of Mental Health. An amino acid–derived metabolite, SAMe is the body's most avid methyl (–CH$_3$) donor, participating in the synthesis and modification of molecules essential for neuronal function, including neurotransmitters, hormones, proteins, phospholipids, and DNA. These pathways are implicated in mood and cognitive function. SAMe has been used for decades as a conventional treatment for depression, arthritis, and cholestasis of pregnancy in European countries; however, it remains an alternative treatment in the United States. In 1998, the U.S. Food and Drug Administration approved SAMe as an over-the-counter nutraceutical. The U.S. Department of Health and Human Services Agency for Healthcare Research and Quality concluded that SAMe was as effective as standard pharmacotherapy for treatment of depression and osteoarthritis and was more effective than placebo for reducing bilirubin and pruritus in cholestasis of pregnancy (Agency for Healthcare Research and Quality 2002). Reviews of SAMe for depression identified more than 50 clinical trials: 17 open-label trials ($N=708$); 19 double-blind, randomized placebo-controlled trials (DBRPCTs; $N=878$); and 21 trials comparing SAMe with other antidepressants ($N=1,591$) (Bottiglieri 2012; Gerbarg and Brown 2015; Sharma et al., in press).

Biochemistry of *S*-Adenosylmethionine

In every living cell, SAMe synthesis entails condensation of the essential amino acid methionine with adenosine triphosphate (ATP), a rate-limiting reaction catalyzed by methionine adenosyltransferase (Figure 4–1). Because the amount of methionine required to sustain SAMe synthesis cannot be obtained from dietary sources alone, cellular de novo synthesis of methionine is required. Methionine synthase (MTR), the enzyme that converts homocysteine to methionine, requires cofactors: 5-methyltetrahydrofolate (5-MTHF) and vitamin B_{12}. The intimate metabolic relationship shared by folate (vitamin B_9), vitamin B_{12}, and SAMe is of intense interest (Bottiglieri 2012) because folate and vitamin B_{12} deficiencies affect mood, cognitive function, neuropathies, and other disorders (Reynolds 2014). Folate and vitamin B_{12} are essential for supporting SAMe synthesis and for keeping intracellular and circulating homocysteine levels low (Refsum et al. 2004). Elevated concentrations of homocysteine are toxic to neuronal and vascular cells (Ansari et al. 2014; Levine et al. 2006; McCully 2015). SAMe contributes to more than 100 methylation-dependent pathways, its primary function being the transfer of methyl groups to molecules such as cytosine residues of DNA, amino acids of proteins and phospholipids, and others (Figure 4–1). The product of SAMe after loss of a methyl group is *S*-adenosylhomocysteine (SAH), which is converted to homocysteine, which in turn may enter the transsulfuration pathway to produce glutathione, a major antioxidant. Alternatively, homocysteine can be converted to methionine. Another role of SAMe is synthesis of polyamines involved in cellular growth, neuronal function, and prevention of bone loss (Li et al. 2007; Nowotarski et al. 2014; Yamamoto et al. 2012).

DNA Methylation in the Central Nervous System

Genomic DNA methylation in the central nervous system affects regulation of gene expression, neural plasticity, and responsivity to neuronal activity and such processes as learning and memory. For example, membrane-bound catechol O-methyltransferase (COMT) promoter DNA is often hypomethylated in frontal lobe brain tissue from patients with schizophrenia and bipolar disorder (Abdolmaleky et al. 2006). Interaction between methylenetetrahydrofolate reductase (MTHFR) C677T and COMT Val108/158Met polymorphisms increases the risk of reduced prefrontal activation and impaired working memory in subjects with schizophrenia, associated with abnormal dopamine signaling (Roffman et al. 2008).

Protein Methylation in the Central Nervous System

Carboxymethylation of amino acids in posttranslational modification of proteins can alter the structure and function of enzymes. Studies show a strong link between methylation of protein phosphatase 2A (PP2A) and key central nervous system proteins involved in the pathogenesis of Alzheimer's disease, for example, phospho-tau (p-tau) and amyloid precursor protein (Sontag and Sontag 2014). Administration to mice of the anti-Parkinsonian drug L-dopa, which rapidly depletes tissue concentra-

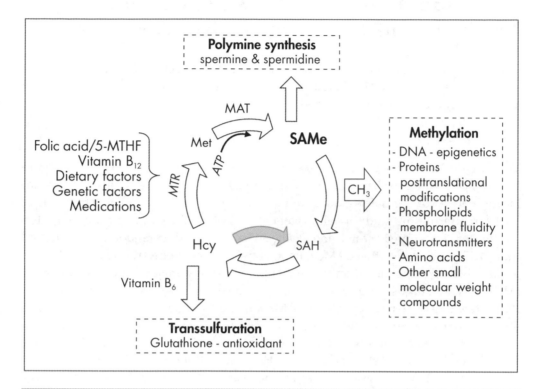

FIGURE 4–1. SAMe metabolism and cellular functions.

Note. ATP=adenosine triphosphate; B$_{12}$=vitamin B$_{12}$; CH$_3$=methyl group; 5-MTHF=5-methyl-tetrahydrofolate; Hcy=homocysteine; MAT=methionine adenosyltransferase; Met=methionine; MTR=methionine synthase; SAH=S-adenosylhomocysteine; SAMe=S-adenosylmethionine.

tions of SAMe, resulted in hypomethylation of a catalytic subunit of PP2A and increased p-tau levels in brain tissue (Bottiglieri et al. 2012), an effect exacerbated by folate deficiency. These and other definitive drug-genome interactions can compromise protein methylation in the brain, leading to p-tau accumulation and possibly contributing to progression of Alzheimer's disease. Methyl donors, such as SAMe, that methylate PP2A are promising treatments for reducing p-tau and preserving cognitive function.

Pharmacological Effect on Neurotransmitters in the Central Nervous System

SAMe increases norepinephrine and serotonin levels in rat brain tissue (Otero-Losada and Rubio 1989). In depressed patients, parenteral SAMe significantly increases metabolites related to dopamine and serotonin (Bottiglieri et al. 1984) and decreases serum prolactin levels, indicating upregulation of the dopaminergic system (Thomas et al. 1987). The mechanisms for SAMe effects on monoamine neurotransmitters are unclear, although methylation is likely involved.

A Perspective on SAMe Studies for Treatment of Depressive Disorders

Since the 2002 report by the Agency for Healthcare Research and Quality, SAMe research has been reviewed by Gerbarg and Brown (2015), Brown et al. (2009), Sarris et al. (2016), and Sharma et al. (in press).

SAMe Monotherapy for Depression

Twelve DBRPCTs found the antidepressant effect of SAMe oral doses (800–1,600 mg) to be significantly greater than placebo (Bottiglieri 2012). In one failed study of a less stable form of SAMe, the tablets oxidized after they were mistakenly removed from blister packs, rendering the study invalid (Fava et al. 1992). A 2002 meta-analysis by the Agency for Healthcare Research and Quality, which included 28 randomized controlled trials (RCTs), concluded that SAMe monotherapy was more effective than placebo and as effective as conventional antidepressants for treating major depressive disorder (MDD; overall effect size=0.65; 95% confidence interval 1.05–0.25). In 18 double-blind RCTs of mild to moderate depression, SAMe was as effective as tricyclic antidepressants (TCAs) and had fewer side effects (Agency for Healthcare Research and Quality 2002).

A recent three-arm DBRPCT ($N=189$ subjects with MDD) conducted at Massachusetts General Hospital (MGH) and Butler Hospital in Rhode Island found no significant difference in response at 12 weeks among subjects given SAMe, escitalopram, or placebo (Mischoulon et al. 2014). The high placebo response rate could reflect problems in patient selection. Post hoc analysis found that among the 144 subjects enrolled at MGH, depression improved significantly in the SAMe and escitalopram groups compared with the placebo group, with no significant difference in response between SAMe and escitalopram. Reanalysis, based on a higher proportion of men at the MGH site, suggested that compared with placebo, men had significantly greater response to SAMe, but women did not (Sarris et al. 2015). Additional studies are needed to validate this finding, particularly because previous research and clinicians in practice have not found gender differences. Differences in efficacy among SAMe preparations may account for lower response rates in more recent studies. Many positive studies of SAMe for depression between 1995 and 2002 used the 1,4-butanedisulfate butyrate form of SAMe, whereas most recent studies use either tosylate disulfate or toluenesulfonate forms of SAMe.

SAMe Augmentation of Other Antidepressants

SAMe can augment antidepressant effects of prescription antidepressants and restore effects that have faded over time (see Brown et al. 2000; Sarris et al. 2016). SAMe significantly enhanced effectiveness of TCAs in three double-blind RCTs in depressed subjects (total $N=350$). An open study of 30 patients with MDD who failed to respond adequately to a selective serotonin reuptake inhibitor (SSRI) or serotonin-norepinephrine reuptake inhibitor (SNRI; venlafaxine) found that within 6 weeks of adding SAMe 800–1,600 mg/day, 50% of patients responded ($P< 0.001$) and 43% attained remission

(Alpert et al. 2004). In an open study of treatment-resistant MDD (N=33), augmentation with SAMe 800 mg/day led to response in 60% and remission in 36% of patients. Significant improvement occurred in 1 week (P< 0.001) and persisted for 8 weeks (De Berardis et al. 2013). A 6-week DBRPCT of 73 MDD patients who had no response or partial response to an SSRI or SNRI found that the rates of response and remission with addition of up to 1,600 mg/day of SAMe (36.1% and 25.8%, respectively) exceeded those of placebo (17.6% and 11.7%; P<0.05) (Papakostas et al. 2010). A multicenter DBRPCT in patients with MDD and inadequate response to antidepressants showed that augmentation with 800 mg/day of a new SAMe formulation, MSI-195 (Strata, MSI Methylation Sciences Inc.), purported to have improved bioavailability resulted in no significant differences between SAMe and placebo. In a subgroup (n=143), excluding those with body mass index >40 and the more unstable patients, MSI-195 led to small but significant improvements on the Montgomery-Åsberg Depression Rating Scale (MADRS) (–3.41, P=0.031) relative to placebo, last observation carried forward/intent to treat (LOCF-ITT) analysis, and effect size=0.36 (Clinical Trials.gov, in process).

Clinicians, researchers, and reviewers agree that SAMe is beneficial for augmentation of antidepressants. More studies using current methodologies are needed to identify patients likely to respond to SAMe monotherapy and preparations with the greatest efficacy. A trial comparing 1,4-butanedisulfonate SAMe with tosylate disulfate or toluenesulfonate SAMe might resolve questions regarding the lack of separation from placebo in some trials.

SAMe for Depression in Patients With Comorbid Medical Illnesses

The use of SAMe in depressed patients with medical conditions has been reviewed (Brown et al. 2009; Gerbarg and Brown 2015). In this section, we briefly discuss the benefits of SAMe in patients with depression and arthritis, fibromyalgia, hepatic dysfunction, and HIV.

Depression and Arthritis

Arthritis and depression are common comorbid conditions. In 12 studies (total N>23,000), 800–1,200 mg/day SAMe demonstrated analgesic and anti-inflammatory effects in patients with osteoarthritis. Seven of these studies were RCTs in which analgesic and anti-inflammatory effects of SAMe were equal to those of nonsteroidal anti-inflammatory drugs, with fewer side effects (Agency for Healthcare Research and Quality 2002). Magnetic resonance imaging documentation of cartilage regeneration indicated that 400–1,200 mg/day SAMe is required for at least 3 months (Konig et al. 1995). Most meta-analyses of SAMe for osteoarthritis are inconclusive because they exclude the largest of these studies, a 2-year German Phase IV study of 20,641 patients with osteoarthritis treated with ademetionine (1,4-butanedisulfonate SAMe) for 8 weeks, which did not include a control group (Berger and Nowak 1987). In six studies of patients with fibromyalgia, 800 mg/day SAMe relieved both pain and depression without causing side effects (Brown et al. 2009; Tavoni et al. 1987).

Depression With Cirrhosis, Hepatitis, or Cholestasis

Depression in patients with hepatic diseases can be difficult to treat with pharmaceutical antidepressants, particularly SSRIs, which can induce or exacerbate liver dysfunction. Alcohol and other toxins cause oxidative damage to the liver; SAMe increases synthesis of the major antioxidant, glutathione (Lieber 2005). Alcohol depletes hepatic SAMe through reduced activity of methionine adenosyltransferase, the catalyst for SAMe synthesis (Figure 4–1). In a DBRPCT of 123 patients with Child Class A and Class B hepatic cirrhosis secondary to alcohol abuse, SAMe (AdoMet) delayed liver transplantation and increased 2-year survival ($P=0.046$) (Mato et al. 1999). The usual dosage for alcoholic cirrhosis is 1,200 mg/day SAMe. For severe hepatitis, cirrhosis, and fibrosis, SAMe 1,200–1,600 mg/day with any or all of the following augmentations may be needed: polyenylphosphatidylcholine to prevent depletion of SAMe; B vitamins, particularly B_6; α-lipoic acid to prevent liver damage; *Bupleurum kaoi* (in Ease 2 or Ease Plus, CraneHerb.com) to reduce inflammation and fibrosis and increase glutathione (Yen et al. 2005); and betaine (trimethylglycine) to increase glutathione (Kharbanda et al. 2005). A 6-month DBRPCT of SAMe 400 mg tid in 37 patients with alcohol-related hepatic disease found SAMe more beneficial than placebo in less severe fibrosis (Medici et al. 2011). Correcting subnormal B_6 levels found in the subjects might have improved outcomes.

Depression in Patients With HIV/AIDS

Depression in people living with HIV/AIDS commonly does not respond well to conventional antidepressant medications. Low levels of SAMe have been found in cerebrospinal fluid in patients with HIV-related neuropathies (Bottiglieri and Hyland 1994). In an 8-week open-label study of 20 HIV-seropositive individuals diagnosed with MDD (DSM-IV; American Psychiatric Association 1994), treatment with SAMe up to 800 mg twice daily (plus 1,000 mcg vitamin B_{12} and 800 mcg folic acid) led to rapid (as soon as 1 week), significant ($P<0.001$) improvements in depression rating scores, with further improvements through week 8 (Shippy et al. 2004).

SAMe Treatment for Cognitive Function and Neurodegenerative Diseases

Alzheimer's Disease and Age-Related Cognitive Decline

Decreased levels of plasma folate and SAMe are associated with increased risk factors for Alzheimer's disease (Gerberg and Brown 2015): increased plasma homocysteine and neurotoxicity, reduced glutathione antioxidant protection, decreased methylation of DNA and increased DNA breakage, and overexpression of presenilin 1 (PS1) leading to increased β-amyloid deposition. In adults without dementia as well as those with early- and late-stage Alzheimer's disease, cognitive function improved in one pilot study and two DBRPCTs in subjects given a vitamin/nutriceutical formulation: 400 mcg folic acid, 6 mcg B_{12}, 30 IU E α-tocopherol, 400 mg SAMe, 600 mg N-acetylcysteine, and 500 mg acetyl-L-carnitine (Chan et al. 2008, 2009, 2010; Remington et al. 2009). SAMe may also be of benefit in brain injury due to stroke or trauma (Brown and Gerbarg 2011; Monaco et al. 1996).

Parkinson's Disease

Deterioration of dopaminergic tracts is believed to underlie symptoms of Parkinson's disease. Patients with Parkinson's disease often become depressed and withdrawn. Levodopa, the mainstay of Parkinson's disease treatment, depletes SAMe in the brain. This may explain why depression in Parkinson's disease tends to be resistant to conventional antidepressants. SAMe supplementation can improve depression in Parkinson's disease but may require up to 4,000 mg/day (Carrieri et al. 1990; Varanese et al. 2011).

Pregnancy, Breast-Feeding, and Pediatric Uses of SAMe

Although safety of conventional antidepressants during pregnancy remains controversial, untreated depression can have serious consequences for mothers and babies in utero. Studies have demonstrated that SAMe treatment for cholestasis in pregnancy caused no adverse effects on neonates, including one study with follow-up to age 1 year (Agency for Healthcare Research and Quality 2002). Normal infants have higher cerebrospinal fluid levels of SAMe than adults. SAMe improves myelination in children with genetic errors of methyl-transfer pathways (Surtees and Hyland 1990; Surtees et al. 1991). Consequently, there are reasons to think that SAMe, a natural metabolite supporting healthy neuronal function, would be less likely to cause adverse effects during pregnancy and breast-feeding compared with conventional antidepressant medications (Gerbarg and Brown 2015). Although no controlled studies of SAMe treatment for depression in children have been published, there are a few case reports in which depressed children between ages 8 and 16 experienced remission with SAMe without side effects (Schaller et al. 2004). Pediatric dosages of SAMe start at 200 mg/day and increase to 600 mg/day (Gerbarg and Brown 2015).

Side Effects, Adverse Reactions, and Contraindications

SAMe has few side effects, causing no weight gain, sexual dysfunction, or impairment of memory or cognitive function (even in elderly patients or those with brain injury) (Lefkovitz et al. 2012). Common side effects are mild nausea, abdominal discomfort, and loose stools; less frequent side effects are severe nausea or vomiting. In anxious patients who are sensitive to stimulating effects, SAMe may temporarily increase anxiety during initiation or dose increases. SAMe is contraindicated in patients with bipolar disorder because, similar to other antidepressants, SAMe can trigger hypomanic or manic symptoms. Anecdotally, in patients with cardiac arrhythmias, stimulative effects of SAMe may occasionally exacerbate the arrhythmia.

SAMe does not cause adverse interactions with other medications. The only case of purported serotonin syndrome described a 71-year-old woman on a constant dose of SAMe who developed shaking 48–72 hours after increasing her clomipramine from 25 to 75 mg/day. No other cases of serotonin syndrome or adverse drug interactions have been documented, including in RCTs using SAMe to augment TCAs, SSRIs, and SNRIs. SAMe is the only antidepressant to have demonstrated no adverse interactions with monoamine oxidase inhibitors (MAOIs). An open trial of SAMe augmentation in 60 patients being treated with MAOIs reported positive improvements and no adverse interactions (Torta et al. 1988). In the same study, SAMe reduced the alcohol- and medication-induced elevated enzyme levels per liver function tests. Theoretically, in extremely severe folate deficiency, SAMe might elevate homocysteine levels; however, no such effect has been documented, and a study of SAMe 1,600 mg/day for 5 days found that serum homocysteine was unchanged (Gören et al. 2004).

Clinical Guidelines for SAMe Treatments

Quality of SAMe Products

To assure efficacy and minimize side effects, best-quality SAMe products are essential. Because SAMe oxidizes on exposure to air, tablets must be carefully manufactured, enteric coated, and protected in individual blister packs. Low-quality SAMe products can lose up to 50% potency while sitting on shelves. Bargain brands may contain inactive isomers. SAMe tablets should not be refrigerated because condensation inside blister packs can degrade tablets. High-quality pharmaceutical-grade SAMe manufactured in Italy is called ademetionina (1,4-butanedisulfonate). Many patients respond well to less expensive brands containing toluenate and tosylate forms. However, for those who do not, a trial of ademetionina is indicated (www.medicamentos.com.mx/dochtm/29997.htm). Anecdotally, the authors find better overall response to 1,4-butanedisulfonate.

SAMe Dosages

SAMe should be taken on an empty stomach to maximize absorption. If nausea occurs, SAMe can be taken with a little food. SAMe is best taken in the morning at least 20 minutes before food. Second doses can be taken at least 20 minutes before lunch or 2 hours after lunch. Taking SAMe, an activating antidepressant, in late afternoon or evening may disturb sleep. Most patients begin with 400 mg SAMe, increasing by 400-mg increments every 3–7 days as tolerated. For mild to moderate depression or antidepressant augmentation, 800–1,200 mg/day is usually sufficient; for more severe cases, 1,600 mg/day; for patients with severe, treatment-resistant depression, up to 2,400 mg/day as tolerated. Elderly, debilitated, or medication-sensitive patients should start at 200 mg/day, titrating upward slowly.

KEY POINTS

- *S*-Adenosylmethionine (SAMe; also referred to as *S*-adenosyl-L-methionine or ademetionine) is a natural metabolite with antidepressant, anti-inflammatory, and analgesic properties.

- Compared with prescription antidepressants, SAMe is low in side effects, causes no weight gain or sexual dysfunction, and has no adverse interactions with other medications.

- SAMe has demonstrated no toxic effects even in doses far exceeding those recommended for routine clinical use.

- The quality of SAMe products varies greatly and is critical for potency and efficacy.

References

Abdolmáleky HM, Cheng KH, Faraone SV, et al: Hypomethylation of MB-COMT promoter is a major risk factor for schizophrenia and bipolar disorder. Hum Mol Genet 15(21):3132–3145, 2006 16984965

Agency for Healthcare Research and Quality: S-Adenosyl-L-metionine for depression, osteoarthritis, and liver disease. Summary, Evidence Report/Technology Assessment: Number 64. AHRQ Publ No 02-E033. Rockville, MD, Agency for Healthcare Research and Quality, August 2002. Available at: https://archive.ahrq.gov/clinic/tp/sametp.htm. Accessed March 3, 2017.

Alpert JE, Papakostas G, Mischoulon D, et al: S-Adenosyl-L-methionine (SAMe) as an adjunct for resistant major depressive disorder: an open trial following partial or nonresponse to selective serotonin reuptake inhibitors or venlafaxine. J Clin Psychopharmacol 24(6):661–664, 2004 15538131

American Psychiatric Association: Diagnostic and Statistical Manual of Mental Disorders, 4th Edition. Washington, DC, American Psychiatric Association, 1994

Ansari R, Mahta A, Mallack E, Luo JJ: Hyperhomocysteinemia and neurologic disorders: a review. J Clin Neurol 10(4):281–288, 2014 25324876

Berger R, Nowak H: A new medical approach to the treatment of osteoarthritis: report of an open phase IV study with ademetionine (Gumbaral). Am J Med 83(5A):84–88, 1987 3318446

Bottiglieri T: Folate, vitamin B12, and S-adenosylmethionine. Psychiatr Clin North Am 36(1):37–47, 2012 23538072

Bottiglieri T, Hyland K: S-adenosylmethionine levels in psychiatric and neurological disorders: a review. Acta Neurol Scand Suppl 154:19–26, 1994 7524260

Bottiglieri T, Laundy M, Martin R, et al: S-Adenosylmethionine influences monoamine metabolism. Lancet 2(8396):224, 1984 6146777

Bottiglieri T, Arning E, Wasek B, et al: Acute administration of L-dopa induces changes in methylation metabolites, reduced protein phosphatase 2A methylation, and hyperphosphorylation of Tau protein in mouse brain. J Neurosci 32(27):9173–9181, 2012 3422683

Brown RP, Gerbarg PL: Complementary and integrative treatments in brain injury, in Textbook of Traumatic Brain Injury, 2nd Edition. Edited by Silver JM, McAllister TW, Yudofsky SC. Washington, DC, American Psychiatric Publishing, 2011, pp 599–622

Brown RP, Gerbarg PL, Bottiglieri T: S-Adenosylmethionine (SAMe) in the clinical practice of psychiatry, neurology, and internal medicine. Clinical Practice of Alternative Medicine 1(4):230–241, 2000

Brown RP, Gerbarg PL, Muskin PR: How to Use Herbs, Nutrients and Yoga in Mental Health Care. New York, WW Norton, 2009

Carrieri PB, Indaco A, Gentile S: S-Adenosylmethionine treatment of depression in patients with Parkinson's disease: a double-blind crossover study versus placebo. Curr Ther Res 48(1):154–160, 1990

Chan A, Paskavitz J, Remington R, et al: Efficacy of a vitamin/nutriceutical formulation for early-stage Alzheimer's disease: a 1-year, open-label pilot study with an 16-month caregiver extension. Am J Alzheimers Dis Other Demen 23(6):571–585, 2008 19047474

Chan A, Tchantchou F, Rogers EJ, Shea TB: Dietary deficiency increases presenilin expression, gamma-secretase activity, and Abeta levels: potentiation by ApoE genotype and alleviation by S-adenosyl methionine. J Neurochem 110(3):831–836, 2009 19457069

Chan A, Remington R, Kotyla E, et al: A vitamin/nutriceutical formulation improves memory and cognitive performance in community-dwelling adults without dementia. J Nutr Health Aging 14(3):224–230, 2010 20191258

De Berardis D, Marini S, Serroni N, et al: S-Adenosyl-L-methionine augmentation in patients with stage II treatment-resistant major depressive disorder: An open label, fixed dose, single-blind study. Scientific World Journal 2013(11):204649, 2013 23766680

Fava M, Rosenbaum JF, Birnbaum R, et al: The thyrotropin response to thyrotropin-releasing hormone as a predictor of response to treatment in depressed outpatients. Acta Psychiatr Scand 86(1):42–45, 1992 1414398

Gerbarg PL, Brown RP: Therapeutic nutrients, herbs, and hormones, in Psychiatric Care of the Medical Patient, 3rd Edition. Edited by Fogel B, Greenberg D. New York, Oxford University Press, 2015, pp 545–608

Gören JL, Stoll AL, Damico KE, et al: Bioavailability and lack of toxicity of S-adenosyl-L-methionine (SAMe) in humans. Pharmacotherapy 24(11):1501–1507, 2004 15537554

Kharbanda KK, Rogers DD, Mailliard ME, et al: A comparison of the effects of betaine and S-adenosylmethionine on ethanol-induced changes in methionine metabolism and steatosis in rat hepatocytes. J Nutr 135(3):519–524, 2005 15735087

Konig H, Stahl H, Sieper J, Wolf KJ: Magnetic resonance tomography of finger polyarthritis: morphology and cartilage signals after ademetionine therapy [in German]. Aktuelle Radiol 5(1):36–40, 1995 7888428

Lefkovitz Y, Alpert JE, Brintz CE, et al: Effects of S-adenosylmethionine augmentation of serotonin-reuptake inhibitor antidepressants on cognitive symptoms of major depressive disorder. J Affect Disord 136(3):1174–1178, 2012 21911258

Levine J, Stahl Z, Sela BA, et al: Homocysteine-reducing strategies improve symptoms in chronic schizophrenic patients with hyperhomocysteinemia. Biol Psychiatry 60(3):265–269, 2006 16412989

Li J, Doyle KM, Tatlisumak T: Polyamines in the brain: distribution, biological interactions, and their potential therapeutic role in brain ischaemia. Curr Med Chem 14(17):1807–1813, 2007 17627518

Lieber CS: Pathogenesis and treatment of alcoholic liver disease: progress over the last 50 years. Rocz Akad Med Bialymst 50:7–20, 2005 16363067

Mato JM, Cámara J, Fernández de Paz J, et al: S-Adenosylmethionine in alcoholic liver cirrhosis: a randomized, placebo-controlled, double-blind, multicenter clinical trial. J Hepatol 30(6):1081–1089, 1999 10406187

McCully KS: Homocysteine metabolism, atherosclerosis, and diseases of aging. Compr Physiol 120(1):471–505, 2015 26756640

Medici V, Virata MC, Peerson JM, et al: S-Adenosyl-L-methionine treatment for alcoholic liver disease: a double-blinded, randomized, placebo-controlled trial. Alcohol Clin Exp Res 35(11):1960–1965, 2011 22044287

Mischoulon D, Price LH, Carpenter LL, et al: A double-blind, randomized, placebo-controlled clinical trial of S-adenosyl-L-methionine (SAMe) versus escitalopram in major depressive disorder. J Clin Psychiatry 75(4):370–376, 2014 24500245

Monaco P, Pastore L, Rizzo S, et al: Safety and tolerability of ademetionine (ADE) SD for inpatients with stroke: a pilot randomized, double-blind, placebo controlled study (abstract). Presented at the Third World Stroke Conference and Fifth European Stroke Conference, Munich, Germany, September 1–5, 1996

Nowotarski SL, Woster PM, Casero RAJr: Polyamines and cancer: implications for chemotherapy and chemoprevention. Expert Rev Mol Med 15:e3, 2013 23432971

Otero-Losada ME, Rubio MC: Acute effects of S-adenosyl-L-methionine on catecholaminergic central function. Eur J Pharmacol 163:353–356, 1989

Papakostas GI, Mischoulon D, Shyu I, et al: S-Adenosyl methionine (SAMe) augmentation of serotonin reuptake inhibitors for antidepressant nonresponders with major depressive disorder: A double-blind, randomized clinical trial. Am J Psychiatry 167(8):942–948, 2010 20595412

Refsum H, Smith AD, Ueland PM, et al: Facts and recommendations about total homocysteine determinations: an expert opinion. Clin Chem 50(1):3–32, 2004 14709635

Remington R, Chan A, Paskavitz J, et al: Efficacy of a vitamin/nutriceutical formulation for moderate-stage to later-stage Alzheimer's disease: a placebo-controlled pilot study. Am J Alzheimers Dis Other Demen 24(1):27–33, 2009 19056706

Reynolds EH: The neurology of folic acid deficiency. Handb Clin Neurol 120:927–943, 2014 24365361

Roffman JL, Gollub RL, Calhoun VD, et al: MTHFR 677C → T genotype disrupts prefrontal function in schizophrenia through an interaction with COMT 158Val → Met. Proc Natl Acad Sci U. S. A. 105(45):17,573–17,578, 2008 18988738

Sarris J, Price LH, Carpenter LL, et al: Is S-adenosyl methionine (SAMe) for depression only effective in males? A re-analysis of data from a randomized clinical trial. Pharmacopsychiatry 48(4–5):141–144, 2015 26011569

Sarris J, Murphy J, Mischoulon D, et al: Adjunctive nutraceuticals for depression: a systematic review and meta-analyses. Am J Psychiatry 173(6):575–587, 2016 27113121

Schaller JL, Thomas J, Bazzan AJ: SAMe use in children and adolescents. Eur Child Adolesc Psychiatry 13(5):332–334, 2004 15490281

Sharma A, Gerbarg PL, Bottiglieri T, et al, Work Group of the American Psychiatric Association Council on Research: S-Adenosylmethionine (SAMe) for neuropsychiatric disorders: a clinician-oriented review of research. J Clin Psychiatry, 2016, in press

Shippy RA, Mendez D, Jones K, et al: S-Adenosylmethionine (SAM-e) for the treatment of depression in people living with HIV/AIDS. BMC Psychiatry 4:38, 2004 15538952

Sontag JM, Sontag E: Protein phosphatase 2A dysfunction in Alzheimer's disease. Front Mol Neurosci 7:1–16, 2014 24653673

Surtees R, Hyland K: Cerebrospinal fluid concentrations of S-adenosylmethionine, methionine, and 5-methyltetrahydrofolate in a reference population: cerebrospinal fluid S-adenosylmethionine declines with age in humans. Biochem Med Metab Biol 44(2):192–199, 1990 2252620

Surtees R, Leonard J, Austin S: Association of demyelination with deficiency of cerebrospinal-fluid S-adenosylmethionine in inborn errors of methyl-transfer pathway. Lancet 338(8782–8783):1550–1554, 1991 1683972

Tavoni A, Vitali C, Bombardieri S, et al: Evaluation of S-adenosylmethionine in primary fibromyalgia: a double-blind crossover study. Am J Med 83(5A):107–110, 1987 3318438

Thomas CS, Bottiglieri T, Edeh J, et al: The influence of S-adenosylmethionine (SAM) on prolactin in depressed patients. Int Clin Psychopharmacol 2:97–102, 1987

Torta R, Zanalda F, Rocca P, et al: Inhibitory activity of S-adenosyl-L-methionine on serum gamma-glutamyl-transpeptidase increase induced by psych drugs and anticonvulsants. Curr Ther Res 44:144–159, 1988

Varanese S, Birnbaum Z, Rossi R, et al: Treatment of advanced Parkinson's disease. Parkinsons Dis 2010:480260, 2011 21331376

Yamamoto T, Hinoi E, Fujita H, et al: The natural polyamines spermidine and spermine prevent bone loss through preferential disruption of osteoclastic activation in ovariectomized mice. Br J Pharmacol 166(3):1084–1096, 2012 22250848

Yen MH, Weng TC, Liu SY, et al: The hepatoprotective effect of Bupleurum kaoi, an endemic plant to Taiwan, against dimethylnitrosamine-induced hepatic fibrosis in rats. Biol Pharm Bull 28(3):442–448, 2005 15744066

CHAPTER 5

Acetyl-L-Carnitine, *N*-Acetylcysteine, and Inositol in the Treatment of Psychiatric and Neuropsychiatric Disorders

Sheng-Min Wang, M.D., Ph.D.
Chi-Un Pae, M.D., Ph.D.

[A]s if, one by one, the memories you used to harbor
decided to retire to the southern hemisphere of the brain...

Billy Collins, Poet Laureate, "Forgetfulness"

The authors wish to thank coeditor Dr. Richard P. Brown for providing clinical case examples for this chapter. Excerpt from "Forgetfulness" from *Questions About Angels*, by Billy Collins, © 1991. Reprinted by permission of the University of Pittsburgh Press.

Acetyl-L-Carnitine

Acetyl-L-carnitine (ALC) has diverse effects in the brain, including modulation of energy and phospholipid metabolism, neurotrophic factors and neurohormones, and synaptic morphology, as well as promotion of synaptic transmission of multiple neurotransmitters (Pettegrew et al. 2000). Finding ALC effects on many central nervous systems led to clinical trials reporting benefits in depression and Alzheimer's disease. Carnitine, an endogenous compound synthesized from amino acids lysine and methionine, is an intermediary metabolite. In biological tissues, high concentrations of carnitine exist as free carnitine or acylcarnitines (Steiber et al. 2004). ALC, the most common natural short-chain acetylcarnitine ester of L-carnitine, is actively transported across the blood-brain barrier.

In depression, the most important mechanism of action is thought to be enhanced neurogenesis in hippocampal and prefrontal regions by upregulation of metabotropic glutamate receptor 2 (mGlu2; Figure 5–1) (Cuccurazzu et al. 2013; Wang et al. 2014). Other possible mechanisms include enhanced neuroplasticity by increased neurotrophic factors such as brain-derived neurotrophic factor (BDNF), glial-derived factor artemin, and nerve growth factor (NGF; Nasca et al. 2013). Membrane molecular and lipid metabolism are important in pathophysiology of depression. ALC may reduce depression by improving brain energy metabolism via increasing myoinositol levels and altering glucose metabolism (Smeland et al. 2012). It may also enhance dopamine and serotonin output in mesocorticolimbic areas. Seven mechanism of action have been proposed for Alzheimer's disease (Pettegrew et al. 2000): restoration of cell membranes, restoration of synaptic function, restoration of brain energy, augmentation of cholinergic activity, protection against toxins, stimulation of NGF, and protein acetylation.

Clinical Trials of Acetyl-L-Carnitine

Reviews of ALC for depression (Wang et al. 2014), mild cognitive impairment (MCI), and Alzheimer's disease (Hudson and Tabet 2003) contain references for studies described below and in Table 5–1.

DEPRESSIVE AND MOOD DISORDERS

The efficacy of ALC for depression, first reported in an open study in geriatric patients, has been studied in nine double-blind, randomized placebo-controlled trials (DBRPCTs; Table 5–1). Three studies showed superior efficacy of ALC monotherapy over placebo in unipolar depression (Garzya et al. 1990; Gecele and Meluzzi 1991; Villardita et al. 1983). One study showed ALC to be more effective than placebo as augmentation in geriatric depression (Nasca et al. 1989). In a randomized controlled trial (RCT) in bipolar depression, ALC failed to show superiority over placebo (Brennan et al. 2013). Two studies found ALC better than placebo for persistent depressive disorder (dysthymia) (Bella et al. 1990; Fulgente et al. 1990), and two found it as effective as fluoxetine or amisulpride in persistent depressive disorder (Bersani et al. 2013; Zanardi and Smeraldi 2006). These RCTs suggest that ALC is generally safe and well tolerated. Adverse events were generally mild. Tolerability of ALC was comparable to that of pla-

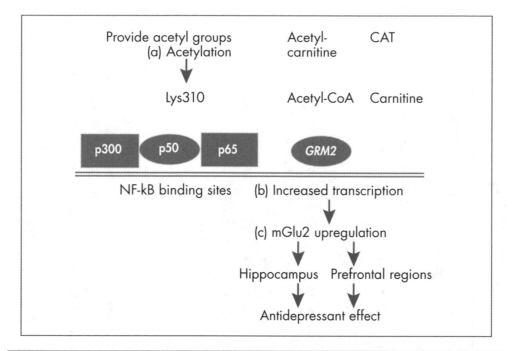

FIGURE 5–1. Putative mechanism of acetyl-L-carnitine-induced antidepressant effect via improving neuroplasticity.

(a) ALC provides acetyl groups for acetylation of p65 at Lys310 located in NF-kB binding sites. This would (b) lead to transcription of *GRM2* and (c) result in upregulation of type 2 mGlu2 and promotion of neurogenesis in hippocampus and prefrontal regions.

ALC=acetyl-L-carnitine; CAT=carnitine acetyl-carnitine translocase; CoA=coenzyme A; mGlu2=type 2 metabotropic glutamate receptor; NF-kB=nuclear factor kappa light chain enhancer.

cebo in patients with bipolar depression. The most common side effects with ALC versus placebo were diarrhea (30% ALC or α-lipoic acid vs. 15% placebo), foul-smelling urine (25% vs. 5%), rash (20% vs. 0%), constipation (15% vs. 5%), and dyspepsia (15% vs. 0%). ALC had fewer significant side effects (6/41) than fluoxetine (18/36).

MILD COGNITIVE IMPAIRMENT, ALZHEIMER'S DISEASE, AND ATTENTION-DEFICIT/HYPERACTIVITY DISORDER

Prior to 2000, many studies suggested that ALC could improve cognitive deficits or delay progressive decline in patients with MCI or Alzheimer's disease (Table 5–1). In one study, the ALC group had a slower rate of deterioration in 13 of 14 measures, such as the Blessed Dementia Scale, logical intelligence, buccofacial apraxia, and selective attention (Spagnoli et al. 1991). In another study, ALC was associated with less deterioration in timed cancellation and digit span tasks (Sano et al. 1992). However, two large studies detected no difference from placebo (Thal et al. 1996, 2000). A meta-analysis of 21 DBRPCTs revealed significant advantage for ALC compared with placebo in MCI and Alzheimer's disease on composite effect size (ES all scales=0.201; 95% confidence

TABLE 5–1. Summary of double-blind, randomized placebo- or comparator-controlled trials of acetyl-L-carnitine in treatment of neuropsychiatric disorders

Author (year)	Diagnosis	Length	ALC dosage	Comparator	Efficacy results
Depressive disorders					
Bersani et al. (2013)	DD elderly	7 weeks	ALC 3 g (N=41)	FOX 20 mg; N=39	ALC=FOX in HDS-21, Ham-A, and BDI
Brennan et al. (2013)	BD	12 weeks	ALC 1–3 g+ALA 0.6~1.8 g (N=20)	PBO; N=20	ALC+ALA=PBO in MADRS, HDS-21, YMRS, and CGI
Zanardi and Smeraldi (2006)	PDD	12 weeks	ALC 1 g (N=99)	ASP 100 mg; N=94	ALC=ASP in HDS-21, MADRS, CDRS, and CGI
Villardita et al. (1983)	MDD	6 weeks	ALC 1.5 g (N=14)	PBO	ALC>PBO in Ham-D
Gecele and Meluzzi (1991)	MDD elderly	6 weeks	ALC 2 g (N=14)	PBO; N=14	ALC>PBO in HDS-17
Fulgente et al. (1990)	PDD	8 weeks	ALC 3 g (N=30)	PBO; N=30	ALC>PBO in HDS-17
Garzya et al. (1990)	MDD elderly	8 weeks	ALC 1.5 g (N=14)	PBO; N=14	ALC>PBO in HDS-17
Bella et al. (1990)	PDD elderly	8 weeks	ALC 3 g (N=30)	PBO; N=30	ALC>PBO in HDS-17
Nasca et al. (1989)	MDD	8 weeks	MIA+ALC 2 g (N=10)	MIA+PBO; N=10	MIA+ALC>MIA+PBO in Ham-D
Alzheimer's disease					
Thal et al. (2000)	Probable AD	12 months	ALC 3 g (N=112)	PBO; N=117	ADAS-Cognitive subscale and CDR: no significance
Thal et al. (1996)	Probable AD	12 months	ALC 3 g (N=207)	PBO; N=212	ADAS-Cognitive subscale and CDR: no significance
Sano et al. (1992)	Probable AD	6 months	ALC 2.5~3 g (N=13)	PBO; N=14	Less deterioration in timed cancellation tasks and digit span (forward)

TABLE 5–1. Summary of double-blind, randomized placebo- or comparator-controlled trials of acetyl-L-carnitine in treatment of neuropsychiatric disorders *(continued)*

Author (year)	Diagnosis	Length	ALC dosage	Comparator	Efficacy results
Alzheimer's disease (continued)					
Spagnoli et al. (1991)	AD	12 months	ALC 2 g (*N*=42)	PBO; *N*=50	Slower deterioration in 13/14 outcome measures with ALC
Rai et al. (1990)	AD	6 months	ALC 2 g (*N*=7)	PBO; *N*=13	No significant difference
Passeri et al. (1990)	MCI	3 months	ALC 2 g (*N*=30)	PBO; *N*=28	ALC>PBO behavior, verbal fluency memory, attention

Note. AD=Alzheimer's disease; ADAS=Alzheimer's Disease Assessment Scale; ALA=α-lipoic acid; ALC=acetyl-L-carnitine; ASP=amisulpride; BD=bipolar depression; BDI=Beck Depression Inventory; CDR=Clinical Dementia Rating Scale; CDRS=Cornell Dysthymia Rating Scale; CGI=Clinical Global Impression Scale; FOX=fluoxetine; Ham-A=Hamilton Anxiety Rating Scale; Ham-D=Hamilton Depression Rating Scale; HDS= Hamilton Depression Scale; MADRS=Montgomery-Åsberg Depression Rating Scale; MCI=mild cognitive impairment; MDD=major depressive disorder; MIA=mianserine; PBO=placebo; PDD=persistent depressive disorder (dysthymia); YMRS=Young Mania Rating Scale.

interval [CI], 0.107–0.295) and clinician assessment of improvement (effect size) on the Clinical Global Impression Scale (ES_{CGI-CH}=0.32; 95% CI, 0.18–0.47) (Montgomery et al. 2003). The meta-analysis confirmed that ALC was well tolerated. Severity of adverse events and dropout rates for ALC and placebo were comparable. However, some studies reported more frequent gastrointestinal side effects, insomnia, agitation, and increased appetite with ALC. Several studies reported benefits for MCI and Alzheimer's disease using ALC with N-acetylcysteine (NAC) and S-adenosylmethionine (SAMe; see Chapter 4, "S-Adenosylmethionine").

The efficacy and safety of carnitine in children were demonstrated in a DBRPCT of 26 boys (ages 6–13 years) with attention-deficit/hyperactivity disorder (ADHD), in whom ALC significantly decreased attention problems and aggressive behavior. Another DBRPCT (n=61) showed greater decline in hyperactivity and improvement in social behavior in patients with ADHD who were treated with ALC than in those receiving placebo (Torrioli et al. 2008). In contrast, a 16-week pilot DBRPCT of 112 children with ADHD failed to separate ALC from placebo on Conners' parent and teacher scales (Arnold et al. 2007). ALC was safe, with adverse events comparable between groups. A 6-week DBRPCT of 40 children (ages 7–13 years) with ADHD comparing ALC plus methylphenidate with placebo plus methylphenidate found no benefit from adjunctive ALC. The ALC group had fewer side effects, particularly headache and irritability.

Case Examples of Acetyl-L-Carnitine

In contrast to subjects in most clinical trials, patients seen in psychiatric practice often have more than one diagnosis. Unlike researchers, clinicians are free to combine synergistic treatments to optimize outcomes, and there is no limit to the number of trials they can offer patients. These cases exemplify the complexity of patients seen in practice and the potential for innovative integrative treatments for those whose conditions are characterized as treatment-resistant.

Case 1: Treatment-Resistant Severe Major Depressive Disorder in Patient With Ovarian Cancer

An occupational therapist developed episodes of severe major depressive disorder (MDD) during her battle with recurrent ovarian cancer starting at age 52. After the patient did not respond to many trials of serotonin reuptake inhibitors (SRIs), serotonin-norepinephrine reuptake inhibitors (SNRIs), and tricyclic antidepressants, she partially responded to buspirone 60 mg daily. At age 69, she began a trial of antidepressant augmentation with ALC 1,500 mg twice daily, which resulted in full remission of depression. Free of depression and cancer for 5 years, and despite exposure to neurotoxic cancer chemotherapy for many years, she continues to work without cognitive impairment.

Case 2: Acetyl-L-Carnitine for Alzheimer's Disease in Apolipoprotein E4+ Patient With Depression

Myron, a business executive, feared developing Alzheimer's disease because his father and maternal aunt died after years of deterioration from Alzheimer's disease. Testing showed he was positive for two apolipoprotein E4 (*APOE4*) alleles, polymorphisms associated with increased risk of Alzheimer's disease. He was taking nefazodone for depression, after he did not respond to many trials of SRIs and SNRIs. At age 59, Myron consulted an integrative psychiatrist who prescribed ALC on the basis of research suggesting preventive benefits if ALC is started before age 60 (Spagnoli et al. 1991). He began additional cognitive enhancers: NAC, B vitamins, SAMe, *Rhodiola rosea*, curcumin, low-dose selegiline 5 mg/day, and optimized saffron. Reevaluation at age 65 showed no signs of cognitive deterioration. Still worried, Myron sought evaluation for a long-term study on Alzheimer's disease but was rejected as a subject because his cognitive test scores were too high for his age.

Although combinations of cognitive protectors are difficult to study, they may provide synergistic benefits through multiple mechanisms. SAMe with ALC, NAC, and B vitamins shows benefits for MCI and Alzheimer's disease (see Chapter 4). These may be augmented with selegiline to delay deterioration from Parkinson's disease and Alzheimer's disease (Ebadi et al. 2006). At low doses (≤10 mg per day), selegiline does not cause monoamine oxidase A inhibition and is therefore safe to use with other medications. *Rhodiola rosea* (Chapter 8, "Adaptogens in Psychiatric Practice," and Chapter 9, "Integrating *Rhodiola rosea* in Clinical Practice") and curcumin may further enhance cognitive function (Jagetia and Aggarwal 2007).

N-Acetylcysteine

NAC, an acetyl derivative of the amino acid cysteine with antioxidant properties, is a U.S. Food and Drug Administration–approved antidote for acetaminophen overdose (Deepmala et al. 2015). NAC is also used as a mucolytic in chronic obstructive pulmonary disease, a renal protectant, and a therapeutic agent for HIV. It has been tested in substance-related disorders, autism spectrum disorder, schizophrenia, mood disorder, and other neuropsychiatric conditions. NAC modulates key neurotransmitter systems, including serotonin, glutamate, and dopamine (Berk et al. 2012). It reduces oxidative stress by providing cysteine, a rate-limiting amino acid in glutathione production. Glutathione reduces reactive oxygen species to hydrogen peroxide, which can be neutralized to water. NAC is also associated with reduced inflammatory cytokines, exerts synaptic potentiation, and has neuroplastic properties (Berk et al. 2008a).

Clinical Trials of *N*-Acetylcysteine

A review by Deepmala et al. (2015) contains references for studies in this section and in Tables 5–2 and 5–3.

SUBSTANCE-RELATED AND ADDICTIVE DISORDERS

The first NAC study in addictive disorders was a crossover DBRPCT in 15 nontreatment-seeking individuals with cocaine dependence (American Psychiatric Association 2000; LaRowe et al. 2007). Patients received either NAC or placebo during a 3-day hospitalization. Four days later, they were crossed over to receive the opposite condition during an identical 3-day hospitalization. In the presence of cocaine-related cues, NAC reduced the desire to use cocaine, interest in cocaine, and cue viewing time. In a pilot study, 24 patients with pathological gambling (American Psychiatric Association

TABLE 5–2. Double-blind, randomized placebo- or comparator-controlled trials: *N*-acetylcysteine in treatment of substance-related and addictive disorders

Author (year)	Primary diagnosis	Age	Length	Study design	NAC dosage	Comparator	Primary outcome measure and efficacy results
Gray et al. (2012)	Cannabis use disorder	15~21 years	8 weeks	DBRPC	2.4 g/day (*N*=58)	PBO; *N*=58	Urine cannabinoid: NAC>PBO (odds ratio, 2.4; 95% CI, 1.1–5.2)
LaRowe et al. (2013)	Cocaine use disorder	Adults	8 weeks	DBRPC	1.2 g/day (*N*=40), 2.4 g/day (*N*=33)	PBO; *N*=38	Urine cocaine metabolite: no difference
LaRowe et al. (2007)	Cocaine use disorder	Mean 37.4 years	3 days	DBRPC-crossover	1.2 g/day (*N*=13)	PBO; *N*=13	Reactivity to cocaine-related stimuli: less with NAC
Mousavi et al. (2015)	Stimulant use disorder	18–65 years	8 weeks	DBRPC-crossover	1.2 g/day for 2 wk → 2.4 g/day (*N*=23)	PBO; *N*=23	Cocaine Craving Questionnaire—Brief: significant effect with NAC but no carryover effects
Grant et al. (2010)	Stimulant use disorder	18–65 years	8 weeks	DBRPC	2.4 g/day +NTX 200 mg/day (*N*=14)	PBO+NTX 200 mg/day; *N*=17	Penn Craving Scale (modified for methamphetamine dependence): no difference
Prado et al. (2015)	Tobacco use disorder	Adults	12 weeks	DBRPC	3 g/day (*N*=17)	PBO; *N*=14	Daily cigarette use: significantly less with NAC (mean change –10.9±7.9 for NAC vs. –3.2±6.1 for PBO)
McClure et al. (2014)	Cannabis use disorder	15–21 years	8 weeks	DBRPC	2.4 g/day (*N*=34)	PBO; *N*=34	Qualitative urinary cotinine: 59% of enrolled were smokers; results: no group difference

TABLE 5–2. Double-blind, randomized placebo- or comparator-controlled trials: *N*-acetylcysteine in treatment of substance-related and addictive disorders *(continued)*

Author (year)	Primary diagnosis	Age	Length	Study design	NAC dosage	Comparator	Primary outcome measure and efficacy results
Grant et al. (2014)	Tobacco use and gambling	Adults	12 weeks	DBRPC	BT+1.2 g/day ~3.0 g/day (*N*=13)	BT+PBO; *N*=15	Fagerström Test for Nicotine Dependence total scores: improvement week 6 but not week 12; PG-YBOCS: NAC>PBO (*t*=2.069; *P*=0.043)
Schmaal et al. (2011)	Tobacco use disorder	College student	3.5 days	DBRPC	3.6 g/day (*N*=10)	PBO; *N*=12	VAS reward cigarette: significantly lower in the NAC group (*P*<0.05)
Bernardo et al. (2009)	BPD	Adults	24 weeks	DBRPC	2.0 g/day (*N*=38)	PBO,;*N*=37	CGI-SU: no difference
Grant et al. (2007)	Gambling disorder	18–75 years	14 weeks	OL (8 wk) → DBPC	1.8 g/day (*N*=6)	PBO; *N*=7	PG-YBOCS: response rate numerically higher for NAC in DBPC phase

Note. BPD=bipolar disorder; BT=behavior therapy; CGI-SU=Clinical Global Impression–Substance Use; CI=confidence interval; DBRPC=double-blind, randomized placebo-controlled; NAC=*N*-acetylcysteine; NTX=naltrexone; OL=open label; PBO=placebo; PG-YBOCS=Yale-Brown Obsessive Compulsive Scale Modified for Pathological Gambling; VAS=Visual Analog Scale.

TABLE 5–3. Double-blind, randomized placebo- or comparator-controlled trials of *N*-acetylcysteine treatment of other neuropsychiatric disorders

Author (year)	Primary diagnosis	Age	Length, weeks	Study design	NAC dosage	Comparator	Primary outcome measure and efficacy results
Nikoo et al. (2015)	Autism spectrum disorder	4–12 years	10	DBRPC	RPR+0.6~0.9g/day (*N*=20)	RPR+PBO; *N*=20	ABC Irritability subscale: NAC>PBO in reduction
Ghanizadeh et al. (2013)	Autism spectrum disorder	3.5–16 years	8	DBRPC	RPR+1.2 g/day (*N*=20)	RPR+PBO; *N*=20,	ABC Irritability subscale: NAC>PBO in reduction ($F1, 29=4.9, P<0.035$)
Hardan et al. (2012)	Autism spectrum disorder	3–12 years	12	DBRPC	0.9 g ~ 2.7 g/day (*N*=14)	PBO; *N*=15	ABC Irritability subscale: NAC>PBO in reduction ($F=6.80; P<0.001; d=0.96$)
Farokhnia et al. (2013)	SPR	18–50 years	8	DBRPC	RPR+2.0 g/day (*N*=23)	RPR+PBO; *N*=23	PANSS: NAC>PBO in reduction ($P=0.006$)
Berk et al. (2008b)	SPR	18–65 years	24	DBRPC	AAP+2.0 g/day (*N*=69)	AAP+PBO; *N*=71	PANSS: NAC>PBO in reduction ($P=0.009$); NAC>PBO in akathisia ($P=0.004$)
Berk et al. (2012)	BPD (≥12 in MADRS)	Adults	32	OL (8 weeks) → DBPC	Usual treatment+ 2.0 g/day (*N*=76)	Usual treatment +PBO *N*=73	Time to interventions for mood symptoms: no difference
Berk et al. (2008b)	BPD	Adults	24	DBRPC	Usual treatment + 2.0 g/day (*N*=38)	Usual treatment +PBO *N*=37	MADRS: NAC>PBO (least squares mean difference=−8.05, $P=0.002$)

TABLE 5–3. Double-blind, randomized placebo- or comparator-controlled trials of *N*-acetylcysteine treatment of other neuropsychiatric disorders *(continued)*

Author (year)	Primary diagnosis	Age	Length, weeks	Study design	NAC dosage	Comparator	Primary outcome measure and efficacy results
Berk et al. (2014)	Major depression	≥18 years	12	DBRPC	Usual treatment +1.0 g/day (*N*=127)	Usual treatment+PBO; *N*=125	MADRS: no difference; response and remission: NAC>PBO at week 16 but not at week 12
Bloch et al. (2013)	Trichotillomania	8–17 years	12	DBRPC	Max 2.4 g/day (*N*=20)	PBO; *N*=20	MGH-HPS: no difference
Grant et al. (2009)	Trichotillomania	18–65 years	12	DBRPC	Max 2.4 g/day (*N*=2)	PBO; *N*=25	MGH-HPS: NAC>PBO in reduction (*P*<0.001)
Ghanizadeh et al. (2013)	Nail biting	Children	8	DBRPC	0.8 g/day (*N*=21)	PBO; *N*=21	Nail length: NAC>PBO (5.21 [5.75] vs. 1.18 [3.02] mm, *P*<0.05) at week 4 but not week 8
Adair et al. (2001)	Probable AD	Elderly	24	DBRPC	50 mg/kg/day (*N*=23)	PBO; *N*=20	Cognitive functions: improvement observed with NAC in some cognitive domains

Note. AAP=antipsychotics; ABC=Aberrant Behavior Checklist; AD=Alzheimer's dementia; BPD=bipolar disorder; DBRPC=double-blind, randomized placebo-controlled; MADRS=Montgomery-Åsberg Depression Rating Scale; MGH-HPS=Massachusetts General Hospital Hair Pulling Scale; NAC=*N*-acetylcysteine; OL=open label; PANSS=Positive and Negative Syndrome Scale; PBO=placebo; RPR=risperidone; SPR=schizophrenia.

2000) were first treated in an 8-week open-label trial with NAC, followed by a 6-week double-blind RCT of NAC ($n=6$) or placebo ($n=7$) (Grant et al. 2007). Although the study failed to show significant superiority of NAC over placebo on the Yale-Brown Obsessive Compulsive Scale Modified for Pathological Gambling (PG-YBOCS), a higher percentage of patients given NAC (83.3%) responded at the end of the second phase compared with those given placebo (28.6%). Numerous DBRPCTs investigated efficacy of NAC in patients with substance use disorders (Table 5–2). A DBRPCT ($N=116$) showed that adolescents and young adults (ages 15–21 years) with cannabis dependence given NAC 2.4 g/day had more than twice the odds of a negative urine cannabinoid test than did those given placebo (Gray et al. 2012). Subsequent analysis of 89 participants found a nonsignificant difference in decreased self-reported (Marijuana Craving Questionnaire) marijuana craving between groups, suggesting that the reduced cannabis use associated with NAC treatment may be mediated by effects other than craving (Roten et al. 2013). Overall, NAC has not been proven effective in trials for cannabis use disorder (McClure et al. 2014), although it may be beneficial in a subgroup (see Case 3 below). Studies of NAC in tobacco use disorder show inconsistent results (Bernardo et al. 2009). One 12-week DBRPCT in 34 treatment-resistant cigarette smokers found that NAC 3 g/day significantly reduced the number of cigarettes used and amount of exhaled carbon monoxide compared with placebo (Prado et al. 2015).

BIPOLAR DISORDER AND MAJOR DEPRESSIVE DISORDER

In a multicenter DBRPCT of 75 patients in the maintenance phase of bipolar disorder, those given NAC had significantly greater improvement on the Montgomery-Åsberg Depression Scale (MADRS; $P=0.002$), Bipolar Depression Rating Scale (BDRS; $P=0.012$), and 9 out of 12 measures of bipolar disorder, compared with those given placebo (Berk et al. 2008a). A subgroup analysis of Berk's data showed the following: 1) There were no significant differences between NAC and placebo on measures of cognitive function (Dean et al. 2011). 2) Among 14 patients with bipolar II disorder, a higher percentage achieved full remission with NAC than with placebo (Magalhães et al. 2011a). 3) In 15 patients with baseline manic or hypomanic episode, manic symptoms improved in the NAC group, whereas depressive symptoms worsened in the placebo group (Magalhães et al. 2013). 4) Patients with baseline major depression had higher response rates with NAC compared with placebo (Magalhães et al. 2011b). 5) Subjects with medical comorbidities given NAC had greater improvement in quality of life versus those given placebo (Magalhães et al. 2012). In a DBRPCT, 149 depressed patients (MADRS ≥12 at baseline) with bipolar disorder who received adjunctive NAC or placebo showed substantial decrease in symptoms during an 8-week open-label phase, but in the double-blind phase NAC was no better than placebo in preventing recurrence of a mood episode (Berk et al. 2012).

Limited data support adjunctive NAC in MDD (Berk et al. 2014). A double-blind RCT in MDD found that MADRS scores improved significantly with NAC compared with placebo at week 16 ($P=0.036$). Moreover, in those with baseline MADRS ≥25, NAC separated from placebo at weeks 6, 8, 12, and 16 ($P<0.05$). Remission and response rates were greater in the NAC group at week 16 but not week 12, indicating a need for a longer treatment period for NAC benefits to emerge. This is consistent with slow effects on neuroplasticity and neurogenesis and may also explain negative findings in studies of less than 16 weeks. Dose may also be an issue because a considerably higher dose of NAC (2 g) was used to show its superior benefit over placebo in bipolar depression (Berk et al. 2008a). Thus, inadequate dosing may account for some negative findings.

AUTISM SPECTRUM DISORDER

Three DBRPCTs showed that NAC improves irritability in children with autism spectrum disorder better than placebo (Table 5–3). In the first study (Hardan et al. 2012), the NAC group had significant improvements on the Aberrant Behavior Checklist (ABC) Irritability subscale ($F=6.80$; $P<0.001$; $d=0.96$) compared with placebo at week 12. A DBRPCT found irritability decreased significantly more in patients with autism spectrum disorder given NAC plus risperidone compared with placebo plus risperidone at week 8 (Ghanizadeh and Moghimi-Sarani 2013). A 10-week small DBRPCT also showed NAC to be more effective than placebo as adjunct to risperidone in reducing irritability and hyperactivity (ABC subscales) (Nikoo et al. 2015).

SCHIZOPHRENIA

A DBRPCT of patients with schizophrenia reported that the NAC group had greater improvement than the placebo group in Positive and Negative Syndrome Scale (PANSS) total score ($P=0.009$), PANSS negative ($P=0.018$), PANSS general ($P=0.035$), Clinical Global Impression (CGI)–Severity ($P=0.004$), and CGI-Improvement ($P=0.025$) at week 24 (Berk et al. 2008b). Interestingly, NAC use was associated with improved akathisia ($P=0.022$). Another DBRPCT showed significantly greater improvement in PANSS total ($P=0.006$) and negative subscale ($P<0.001$) scores in NAC-treated patients compared with placebo controls (Farokhnia et al. 2013).

TRICHOTILLOMANIA AND NAIL BITING

A DBRPCT in trichotillomania (hair-pulling disorder) showed greater reduction in hair pulling with adjunctive NAC than with placebo (Massachusetts General Hospital Hair Pulling Scale, $P<0.001$; Psychiatric Institute Trichotillomania Scale, $P=0.001$) (Grant et al. 2009). However, another trichotillomania study found no significant differences between NAC and placebo (Bloch et al. 2013). A DBRPCT for nail biting in children found no significant difference between NAC and placebo (Ghanizadeh et al. 2013).

ALZHEIMER'S DISEASE

A 24-week DBRPCT in 43 elderly subjects with probable Alzheimer's disease reported that NAC improved performance in some cognitive domains more than did placebo (Adair et al. 2001).

Safety and Tolerability of *N*-Acetylcysteine

Overall, NAC is well tolerated, with rare discontinuation due to adverse events and no significant difference in adverse events compared with placebo (Deepmala et al.

2015). In two studies, severe adverse events—a full body rash in one child with trichotillomania and aggression in one child with nail biting—led to discontinuation (Bloch et al. 2013; Ghanizadeh et al. 2013).

Clinical Case of *N*-Acetylcysteine

Case 3: NAC for Cannabis Use Disorder in a Patient With Posttraumatic Stress Disorder

A 30-year-old single IT manager, Joseph, sought treatment for anxiety and irritability 3 weeks after stopping cannabis. The previous year, he was abstinent for 9 months but relapsed. Joseph was smoking "weed" heavily, four times a day by age 17. Cannabis cost him $60 a day and interfered with his functioning at work and school. On bupropion 150 mg/day with weekly psychotherapy, he was not making progress. Joseph was traumatized at age 8 when his family's home burned down. The following year, his mother died of cancer. He was never diagnosed or treated for posttraumatic stress disorder. Joseph was rated hyperactive and impulsive at school at age 10, and neuropsychological testing indicated ADHD. Ritalin and Concerta trials caused facial tics. Adderall 5 mg/day helped slightly, but higher doses caused tics, anxiety, and agitation. In adulthood, Joseph was treated on and off for anxiety, depression, and ADHD with alprazolam and bupropion. Undiagnosed bipolar disorder was also suspected. To reduce cannabis craving, anxiety, and insomnia, Joseph was started on NAC 1,800 mg twice a day, divalproex 1,000 mg at bedtime (Levin et al. 2004), and cranial electrotherapy stimulation (Alpha-Stim) (see Chapter 27, "Cranial Electrotherapy Stimulation in the Psychiatric Setting") 1 hour/day for 3 weeks, then 30 minutes/day. Bupropion was increased to 300 mg/day. Switching from 5 mg regular Adderall to 10 mg extended-release Adderall improved mental focus without side effects. In psychotherapy, Joseph talked more about the loss of his mother. Within 2 months, anxiety, insomnia, depression, and concentration improved. At 2-year follow-up, still abstinent from cannabis, Joseph was working part time while earning a graduate degree.

Inositol

Inositol, $C_6H_{12}O_6$, an isomer of glucose, is present in the diet (about 1 g/day) (Eden Evins et al. 2006). It is a constituent of the intracellular phosphatidylinositol second-messenger system linked to neurotransmitter receptors such as serotonin, dopamine, and glutamate receptors (Mukai et al. 2014). It also serves in a second-messenger system for 5-hydroxytryptamine-2 (5-HT$_2$) receptors. Hypothetically, inositol abnormalities may be related to depression. Reduced inositol levels have been found in cerebrospinal fluid of patients with unipolar and bipolar depression. Decreased inositol in the anterior cingulate occurs in adults with unipolar depression. Mood stabilizers (e.g., lithium, valproate, carbamazepine) may share a mechanism of action: stabilization of inositol signaling (Wolfson et al. 2000). Hence, most inositol research focuses on mood disorders, including unipolar and bipolar depression.

Clinical Trials of Inositol

For references on inositol trials for depression and anxiety disorders (Table 5–4), see the meta-analysis by Mukai et al. (2014).

TABLE 5–4. Double-blind, randomized placebo- or comparator-controlled trials of inositol in treatment of neuropsychiatric disorders

Author (year)	Diagnosis	Length	Inositol dosage	Comparator	Efficacy results
Depressive disorders					
Gianfranco et al. (2011)	PMDD	6 months	12 g/day gel (N=18); 12 g/day pwd (N=19)	PBO pwd; N=12	DSR reduction; improvement of Ham-D and CGI-S: INO gel and pwd>PBO
Eden Evins et al. (2006)	BD	6 weeks	12 g/day+MS (N=9)	PBO+MS; N=8	Ham-D responder: INO versus PBO (44% vs. 0%, P=0.053)
Nemets et al. (2002)	PMDD	6 months	12 g/day (N=11)	PBO; N=11	24-item Ham-D: INO=PBO
Chengappa et al. (2000)	BD	6 weeks	12 g/day+MS (N=12)	PBO+MS; N=12	Responder (MADRS and Ham-D): INO+MS=PBO+MS
Nemets et al. (1999)	MDD	4 weeks	12 g/day+SSRI (N=23)	PBO+SSRI; N=19	Ham-D improvement: INO+SSRI=PBO+SSRI
Levine et al. (1999)	MDD	4 weeks	12 g/day+SSRI (N=13)	PBO+SSRI; N=14	Ham-D improvement: INO+SSRI=PBO+SSRI
Levine et al. (1995)	MDD or BD	4 weeks	12 g/day (N=13)	PBO; N=15	Ham-D improvement: INO>PBO
Anxiety disorders					
Fux et al. (1999)	OCD	6 weeks	12 g/day+SSRI (N=10)	PBO+SSRI or CLO; N=10	Y-BOCS: INO+SSRI=PBO+SSRI
Fux et al. (1996)	OCD	6 weeks	12 g/day+SSRI (N=13)	PBO+SSRI or CLO; N=13	Y-BOCS: INO+SSRI>PBO+SSRI

TABLE 5–4. Double-blind, randomized placebo- or comparator-controlled trials of inositol in treatment of neuropsychiatric disorders *(continued)*

Author (year)	Diagnosis	Length	Inositol dosage	Comparator	Efficacy results
Anxiety disorders (continued)					
Benjamin et al. (1995)	PD	4 weeks	12 g/day+LZP (*N*=21)	12 g/day+PBO: *N*=21	Number of panic attacks declined: LZP+INO>LZP+PBO
Kaplan et al. (1996)	PTSD	4 weeks	12 g/day+LZP (*N*=21)	12 g/day+PBO; *N*=21	IES, Ham-D, Ham-A: INO=PBO

Note. BD=bipolar depression; CGI-S=Clinical Global Impression–Severity of Illness scale; CLO=clomipramine; DSR=Daily Symptoms Records Scale; Ham-A=Hamilton Anxiety Rating Scale; Ham-D=Hamilton Depression Rating Scale; IES=Impact of Event Scale; INP=inositol; LZP=lorazepam; MADRS=Montgomery-Åsberg Depression Rating Scale; MS=mood stabilizer; MDD=major depressive disorder; OCD=obsessive-compulsive disorder; PBO=placebo; PD=panic disorder; PMDD=premenstrual dysphoric disorder; pwd=powder; PTSD=posttraumatic stress disorder; SSRI=selective serotonin reuptake inhibitor; Y-BOCS=Yale-Brown Obsessive-Compulsive Scale.

DEPRESSIVE AND MOOD DISORDERS

A small 4-week DBRPCT, the first to use a second messenger, inositol, rather than a neurotransmitter modulator for depression, showed significantly greater improvement in Hamilton Depression Rating Scale (Ham-D; $P=0.04$) scores in patients given inositol versus placebo (Levine et al. 1995). However, two studies in unipolar depression (Levine et al. 1999; Nemets et al. 1999) and one in bipolar depression (Chengappa et al. 2000) did not find inositol to be superior to placebo. A DBRPCT of 90 patients with premenstrual dysphoric disorder showed that compared with placebo, myoinositol (gel or powder) reduced scores more on Ham-D, Penn Daily Symptoms Records scale, and Clinician's Global Impression–Severity of Illness (CGI-S). Moreover, no subjects experienced severe side effects. Only one patient in the myoinositol powder group reported mild gastrointestinal side effects, but these side effects did not result in discontinuation (Gianfranco et al. 2011).

OBSESSIVE-COMPULSIVE AND ANXIETY DISORDERS

In a 6-week crossover DBRPCT, 13 patients with obsessive-compulsive disorder were given 18 g inositol or placebo added to a selective serotonin reuptake inhibitor or clomipramine (Fux et al. 1996). Compared with placebo, patients given inositol had significantly lower scores on the Yale-Brown Obsessive Compulsive Scale (Y-BOCS). However, in a repeat study, inositol had no greater efficacy than placebo on Y-BOCS, Ham-D, and Hamilton Anxiety Rating Scale (Ham-A; Fux et al. 1999). One crossover DBRPCT found that frequency and severity of panic attacks and agoraphobia declined more significantly with inositol than with placebo (Benjamin et al. 1995). Another crossover study did not separate inositol from placebo in posttraumatic stress disorder (Table 5–4).

Efficacy and Tolerability of Inositol

A meta-analysis did not find sufficient evidence for greater efficacy of inositol over placebo in depressive or anxiety disorders (Mukai et al. 2014). However, for depression, inositol trended toward a higher percentage of responders ($P=0.06$) and improved depressive symptoms in premenstrual dysphoric disorder ($P=0.07$). Inositol was well tolerated; discontinuation rate was comparable to placebo.

KEY POINTS

- Acetyl-L-carnitine (ALC) effects include neuroplasticity, membrane modulation, neurotransmitter regulation, antioxidant effect, and anti-inflammatory effect.

- ALC has shown potential efficacy in numerous clinical trials for treatment of depression, persistent depressive disorder (dysthymia), and Alzheimer's disease.

- *N*-Acetylcysteine (NAC) warrants investigation as a novel treatment for a range of neuropsychiatric disorders. To date, the results of clinical trials have been mixed.

- Inositol may augment treatment of depression and bipolar disorder.

- ALC, NAC, and inositol were shown to be very safe. Larger controlled trials with adequate doses and durations would provide more guidance for clinical treatment.

References

Adair JC, Knoefel JE, Morgan N: Controlled trial of N-acetylcysteine for patients with probable Alzheimer's disease. Neurology 57(8):1515–1517, 2001 11673605

American Psychiatric Association: Diagnostic and Statistical Manual of Mental Disorders, 4th Edition, Text Revision. Arlington, VA, American Psychiatric Association, 2000

Arnold LE, Amato A, Bozzolo H, et al: Acetyl-L-carnitine (ALC) in attention-deficit/hyperactivity disorder: a multi-site, placebo-controlled pilot trial. J Child Adolesc Psychopharmacol 17(6):791–802, 2007 18315451

Bella R, Biondi R, Raffaele R, et al: Effect of acetyl-L-carnitine on geriatric patients suffering from dysthymic disorders. Int J Clin Pharmacol Res 10(6):355–360, 1990 2099360

Benjamin J, Levine J, Fux M, et al: Double-blind, placebo-controlled, crossover trial of inositol treatment for panic disorder. Am J Psychiatry 152(7):1084–1086, 1995 7793450

Berk M, Copolov DL, Dean O, et al: N-Acetyl cysteine for depressive symptoms in bipolar disorder: a double-blind randomized placebo-controlled trial. Biol Psychiatry 64(6):468–475, 2008a 18534556

Berk M, Copolov D, Dean O, et al: N-Acetyl cysteine as a glutathione precursor for schizophrenia: a double-blind, randomized, placebo-controlled trial. Biol Psychiatry 64(5):361–368, 2008b 18436195

Berk M, Dean OM, Cotton SM, et al: Maintenance N-acetyl cysteine treatment for bipolar disorder: a double-blind randomized placebo controlled trial. BMC Med 10:91, 2012 22891797

Berk M, Dean OM, Cotton SM, et al: The efficacy of adjunctive N-acetylcysteine in major depressive disorder: a double-blind, randomized, placebo-controlled trial. J Clin Psychiatry 75(6):628–636, 2014 25004186

Bernardo M, Dodd S, Gama CS, et al: Effects of N-acetylcysteine on substance use in bipolar disorder: a randomised placebo-controlled clinical trial. Acta Neuropsychiatr 21(6):285–291, 2009 25384734

Bersani G, Meco G, Denaro A, et al: L-Acetylcarnitine in dysthymic disorder in elderly patients: a double-blind, multicenter, controlled randomized study vs. fluoxetine. Eur Neuropsychopharmacol 23(10):1219–1225, 2013 23428336

Bloch MH, Panza KE, Grant JE, et al: N-Acetylcysteine in the treatment of pediatric trichotillomania: a randomized, double-blind, placebo-controlled add-on trial. J Am Acad Child Adolesc Psychiatry 52(3):231–240, 2013 23452680

Brennan BP, Jensen JE, Hudson JI, et al: A placebo-controlled trial of acetyl-L-carnitine and α-lipoic acid in the treatment of bipolar depression. J Clin Psychopharmacol 33(5):627–635, 2013 23948785

Chengappa KN, Levine J, Gershon S, et al: Inositol as an add-on treatment for bipolar depression. Bipolar Disord 2(1):47–55, 2000 11254020

Cuccurazzu B, Bortolotto V, Valente MM, et al: Upregulation of mGlu2 receptors via NF-kB p65 acetylation is involved in the proneurogenic and antidepressant effects of acetyl-L-carnitine. Neuropsychopharmacology 38(11):2220–2230, 2013 23670591

Dean O, Giorlando F, Berk M: N-Acetylcysteine in psychiatry: current therapeutic evidence and potential mechanisms of action. J Psychiatry Neurosci 36(2):78–86, 2011 21118657

Deepmala D, Slattery J, Kumar N, et al: Clinical trials of N-acetylcysteine in psychiatry and neurology: a systematic review. Neurosci Biobehav Rev 55:294–321, 2015 25957927

Ebadi M, Brown-Borg H, Ren J, et al: Therapeutic efficacy of selegiline in neurodegenerative disorders and neurological diseases. Curr Drug Targets 7(11):1513–1529, 2006 17100591

Eden Evins A, Demopulos C, Yovel I, et al: Inositol augmentation of lithium or valproate for bipolar depression. Bipolar Disord 8(2):168–174, 2006 16542187

Farokhnia M, Azarkolah A, Adinehfar F, et al: N-Acetylcysteine as an adjunct to risperidone for treatment of negative symptoms in patients with chronic schizophrenia: a randomized, double-blind, placebo-controlled study. Clin Neuropharmacol 36(6):185–192, 2013 24201233

Fulgente T, Onofrj M, Del Re ML, et al: Laevo-acetylcarnitine (Nicetile) treatment of senile depression. Clin Trials J 27:155–163, 1990

Fux M, Levine J, Aviv A, et al: Inositol treatment of obsessive-compulsive disorder. Am J Psychiatry 153(9):1219–1221, 1996 8780431

Fux M, Benjamin J, Belmaker RH: Inositol versus placebo augmentation of serotonin reuptake inhibitors in the treatment of obsessive-compulsive disorder: a double-blind cross-over study. Int J Neuropsychopharmacol 2(3):193–195, 1999 11281989

Garzya G, Corallo D, Fiore A, et al: Evaluation of the effects of L-acetylcarnitine on senile patients suffering from depression. Drugs Exp Clin Res 16(2):101–106, 1990 2205455

Gecele MFG, Meluzzi A: Acetyl-l-carnitine in aged subjects with major depression: clinical efficacy and effects on the circadian rhythm of cortisol. Dement Geriatr Cogn Disord 2(6):333–337, 1991

Ghanizadeh A, Moghimi-Sarani E: A randomized double blind placebo controlled clinical trial of N-acetylcysteine added to risperidone for treating autistic disorders. BMC Psychiatry 13:196, 2013 23886027

Ghanizadeh A, Derakhshan N, Berk M: N-Acetylcysteine versus placebo for treating nail biting, a double blind randomized placebo controlled clinical trial. Antiinflamm Antiallergy Agents Med Chem 12(3):223–228, 2013 23651231

Gianfranco C, Vittorio U, Silvia B, et al: Myo-inositol in the treatment of premenstrual dysphoric disorder. Hum Psychopharmacol 26(7):526–530, 2011 22031267

Grant JE, Kim SW, Odlaug BL: N-Acetyl cysteine, a glutamate-modulating agent, in the treatment of pathological gambling: a pilot study. Biol Psychiatry 62(6):652–657, 2007 17445781

Grant JE, Odlaug BL, Kim SW: N-Acetylcysteine, a glutamate modulator, in the treatment of trichotillomania: a double-blind, placebo-controlled study. Arch Gen Psychiatry 66(7):756–763, 2009 19581567

Grant JE, Odlaug BL, Kim SW: A double-blind, placebo-controlled study of N-acetyl cysteine plus naltrexone for methamphetamine dependence. Eur Neuropsychopharmacol 20(11):823–828, 2010 20655182

Grant JE, Odlaug BL, Chamberlain SR: A randomized, placebo-controlled trial of N-acetylcysteine plus imaginal desensitization for nicotine-dependent pathological gamblers. J Clin Psychiatry 75(1):39–45, 2014 24345329

Gray KM, Carpenter MJ, Baker NL, et al: A double-blind randomized controlled trial of N-acetylcysteine in cannabis-dependent adolescents. Am J Psychiatry 169(8):805–812, 2012 22706327

Hardan AY, Fung LK, Libove RA, et al: A randomized controlled pilot trial of oral N-acetylcysteine in children with autism. Biol Psychiatry 71(11):956–961, 2012 22342106

Hudson S, Tabet N: Acetyl-L-carnitine for dementia. Cochrane Database Syst Rev 2(2):CD003158, 2003 12804452

Jagetia GC, Aggarwal BB: "Spicing up" of the immune system by curcumin. J Clin Immunol 27(1):19–35, 2007 17211725

Kaplan Z, Amir M, Swartz M, Levine J: Inositol treatment of post-traumatic stress disorder. Anxiety 2(1):51–52, 1996 9160600

LaRowe SD, Myrick H, Hedden S, et al: Is cocaine desire reduced by N-acetylcysteine? Am J Psychiatry 164(7):1115–1117, 2007 17606664

LaRowe SD, Kalivas PW, Nicholas JS, et al: A double-blind placebo-controlled trial of N-acetylcysteine in the treatment of cocaine dependence. Am J Addict 22(5):443–452, 2013 23952889

Levin FR, McDowell D, Evans SM, et al: Pharmacotherapy for marijuana dependence: a double-blind, placebo-controlled pilot study of divalproex sodium. Am J Addict 13(1):21–32, 2004 14766435

Levine J, Barak Y, Gonzalves M, et al: Double-blind, controlled trial of inositol treatment of depression. Am J Psychiatry 152(5):792–794, 1995 7726322

Levine J, Mishori A, Susnosky M, et al: Combination of inositol and serotonin reuptake inhibitors in the treatment of depression. Biol Psychiatry 45(3):270–273, 1999 10023500

Magalhães PV, Dean OM, Bush AI, et al: N-Acetyl cysteine add-on treatment for bipolar II disorder: a subgroup analysis of a randomized placebo-controlled trial. J Affect Disord 129(1–3):317–320, 2011a 20800897

Magalhães PV, Dean OM, Bush AI, et al: N-Acetylcysteine for major depressive episodes in bipolar disorder. Rev Bras Psiquiatr 33(4):374–378, 2011b 22189927

Magalhães PV, Dean OM, Bush AI, et al: Systemic illness moderates the impact of N-acetyl cysteine in bipolar disorder. Prog Neuropsychopharmacol Biol Psychiatry 37(1):132–135, 2012 22212173

Magalhães PV, Dean OM, Bush AI, et al: A preliminary investigation on the efficacy of N-acetyl cysteine for mania or hypomania. Aust N Z J Psychiatry 47(6):564–568, 2013 23493756

McClure EA, Baker NL, Gray KM: Cigarette smoking during an N-acetylcysteine-assisted cannabis cessation trial in adolescents. Am J Drug Alcohol Abuse 40(4):285–291, 2014 24720376

Montgomery SA, Thal LJ, Amrein R: Meta-analysis of double blind randomized controlled clinical trials of acetyl-L-carnitine versus placebo in the treatment of mild cognitive impairment and mild Alzheimer's disease. Int Clin Psychopharmacol 18(2):61–71, 2003 12598816

Mousavi SG, Sharbafchi MR, Salehi M, et al: The efficacy of N-acetylcysteine in the treatment of methamphetamine dependence: a double-blind controlled, crossover study. Arch Iran Med 18(1):28–33, 2015 25556383

Mukai T, Kishi T, Matsuda Y, et al: A meta-analysis of inositol for depression and anxiety disorders. Hum Psychopharmacol 29(1):55–63, 2014 24424706

Nasca D, Zurria G, Aguglia E: Action of acetyl-l-carnitine in association with mianserine on depressed old people. New Trends in Clinical Neuropharmacology 3:225–230, 1989

Nasca C, Xenos D, Barone Y, et al: L-Acetylcarnitine causes rapid antidepressant effects through the epigenetic induction of mGlu2 receptors. Proc Natl Acad Sci USA 110(12):4804–4809, 2013 23382250

Nemets B, Mishory A, Levine J, et al: Inositol addition does not improve depression in SSRI treatment failures. J Neural Transm (Vienna) 106(7–8):795–798, 1999 10907738

Nemets B, Talesnick B, Belmaker RH, Levine J: Myo-inositol has no beneficial effect on premenstrual dysphoric disorder. World J Biol Psychiatry 3(3):147–149, 2002 12478879

Nikoo M, Radnia H, Farokhnia M, et al: N-Acetylcysteine as an adjunctive therapy to risperidone for treatment of irritability in autism: a randomized, double-blind, placebo-controlled clinical trial of efficacy and safety. Clin Neuropharmacol 38(1):11–17, 2015 25580916

Passeri M, Cucinotta D, Bonati PA, et al: Acetyl-L-carnitine in the treatment of mildly demented elderly patients. Int J Clin Pharmacol Res 10(1–2):75–79, 1990 2201659

Pettegrew JW, Levine J, McClure RJ: Acetyl-L-carnitine physical-chemical, metabolic, and therapeutic properties: relevance for its mode of action in Alzheimer's disease and geriatric depression. Mol Psychiatry 5(6):616–632, 2000 11126392

Prado E, Maes M, Piccoli LG, et al: N-Acetylcysteine for therapy-resistant tobacco use disorder: a pilot study. Redox Rep 20(5):215–222, 2015 25729878

Rai G, Wright G, Scott I, et al: Double-blind, placebo controlled study of acetyl-L-carnitine in patients with Alzheimer's dementia. Curr Med Res Opin 11(10):638–647, 1990 2178869

Roten AT, Baker NL, Gray KM: Marijuana craving trajectories in an adolescent marijuana cessation pharmacotherapy trial. Addict Behav 38(3):1788–1791, 2013 23261493

Sano M, Bell K, Cote L, et al: Double-blind parallel design pilot study of acetyl levocarnitine in patients with Alzheimer's disease. Arch Neurol 49(11):1137–1141, 1992 1444880

Schmaal L, Berk L, Hulstijn KP, et al: Efficacy of N-acetylcysteine in the treatment of nicotine dependence: a double-blind placebo-controlled pilot study. Eur Addict Res 17(4):211–216, 2011 21606648

Smeland OB, Meisingset TW, Borges K, et al: Chronic acetyl-L-carnitine alters brain energy metabolism and increases noradrenaline and serotonin content in healthy mice. Neurochem Int 61(1):100–107, 2012 22549035

Spagnoli A, Lucca U, Menasce G, et al: Long-term acetyl-L-carnitine treatment in Alzheimer's disease. Neurology 41(11):1726–1732, 1991 1944900

Steiber A, Kerner J, Hoppel CL: Carnitine: a nutritional, biosynthetic, and functional perspective. Mol Aspects Med 25(5–6):455–473, 2004 15363636

Thal LJ, Carta A, Clarke WR, et al: A 1-year multicenter placebo-controlled study of acetyl-L-carnitine in patients with Alzheimer's disease. Neurology 47(3):705–711, 1996 8797468

Thal LJ, Calvani M, Amato A, et al: A 1-year controlled trial of acetyl-l-carnitine in early onset AD. Neurology 55(6):805–810, 2000 10994000

Torrioli MG, Vernacotola S, Peruzzi L, et al: A double-blind, parallel, multicenter comparison of L-acetylcarnitine with placebo on the attention deficit hyperactivity disorder in fragile X syndrome boys. Am J Med Genet A 146A(7):803–812, 2008 18286595

Villardita C, Smirni P, Vecchio I: Acetyl-l-carnitine in depressed geriatric patients. Eur Rev Med Pharmacol Sci 6:1–12, 1983

Wang SM, Han C, Lee SJ, et al: A review of current evidence for acetyl-l-carnitine in the treatment of depression. J Psychiatr Res 53:30–37, 2014 24607292

Wolfson M, Bersudsky Y, Zinger E, et al: Chronic treatment of human astrocytoma cells with lithium, carbamazepine or valproic acid decreases inositol uptake at high inositol concentrations but increases it at low inositol concentrations. Brain Res 855(1):158–161, 2000 10650143

Zanardi R, Smeraldi E: A double-blind, randomised, controlled clinical trial of acetyl-L-carnitine vs. amisulpride in the treatment of dysthymia. Eur Neuropsychopharmacol 16(4):281–287, 2006 16316746

CHAPTER 6

Single and Broad-Spectrum Micronutrient Treatments in Psychiatric Practice

Charles Popper, M.D.

Bonnie J. Kaplan, Ph.D.

Julia J. Rucklidge, Ph.D., C.Psych.

Significant improvement in the mental health of many persons might be achieved by the provision of the optimum molecular concentrations of substances normally present in the human body. Among these substances, the essential nutrients may be the most worthy of extensive research.

Linus Pauling (1968)

Micronutrients is a term that refers to all essential minerals and vitamins that are required in small or trace amounts to sustain health. Micronutrients play a role in virtually every biological, chemical, and physiological process. They serve as cofactors required for the activity of enzymes and other regulatory proteins, including transcription factors that modify gene expression. Micronutrients also play essential roles in receptors, transporters, ion channels, and pump mechanisms. They are crucially involved in neurotransmitter synthesis, intracellular signaling, membrane function, mitochondrial function, oxidative damage, inflammation, microbiome profiles, drug metabolism, and many other biological processes (Kaplan et al. 2015a). The role of micronutrients in biology is pervasive and fundamental.

It is often assumed that people in developed countries are adequately nourished, but many are not. Nutritional epidemiological studies show that more than 50% of the American population fails to meet formal "estimated average requirements" for dietary intake of at least one micronutrient (U.S. Department of Agriculture, Agriculture Research Service 2016), and on the basis of biochemical indicators, at least 10% are at risk for a mineral or vitamin deficiency (Centers for Disease Control and Prevention 2012). Although overt micronutrient deficiency diseases (e.g., scurvy) are rare in the developed world, micronutrient deficiencies are not rare.

Numerous factors contribute to micronutrient deficiencies. Modern agriculture and food industry practices have sharply reduced the nutrient density of foods, with 20%–80% reductions over several decades in the micronutrient content of fruits and vegetables (Mayer 1997). These reductions result from insufficient soil replenishment, overgrazing, over-irrigation, herbicides (e.g., glyphosates bind micronutrients, reducing their bioavailability), and varietal trade-offs between nutrient content and market demands (productivity, cost, appearance). Public reliance on low-nutrient processed foods, fast foods, high-fructose corn syrup, and sugary drinks also reduces dietary intake of micronutrients. Individuals may fail to meet nutrient needs because of genetics, age, physical activity, stress, pregnancy, alcohol or drug use, dieting, culturally diverse cuisines and cooking methods, diseases, or medical treatments. Estimates of vitamin and mineral deficiencies probably underestimate true prevalence. See Figure 6–1, which is derived from 2003–2006 data from the National Health and Nutrition Examination Survey. Similar data are available for Canada and England.

Micronutrient *insufficiencies* are less severe and less clinically obvious but are even more prevalent. For example, among American adults, 7% have vitamin D levels in the deficiency range (serum 25-hydroxyvitamin D < 10 ng/mL; normal 40–70 ng/mL), and 64% have levels in the insufficiency range (39% < 20 ng/mL and 64% < 30 ng/mL) (Mitchell et al. 2012).

Suboptimal micronutrient status can compromise physiological functioning and increase symptoms of many disorders through a variety of mechanisms. Fifty genetic disorders entailing structurally distorted enzymes with low binding affinity for their cofactors can be treated simply by increased dietary consumption of micronutrients (Ames et al. 2002). Ames showed that micronutrient deficiencies can increase oxidative damage to nuclear DNA (vitamins B_{12}, B_9, B_6, C, and E; iron, zinc) and mitochondrial DNA (biotin, iron), leading to metabolic changes in multiple organ systems, chronic inflammation, neuronal deterioration, and accelerated aging (Shigenaga et al. 1994). These changes can be reversed in rats with vitamin-like substances (Ames 2010).

These findings imply that a broad spectrum of micronutrients is needed for optimal physiological functioning. An incomplete supply of micronutrients can have diverse health effects. Ames proposed that supplying a broad variety of micronutrients can be used to pervasively optimize physiological functioning—a process he calls "metabolic tune-up" (Ames 2004).

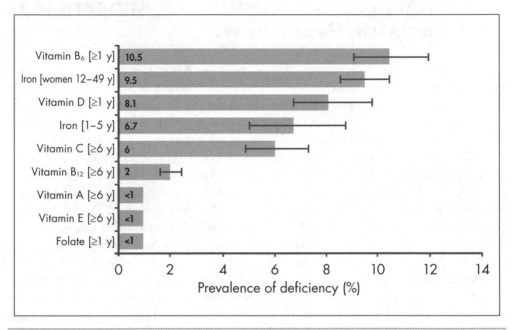

FIGURE 6–1. Prevalence of single-micronutrient deficiencies in the American population based on biochemical indicators of nutritional status.
Source. Centers for Disease Control and Prevention 2012. Reprinted from Popper C: "Single-Micronutrient and Broad-Spectrum Micronutrient Approaches for Treating Mood Disorders in Youth and Adults," *Child and Adolescent Psychiatric Clinics of North America* 23(3):591–672, 2014, with permission from Elsevier.

Do Micronutrient Insufficiencies Lead to Mental Changes or Psychiatric Symptoms?

All classical micronutrient deficiency disorders, including beriberi, pellagra, and scurvy, are associated with psychiatric symptoms (Popper 2014). A very large literature documents correlations between more subtle variations in dietary quality and mental health status. Clinical studies over the past 100 years have shown correlations of mood with dietary intake or with metabolic markers of nutritional status (such as plasma micronutrient levels or endogenous enzyme activities). Correlations with mental health have been demonstrated for vitamins B_1 (thiamine), B_3 (niacin), B_6 (pyridoxine), B_7 (biotin), B_9 (folate), B_{12} (cobalamin), C (ascorbic acid), D (calciferols), and E (tocopherols) as well as numerous individual minerals, including lithium, calcium, magnesium, iron, copper, zinc, chromium, and selenium (Kaplan et al. 2007). Many population-based cross-sectional epidemiological studies show that poor dietary patterns are associated with worse mental health, especially worse mood ratings (although correlations with mood disorders are less clear.) The interpretation of these studies is limited because correlations are ambiguous about causal direction and thus do not allow inferences about mechanism. Prospective studies are more effective for enhancing mechanistic understanding.

Do Dietary Factors Modify the Appearance of Psychiatric Symptoms?

Three large-scale prospective observational studies in adults demonstrate that dietary quality predicts the subsequent rate of depression diagnoses at follow-up. A study of nearly 3,500 women followed for 5 years found that the consumption of whole foods was associated with a reduced risk of depression (odds ratio [OR] 0.74; $P=0.04$) and that eating processed foods was associated with an increased risk of depression (OR 1.6; $P=0.01$) (Akbaraly et al. 2009). A report on more than 10,000 adults followed for a median of 4 years revealed that adherence to a Mediterranean dietary pattern (high intake of fruits, nuts, legumes, and fish; low intake of saturated fatty acids) protected against the development of new-onset depression (Sánchez-Villegas et al. 2009). Another study of almost 9,000 adults found that a higher risk of depression at follow-up (median 6 years) was associated with the consumption of fast foods, whereas there was no correlation with the consumption of baked goods (Sánchez-Villegas et al. 2012).

On the basis of such studies, diet quality appears to be a modifiable lifestyle practice that can protect against and perhaps reduce the prevalence of mental disorders (Jacka et al. 2012). However, a similar outcome in these studies could result from unidentified confounding factors unrelated to diet, such as exercise or sleep habits. Prospective interventional studies are more helpful for establishing a causal link between micronutrient status and mental changes.

Single-Micronutrient Treatments of Psychiatric Disorders

There is a large literature on the use of individual minerals or vitamins for the treatment of psychiatric symptoms (Kaplan et al. 2007). Virtually all of it has negative or modest results, except for lithium (a mineral) and folate (a vitamin). This unsatisfying literature predominantly consists of studies that were methodologically compromised by the usual factors: small sample sizes, poorly defined populations, sampling and randomization problems, blinding and design problems, inadequate outcome measures, weak statistical analysis, clinically insignificant changes, and findings that cannot be replicated. Mood disorders and attention-deficit/hyperactivity disorder (ADHD) have been the most extensively studied. ADHD studies have examined augmentation of psychostimulants with zinc, magnesium, or iron, with mixed but mainly negative findings (Hariri and Azadbakht 2015). Studies of single-micronutrient treatments of depressive disorders have been more promising but are still quite limited.

Folate and Other B Vitamins

FOLIC ACID AND ITS CONGENERS

Folic acid has not been studied in double-blind, randomized, placebo-controlled trials (DBRPCTs) as a monotherapy for major depressive disorder (MDD). However, folate or folate derivatives (vitamin B_9) were efficacious as adjunctive (add-on) treatments to antidepressants (mostly selective serotonin reuptake inhibitors [SSRIs]) in six of seven randomized controlled trials (RCTs; Bedson et al. 2014; Coppen and Bailey 2000; Godfrey et al. 1990; Pan et al. 2017; Papakostas et al. 2012; Resler et al. 2008; Venkatasubramanian et al. 2013). The negative RCT was the largest trial, examining folate in 475 adults, but this study was unique in excluding patients with folate deficiency (Bedson et al. 2014). Even omitting that study, the effect size (ES) of 0.35–0.4 for folate or L-methylfolate adjunctive treatment was small. Conventionally, an ES of 0.2–0.4 is considered small, 0.5–0.7 moderate, and 0.8 or more large. In an RCT designed to test whether folate could prevent mood disorders in high-risk 14- to 24-year-olds treated for a mean of 20 months, folate did not reduce the incidence of mood disorders but might have slightly delayed the onset of illness (Sharpley et al. 2014). Folate did appear to be effective in an RCT for treating acute bipolar I mania as an adjunct to valproate (Behzadi et al. 2009).

L-Methylfolate, the main biologically active form of folate, may be more effective than folate (Sarris et al. 2016). An RCT found that the addition of L-methylfolate was beneficial for patients who had not responded to 8 weeks of fluoxetine (Papakostas et al. 2012), with a better clinical response linked to obesity and to specific genetic and biological markers related to inflammation and folate metabolism (Shelton et al. 2015).

A study found that 12 of 33 patients with treatment-resistant depression had a cerebral folate deficiency, diagnosed by folate metabolite abnormalities in cerebrospinal fluid (typically 5-methyltetrahydrofolate <40 nmol/L) in the presence of normal serum folate levels (Pan et al. 2017). Ten of the 12 patients completed at least 6 weeks of open-label treatment with folinic acid (1–2 mg/kg daily) added to ongoing antidepressant therapy. All 10 patients with treatment-resistant depression and central folate deficiency showed significant mood improvements with adjunctive folinic acid, although full response may take several months to 1–3 years.

Folic acid and its congeners appear to be the most likely of the single micronutrients to gain a role in treating depression, albeit as an augmentation therapy with a small clinical effect, except perhaps for cases of cerebral folate deficiency. A meta-analysis found that the effect size for folic acid was unimpressive and that L-methylfolate and folinic acid appeared better for antidepressant augmentation (Sarris et al. 2016). Folinic acid may be preferable to L-methylfolate because it can correct a wider range of folate-related metabolic disorders (Pan et al. 2017). However, the L-methylfolate and folinic acid studies were conducted in patients with known folate abnormalities, whereas no RCT has examined folic acid in a sample of patients selected for low folate levels or other folate abnormalities. Therefore, it remains unsettled which folate congener is preferable.

VITAMIN B_{12}

Vitamin B_{12} (cobalamin) was ineffective in two monotherapy RCTs for MDD (Hvas et al. 2004; Oren et al. 1994) but was found to augment tricyclic and SSRI antidepressant effects (Syed et al. 2013). Speculatively, vitamin B_{12} might help treat depression in patients with gastrointestinal disease and impaired absorption, but RCTs are not available.

VITAMIN B_6

Pyridoxine (vitamin B_6) serves many functions, including as a cofactor for decarboxylase enzymes that play a crucial role in the synthesis of dopamine, norepinephrine, serotonin, melatonin, and γ-aminobutyric acid. There are no rigorous RCTs of pyridoxine monotherapy in mood disorders or of solo pyridoxine augmentation of antidepressants (i.e., in the absence of other B vitamins). Pyridoxine monotherapy has been examined for effects on premenstrual mood and autism spectrum disorder. Reviews (Kleijnen et al. 1990) and meta-analyses (Bendich 2000; Wyatt et al. 1999) of the many early trials found conflicting or weakly supported positive effects on premenstrual mood. In autism, the questionable claims of pyridoxine benefits have been largely dismissed (Findling et al. 1997; Pfeiffer et al. 1995); mood effects were not evaluated.

VITAMIN B_1

Thiamine (vitamin B_1) monotherapy trials for treating mood disorders are not available. Thiamine augmentation of fluoxetine was described in an RCT in 51 adults with MDD, but the effect was temporary (Ghaleiha et al. 2016). Thiamine was effective in two monotherapy trials in improving mood and sense of well-being in nonclinical volunteers (Benton et al. 1997; Smidt et al. 1991).

VITAMIN B COMPLEX

With folate congeners, vitamin B_{12}, and vitamin B_1 showing some capacity to augment antidepressants, it would be sensible to examine the combined effect of several B vitamins. An RCT in 330 adults found vitamin B complex (in combination with other micronutrients) beneficial in treating MDD associated with certain methylenetetrahydrofolate reductase polymorphisms (Mech and Farah 2016). Another RCT found that adjunctive treatment with a combination of folic acids, vitamin B_{12}, and vitamin B_6 did not improve response to antidepressants over 12 weeks, but compared to placebo did reduce relapse over 1 year (Almeida et al. 2014). For additional details on B vitamins, see Chapter 4, "S-Adenosylmethionine."

Calciferols (Vitamin D)

Vitamin D, no longer viewed as merely a "bone vitamin," has been implicated in the pathophysiology of numerous diseases in multiple organ systems. Vitamin D (calcitriol) receptors are distributed diffusely in the brain, and low vitamin D levels have been linked to depression, bipolar disorder, schizophrenia, autism spectrum disorder, epilepsy, Alzheimer's disease, and chronic pain. Psychiatric patients, especially those with psychosis or suicidality, appear to be at increased risk for hypovitaminosis D (Popper 2014). Vitamin D was found to be helpful for MDD in 6 of 10 RCTs, but the methodology was weak, and the two best-designed studies had opposite outcomes. The most rigorous RCT suggested that vitamin D_3 (1,500 IU daily) augmentation of fluoxetine enhanced outcome in 42 adults starting at week 4, with an ES of 0.5 (Khoraminya et al. 2013). In contrast, an RCT of 243 adults with MDD and low baseline vitamin D levels treated with high-dose vitamin D (40,000 IU weekly for 6 months) showed no improvement relative to placebo (Kjærgaard et al. 2012). Two systematic reviews found that the studies on vitamin D for MDD are inconclusive (Li et al. 2014; Qureshi and Al-Bedah 2013).

Although current evidence does not support vitamin D supplementation in the treatment or prevention of depression, additional studies are warranted. Given the relatively low toxicity of vitamin D, supplementation can still be justified for "general health" reasons in patients with demonstrated vitamin D insufficiency. Risk factors include low sunlight exposure (northern climes, winter months, indoor workers, dark skin tone, bedridden status), obesity, advanced age, and chronic illness. A chart review found that 75% of 544 psychiatric adult inpatients in the northern city of Chicago were at risk for vitamin D insufficiency (<30 ng/mL), with a mean level of 22 ng/mL (Rylander and Verhulst 2013). Adverse effects are mostly related to hypercalcemia, and nutrient-drug interactions include vitamin D reduction of calcium channel blocker activity and reduction of vitamin D effects by valproate or carbamazepine. Adequate dosing is clinically determined by plasma levels.

Other Single Micronutrients

Several other micronutrients have been examined for mood effects in RCTs, mostly with conflicting or negative effects. Table 6–1 summarizes the best available studies, although most are flawed (for full citations, see Popper 2014).

Chromium was found to have no benefit for MDD in two RCTs (Davidson et al. 2003; Docherty et al. 2005), but Docherty and colleagues found a subgroup of patients with atypical depression showing improvement in carbohydrate craving and mood, although this post hoc finding needs replication. Zinc appeared effective as adjunctive treatment for MDD in three small RCTs (Nowak et al. 2003; Sawada and Yokoi 2010), including an unreplicated post hoc finding that suggested benefit for a subgroup with treatment-resistant MDD (Siwek et al. 2010). Selenium monotherapy was found in a RCT to improve symptoms of postpartum depression if initiated during the first trimester (Mokhber et al. 2011). Magnesium appeared effective for treating mania in a preliminary RCT as an adjunct to verapamil, a calcium channel blocker (Giannini et al. 2000).

Clinical Impact of Single-Micronutrient Treatments

Apart from lithium, the only clearly positive evidence for single-micronutrient interventions for psychiatric disorders supports folate congeners as an adjunctive therapy for MDD; these effects appear to have only modest effect sizes (0.35–0.40), except for cerebral and perhaps systemic folate deficiency. Vitamin B_{12} might be useful for geriatric depression and for MDD associated with chronic gastrointestinal diseases and impaired absorption. Vitamin D shows mixed findings in MDD but is a good health measure in patients with documented insufficiency. Additional research is needed to determine whether chromium has a niche for treating atypical depression with carbohydrate craving, whether zinc might have an augmentation role for MDD (or perhaps specifically treatment-resistant MDD), and whether selenium might prevent postpartum depression.

Single micronutrients are powerful in treating the classical single-micronutrient deficiency diseases, but in treating DSM-5 (American Psychiatric Association 2013) psychiatric disorders, it is striking that single-micronutrient studies show so few pos-

TABLE 6–1. Effects of randomized controlled trials of single micronutrients on mood (excluding folic acid, vitamin D, and pyridoxine)

Treatment	Concurrent treatment	Design	Population	Outcome measures	Statistically significant change vs. placebo ($P<0.05$)	Citation
Chromium	Monotherapy	DBRPCT, 2 months, N=113	Atypical depression, mean age 46	Ham-D, CGI-I	No overall improvement, but subgroup of carbohydrate cravers had ↑mood, ↓ craving	Docherty et al. (2005)
Chromium	Monotherapy	DBRPCT, 2 months, N=15	Atypical depression, mean age 46	Ham-D, CGI-I	Nonsignificant ↓ in depression, but perhaps more in overeaters	Davidson et al. (2003)
Chromium	Monotherapy	DBRPCT, 6 months, N=24	Binge eating disorder, overweight, mean age 36	QIDS-SR, EDE-Q	Nonsignificant ↓ in depression, binge frequency, and weight	Brownley et al. (2013)
Zinc	Imipramine	DBRPCT, 12 weeks, N=60	DSM-IV MDE unipolar, ages 18–55	CGI, BDI, Ham-D, MADRS	Zinc add-on: ↓ depression in treatment-resistant patients, but no benefit in nonresistant patients	Siwek et al. (2009, 2010)
Zinc	TCA or SSRI	DBRPCT, 12 weeks, N=20	DSM-IV MDE unipolar, ages 25–57	Ham-D, BDI	Zinc add-on ↓ depression	Nowak et al. (2003)
Zinc	Multivitamins	DBRPCT, 10 weeks, N=30	Healthy volunteers, mean age 19	POMS, CMI	Zinc add-on ↓ depression and anger	Sawada and Yokoi (2010)
Thiamine	Monotherapy	DBRPCT, 2 months, N=120	Healthy students, mean age 20	POMS, GHQ	Better mood, trend toward ↑ clear headedness	Benton et al. 1997
Thiamine	Monotherapy	DBRPCT, 6 weeks, N=80	Healthy, ages 65–92; in thiamine-deficient area: 65% insufficiency	Subjective assessment	↑ Well-being, energy, and appetite	Smidt et al. (1991)

TABLE 6–1. Effects of randomized controlled trials of single micronutrients on mood (excluding folic acid, vitamin D, and pyridoxine) *(continued)*

Treatment	Concurrent treatment	Design	Population	Outcome measures	Statistically significant change vs. placebo ($P<0.05$)	Citation
Thiamine	SSRI	DBRPCT, 12 weeks, N=51	DSM-5 MDD, mean age 35	Ham-D	↓ Depression	Ghaleiha et al. (2016)
Selenium	A few on folate or iron	DBRPCT, 8 months, N=166	Postpartum depression, ages 16–35	EPDS	Prenatal (starting first trimester) treatment ↓ postpartum depression	Mokhber et al. (2011)
Selenium	Monotherapy	DBRPCT, 5 weeks, N=50	Healthy, ages 14–72	POMS	Improved mood, ↓ anxiety; more mood change in subgroup with lower baseline selenium	Benton and Cook (1990, 1991)
Selenium	Monotherapy	RDB, 4 months, 2 doses, N=11	Healthy, ages 20–45	POMS-BI	No change in mood; more change in patients with lower baseline selenium	Hawkes and Hornbostel (1996)
Selenium	Monotherapy	R, 14 weeks, 2 doses, N=30	Healthy, ages 18–45	POMS-BI	Better mood, ↑ clear headedness with high-dose selenium	Finley and Penland (1998)
Selenium	Monotherapy	DBRPCT, 6 months, N=448	Healthy, ages 60–74	POMS-BI	No benefit	Rayman et al. (2006)
Selenium	Monotherapy	DBRPCT, 12 months, N=115	HIV+ drug users, 25% likely MDE, ages 24–53	BDI, STAI POMS-BI	↑ Vigor, ↓ anxiety; no change in mood	Shor-Posner et al. (2003)
Magnesium	Monotherapy	DBRPCT, 2 months, N=32	PMS, ages 24–39	Moos	↓ Premenstrual mood symptoms	Facchinetti al. (1991)

TABLE 6–1. Effects of randomized controlled trials of single micronutrients on mood (excluding folic acid, vitamin D, and pyridoxine) *(continued)*

Treatment	Concurrent treatment	Design	Population	Outcome measures	Statistically significant change vs. placebo (*P*<0.05)	Citation
Magnesium	Monotherapy	DBRPCT, 2 months, *N*=38	PMS, ages 18–50 (mostly 18–25)	Moos	No effect on mood	Walker et al. (1998)
Magnesium	Monotherapy	DBRPCT, 1 month, *N*=44	PMS, mean age 32	Moos	No mood improvement; ↓ anxiety if combined with pyridoxine	De Souza et al. (2000)

Note. BDI=Beck Depression Inventory; BI=bipolar; CGI=Clinical Global Impression; CGI-I=Clinical Global Impression–Improvement; CMI=Cornell Medical Index; DBRPCT=double-blind, randomized, placebo-controlled trial; EDE-Q=Eating Disorder Examination–Questionnaire; EPDS=Edinburgh Postnatal Depression Scale; GHQ=General Health Questionnaire; HADRS=Hospital Anxiety and Depression Rating Scale; Ham-D=Hamilton Depression Rating Scale; MADRS=Montgomery-Åsberg Depression Rating Scale; MDD=major depressive disorder; MDE=major depressive episode; MMSE=Mini-Mental State Examination; Moos=Moos Menstrual Distress Questionnaire; PMS=premenstrual syndrome; POMS=Profile of Moods State; QIDS-SR=Quick Inventory of Depressive Symptomatology–Self Report; R=randomized; RDB=randomized, double-blind; SSRI=selective serotonin reuptake inhibitor; STAI=State-Trait Anxiety Inventory; TCA=tricyclic antidepressant; ↑=increased; ↓=decreased.

Source. Modified from Popper C: "Single-Micronutrient and Broad-Spectrum Micronutrient Approaches for Treating Mood Disorders in Youth and Adults," *Child and Adolescent Psychiatric Clinics of North America* 23(3):591–672, 2014, with permission from Elsevier.

itive findings with mostly minor clinical improvements. At best, some single micronutrients might serve as adjunctive treatments. Except for lithium, no single-micronutrient treatment stands up to conventional psychiatric medications as a monotherapy for any psychiatric disorder.

Why are most single-micronutrient interventions so weak? Adjusting a single micronutrient may not have much impact because 1) micronutrients typically act together physiologically (e.g., B complex) rather than as single actors; 2) many enzymes have multiple cofactors, so adjusting one may have little effect; and 3) treating with a single micronutrient can be disruptive by creating imbalances among micronutrients (relative micronutrient insufficiencies).

Broad-Spectrum Micronutrient Interventions for Mental Health

A more physiologically sensible approach is to examine the effects of multiple micronutrients acting in concert. A broader range of micronutrients is more likely to provide more pervasive physiological changes, including more wide-ranging enhancements of central nervous system (CNS) activity. Broad-spectrum mineral-vitamin combinations have been evaluated for treating violent behavior and conduct problems, ADHD, mood disorders, anxiety disorders, obsessive-compulsive disorder, autism spectrum disorder, and substance use disorders. Broad-spectrum interventions have also been examined in nonclinical ("normal") populations for improving mood, cognition, sense of well-being, and stress tolerance. None of the research on broad-spectrum treatments for psychiatric indications was supported by commercial funding, whereas several studies in nonclinical populations received industry funding.

Broad-Spectrum Micronutrient Treatment of Psychiatric Symptoms and Disorders

AGGRESSIVE BEHAVIORS AND CONDUCT VIOLATIONS

Aggressive behaviors and conduct violations have been studied in underprivileged preadolescent and adolescent students in working-class public schools (Schoenthaler and Bier 2000; Tammam et al. 2016) and incarcerated adolescents (Schoenthaler et al. 1997) and young adults (Gesch et al. 2002; Zaalberg et al. 2010). All five RCTs (total $N=790$) involved concurrent administration of 23–25 micronutrients and showed marked statistically and clinically significant changes: 26%–47% reductions in disciplinary violations and aggressive behaviors after 2–12 weeks (Gesch et al. 2002; Schoenthaler and Bier 2000; Schoenthaler et al. 1997; Tammam et al. 2016; Zaalberg et al. 2010). Three formulations included omega fatty acids, and two did not; the results were comparable. These five positive RCTs (with no negative RCTs) justify implementation of broad-spectrum micronutrient interventions in correctional settings, but more data are needed before recommendations are made for public school students.

ATTENTION-DEFICIT/HYPERACTIVITY DISORDER

ADHD was effectively treated with broad-spectrum micronutrients in one RCT in adults (Rucklidge et al. 2014) and appeared to be effective in nine open-label studies in youth and adults. In the RCT on 80 adults by Rucklidge et al. (2014), micronutrients produced greater changes than placebo in hyperactivity/impulsivity (intent to treat ES 0.46–0.67) and inattention (ES 0.33–0.62) on patient and family ratings. At 8 weeks, improvement (30% reduction in ADHD symptoms) was observed in the self-reports of 64% of subjects receiving micronutrients (vs. 37% of those receiving placebo). Clinician ratings were mixed, with reports of "much" or "very much" improvement in global functioning in 48% of micronutrient subjects, compared with 21% of subjects receiving placebo (ES 0.53–0.57). Global ratings also showed improvements in sleep, anxiety, and irritability. In youths, two open-label within-subject crossover studies of 8- to 15-year-olds with ADHD showed significant on-off symptom control (ABAB) in ADHD, conduct, and mood measures (Gordon et al. 2015; Kaplan et al. 2004).

MOOD DISORDERS

Mood disorders have not been directly examined in RCTs, but a post hoc analysis of the ADHD RCT examined a subsample with comorbid MDD (Rucklidge et al. 2014). Among 21 adults with baseline moderate or severe depression (Montgomery-Åsberg Depression Rating Scale score ≥20, a cutoff often used in U.S. Food and Drug Administration registration trials), the antidepressant effect of broad-spectrum micronutrients (ES 0.64; $P < 0.04$) was comparable in strength to conventional antidepressants. In databases on patients transitioned from psychiatric medications to micronutrients in open-label treatments, about 50% of 358 adults and 120 youths with self- or parent-reported diagnoses of bipolar disorder showed a clinical response of >50% symptom reduction on depression or mania scales at 3 months, with this improvement sustained at 6 months (Gately and Kaplan 2009; Rucklidge et al. 2010). Drug-naïve patients appeared to respond faster and more fully, but most patients taking conventional drugs were able to completely discontinue the medications for at least 6 months once they were stabilized on micronutrients. A case report of a 12-year-old child has been well described (Frazier et al. 2009).

In these studies, broad-spectrum micronutrients and psychiatric medications appear comparable in both antidepressant and anti-manic effects, but the micronutrients had far fewer and less severe side effects and much lower relapse rates. Compared with conventional psychotropics, patients stabilized on broad-spectrum micronutrients have fewer residual symptoms and mood fluctuations, fewer necessary dose changes, less need for monthly medication checks, rare hospitalizations, and lower treatment costs (Kaplan et al. 2017; Rodway et al. 2012).

Broad-Spectrum Micronutrient Interventions in Nonclinical Community Populations

MOOD

Mood in nonclinical samples has been examined in many studies. No consistent effects are observed at recommended daily allowance (RDA) dosing levels; however, a meta-analysis found that formulations with higher doses of B vitamins had more effect on mood ratings, especially when the vitamin B doses were 5–10 times above RDA levels (Long and Benton 2013).

COGNITION

Cognition has been investigated in many nonclinical populations. Although single (and narrow-spectrum) micronutrients have little effect on cognition (Forbes et al. 2015), a meta-analysis (Grima et al. 2012) of the 10 highest-quality RCTs in 3,200 adults concluded that broad-spectrum micronutrients induce a small but consistent improvement in immediate free recall memory, with ES 0.32 ($P<0.01$). An RCT of 4,447 middle-aged adults (ages 45–60) treated with broad-spectrum micronutrients for several years showed a slowing of age-related declines in executive functioning and verbal memory (Kesse-Guyot et al. 2011), a notable "anti-aging" effect. Unfortunately, elderly subjects taking micronutrients show inconsistent changes in cognition, possibly due in part to senescent gastrointestinal absorption of nutrients. In youth, a meta-analysis (Eilander et al. 2010) of RCTs in children (5–16 years old) found no effect on processing speed, working memory, longer-term memory, or sustained attention, but the four highest-quality trials showed a benefit for overall academic performance, again with ES 0.30 ($P=0.04$).

SENSE OF WELL-BEING

Sense of well-being is an operationalized concept measurable by several instruments. The RCTs of broad-spectrum micronutrients show small but statistically significant improvements in ratings of well-being, general energy, clear headedness, and "agreeable feelings," all with ES 0.23–0.35 ($P<0.05$).

MOOD, COGNITION, AND WELL-BEING IN HEALTHY ADULTS

"Enhanced normalcy," as reflected in improved mood, cognition, and well-being, has been shown in healthy adults with broad-spectrum micronutrients in RCTs and meta-analyses, all with ES of about 0.3. In treating a medical disorder, ES of 0.3 is considered weak, but as an easy, inexpensive life enhancement, ES of 0.3 could be viewed as a valuable improvement in brain functioning and the quality of life of typical adults, that is, an enhancement beyond normal levels of mental performance.

ANXIETY AND STRESS REDUCTION

Reductions in anxiety and stress reactions were reported in all 11 RCTs using broad-spectrum micronutrients in typical individuals in a variety of situations, including survivors in the aftermath of natural disasters, adults living in inner-city poverty districts, people in stress-related work settings, men in military basic training (Li et al. 2013), and adults and youth volunteers in the community (Long and Benton 2013; Rucklidge and Kaplan 2013). Two RCTs conducted after earthquakes (Rucklidge et al. 2012) and floods (Kaplan et al. 2015b) showed reduced acute stress and anxiety scores with micronutrients; in one, the prevalence of probable posttraumatic stress disorder was reduced from 65% to 19% after 1 month of treatment (control group remained unchanged). These two RCTs suggest that broad-spectrum micronutrients could be an innovative and inexpensive public health intervention for normal populations following natural disasters.

It is notable that the RCTs in these high-stress situations show much stronger effect sizes (ES 0.69–1.3) than RCTs on normal stress tolerance, mood, cognition, and sense of well-being (ES 0.3). This suggests that broad-spectrum micronutrients are especially useful in high-stress and high-performance situations associated with greater metabolic demand, elevated micronutrient utilization, and increased vulnerability to micronutrient deficiency.

DIVERSE MENTAL HEALTH TARGETS FOR BROAD-SPECTRUM MICRONUTRIENTS

Targets for broad-spectrum micronutrients include psychiatric disorders and normal (nonclinical) brain functions. Evidence for psychiatric indications includes five RCTs on violent and nonviolent conduct problems; one RCT on ADHD; strongly suggestive data on mood disorders; and open-label reports on anxiety disorders, obsessive-compulsive disorder, autism spectrum disorder, emotional regulation in traumatic brain injury, psychotic disorders, and substance use disorders. Evidence in nonclinical samples includes RCTs on mood improvement, cognitive enhancement, better sense of well-being and general energy, and improved stress tolerance. Except for lithium, single micronutrients show limited promise, and only as weak augmentation agents. In contrast, broad-spectrum micronutrients may have greater potential to modify CNS function in more pervasive and potent ways.

Using Broad-Spectrum Micronutrients in Clinical Practice

Clinical principles for using broad-spectrum micronutrient treatments in psychiatric patients were initially developed by David Hardy (Hardy Nutritionals) and Anthony Stephan (Truehope Nutritional Support). Hardy and Stephan marketed the commercial products used in these treatments but never published their informal findings in the scientific literature. Scientists then conducted independent studies (without commercial funding) to examine these unpublished findings. Some aspects of clinical management have not yet been formally evaluated. The management recommendations described here reflect the work of Hardy and Stephan, as confirmed by published RCT and open-label data as well as the authors' clinical experience.

Treating Drug-Naïve or Drug-Free Individuals

Broad-spectrum micronutrient treatments are straightforward for psychiatric patients who are drug-naïve as well as for individuals who are seeking benefits for normal brain functioning, assuming they are not using other CNS-active drugs. Micronutrient use is usually not complicated for patients who have been free of CNS drugs for several weeks or months, except if those medications have significant withdrawal syndromes.

In contrast, cross-tapering patients from ongoing psychiatric drug regimens to broad-spectrum micronutrients generally requires gradual and skillful management because of apparent interactions between broad-spectrum micronutrients and CNS-active drugs. It is strongly urged that clinicians who are learning to use broad-spectrum micronutrient treatments begin with a drug-naïve patient in order to get a feeling for the treatment without the micronutrient-drug interactions.

Dosing depends on the particular micronutrient product, so it is sensible to consult the manufacturer for guidance. A typical dosage range for high-quality formulations may involve 6–12 capsules daily for psychiatric indications (or 4–6 capsules for nonclinical lifestyle enhancement). The large number of pills results from the use of bulky chelated forms of minerals that enhance their absorption and the inclusion of macrominerals, such as calcium, magnesium, and phosphorus, which are often underrepresented in American diets and are required in large bulk quantities. Products containing chelated microminerals and bulky macrominerals are more expensive but are much more effective than regular low-bioavailability formulations.

For drug-naïve or drug-free patients treated with formulations such as Daily Essential Nutrients (Hardy Nutritionals) or EMPowerplus (Truehope Nutritional Supports), doses can be rapidly raised from one pill three times daily on day 1, to two pills three times daily on day 2, to three pills three times daily on day 3, to a final dose of four pills three times daily on day 4. Dividing the dose into three or four daily administrations optimizes nutrient absorption and maintains a sustained effect; two daily doses are usually not adequate. The dosing appears to be independent of body weight or age (>8 years old). If adverse effects emerge, the dose can be temporarily lowered and then increased more slowly. It is sensible to go slower in patients with autism spectrum disorder or known brain damage because they tend to have more adverse CNS effects (as with conventional drugs). Generally, it is best to take the micronutrients with food (optimally, in the middle of a meal) to aid absorption and reduce gastrointestinal side effects. Doses should be a minimum of 2 hours apart because calcium absorption is rate-limited. Missed doses can be made up the next day.

Treating Individuals Taking Psychiatric Medications or Other CNS-Active Drugs

The treatment of individuals who are already taking CNS drugs is considerably more complicated. Transitioning from conventional medications to micronutrients involves a cross-tapering process, during which clinically prominent drug-nutrient interactions usually emerge. This transitioning process can be difficult because of 1) potentiated psychiatric drug side effects; 2) increased psychiatric symptoms as drug doses are tapered down; 3) potentiated, protracted, or delayed drug discontinuation symptoms (including anxiety); and 4) situational anxiety that accompanies the transition. Patients and families need to be warned that there may be a period of symptom regression and anxiety during the transition. It is strongly advised that clinicians obtain training and/or supervision before attempting to transition patients taking conventional psychiatric medications to broad-spectrum micronutrients. Individuals who consume caffeine, nicotine, alcohol, or recreational drugs also may notice interactions with broad-spectrum micronutrients. People who ingest large amounts of these substances (e.g., four cups of coffee daily, marijuana twice weekly) are likely to notice weaker therapeutic effects of micronutrients.

Safety and Minimizing Adverse Effects of Single and Broad-Spectrum Micronutrients

Adverse effects of single vitamins and minerals are well established, but government-issued guidelines for safe upper dose limits for individual nutrients do not directly address micronutrient combinations. Although individual and combination products are "generally recognized as safe" by the U.S. Food and Drug Administration, safety studies are advisable for multinutrient formulations containing ingredients above RDA levels, even if they are within defined safety limits, because of possible nutrient-nutrient potentiation.

Certain forms of micronutrient toxicity can be decreased *or* increased by adjusting their balance with other micronutrients. For example, proper balancing of calcium, magnesium, and phosphorus can prevent constipation from excessive calcium and diarrhea from excessive magnesium. Similarly, zinc-copper balance is critical and is strongly influenced by iron, magnesium, and manganese. A high-quality micronutrient product is more likely to be carefully formulated to reduce potential adverse effects and improve the benefits of its ingredients.

ADVERSE EFFECTS

The adverse effects of well-designed micronutrient products are generally mild and markedly fewer than the adverse effects of psychiatric drugs. Insomnia, headache, and loose stools are infrequent and transient. Urine may turn "neon" yellow, a harmless effect of riboflavin (vitamin B_2) excretion. More significantly, worsening of preexisting *Candida* (yeast) infections, anxiety, agitation, impulsivity, or depression may, in some situations, indicate that a micronutrient dose is too high. Numerous clinical reports on broad-spectrum micronutrients document the absence of sedation, fatigue, carbohydrate or lipid problems, weight changes, sexual side effects, seizures, blood pressure or heart rate changes, motor side effects, tremor, liver or thyroid changes, dry mouth, constipation, and blurred vision (Frazier et al. 2013; Rucklidge et al. 2014; Simpson et al. 2011). Electrocardiogram (ECG) data have not been reported; anecdotally, there is no suggestion of ECG or rhythm change.

LABORATORY TESTING

Laboratory testing has revealed an uncommon, asymptomatic, clinically insignificant increase in prolactin levels well within normal limits in all cases (Rucklidge et al. 2014). No other changes have been found in standard blood or urine measures.

CONTRAINDICATIONS

Contraindications include Wilson's disease (copper), hemochromatosis (iron), phenylketonuria (phenylalanine), and trimethylaminuria (choline). Prostate cancer might be another contraindication. A prospective study of 295,000 men found that using above-recommended doses of three common commercial multivitamins was associated with an increased rate of spread of prostate cancer but not in the incidence of de novo cancer (Lawson et al. 2007). A 32% increase in metastases and a 98% increase in fatalities were observed mainly in men with a family history of prostate cancer. This effect was observed only when commercial once-daily multivitamins were taken more than once daily, potentially exceeding safe levels of some ingredients. Nonetheless, pending more data, broad-spectrum micronutrient treatment could be considered strictly contraindicated in men with prostate cancer, probably contraindicated in men with elevated prostate-specific antigen, and possibly contraindicated in older men with a family history of prostate cancer. The implications of this finding for other cancers are not known.

Relative contraindications include 1) inability to reduce recreational drug use or high intake of caffeine, nicotine, or alcohol; 2) recent use of medications with discontinuation syndromes; 3) treatment-resistant *Candida*; 4) some thyroid diseases (iodine); 5) severe hyperlipidemia or severe protein malnutrition, which are associated with increased susceptibility to vitamin A toxicity; and 6) some liver or renal diseases, especially alcohol-related disease.

Pregnancy is not a contraindication because it is well established that broad-spectrum micronutrients are healthful for the fetus and are routinely recommended to pregnant mothers.

General Clinical Management

INITIAL EVALUATION

Initial evaluation of patients includes standard psychiatric evaluation, medication history (duration and last use of CNS-active agents, marijuana, other recreational drugs, caffeine, alcohol, nicotine), assessment of the individual's willingness to reduce his or her usage of these drugs, contraindications (*Candida* infection, prostate cancer), and antibiotic usage. If the patient will be transitioning from a psychiatric drug regimen, the patient and family need preparation for clinical regression and anxiety during the transition. No specific laboratory testing is required, but prolactin, vitamin A level, and ECG might be considered. Occupational exposure to heavy metals is an indication for evaluation for potential micronutrient toxicities (manganese, iron, zinc, copper, lead).

INFORMED CONSENT

Informed consent should be thorough and well documented for any nonestablished treatment. The informed consent may include explicit statements that 1) this is not an established treatment; 2) established treatments are available; 3) limited RCTs are available to evaluate safety or efficacy; 4) if transitioning from psychiatric drugs, anxiety and some symptom relapse are expected; 5) adverse effects include potential worsening of *Candida* infections and speculatively of prostate cancer (and, even more speculatively, other cancers); 7) nutrient interactions with psychiatric and nonpsychiatric medications can occur; 8) the prescriber should be contacted when starting any new drug, especially an antibiotic; and 9) reducing or preferably stopping recreational drugs, caffeine, alcohol, and smoking will enhance treatment effectiveness and safety. Documentation should specify reasons for using a nonestablished treatment, such as patient preference and potential for fewer adverse effects or better clinical response. If transitioning a patient from psychiatric drugs, the medical record should explain the reason each time a psychiatric drug dose is lowered, such as adverse effects detected, withdrawal symptoms, or other specific clinical observations in the individual patient; it is not sufficient to appeal to a general protocol.

ORAL ANTIBIOTICS

Oral antibiotics and antifungal treatments usually require an adjustment in micronutrient dosing. The intestinal microbiome is crucially involved in micronutrient absorption (and for some vitamins, synthesis), so antibiotics sharply reduce nutrient absorption and can lead to a return of psychiatric symptoms. This problem is avoided by increasing the micronutrient dose by 40%–50% during the antibiotic therapy plus 4 additional days. For chronic antibiotic treatment (e.g., acne), the micronutrient dose can be adjusted around the antibiotic dose.

RESIDUAL SYMPTOMS

Unresolved residual symptoms may respond to certain natural compounds in combination with micronutrients. Lithium may be used for residual symptoms of mania; however, when combined with micronutrient formulas, the lithium dose must not exceed 25 mg daily because of the risk of marked potentiation as observed by the authors. Choline also can be used for residual mania, 5-hydroxytryptophan or *S*-adenosylmethionine for residual depression, and inositol or L-theanine for residual anxiety.

TREATMENT DISCONTINUATION

Discontinuation by patients usually results from 1) the uninsured cost of treatment (about $135 monthly), most commonly; 2) inability to tolerate the transition process, usually because of drug withdrawal effects, especially when use of abusable drugs is not disclosed to the prescriber; 3) lack of benefit; and 4) inability to swallow many pills. Techniques to facilitate pill swallowing may be helpful (Kaplan et al. 2010; see also video at http://research4kids.ucalgary.ca/pillswallowing). When micronutrients are stopped after brief treatment, they can be discontinued without tapering, and medication can be restored as tolerated. If treatment lasted more than 2 weeks, it is preferable to taper the nutrients and increase drug doses gradually over days or weeks as nutrient-drug interactions subside.

FIRST-LINE TREATMENT

First-line treatment may be considered prior to using established treatments in some circumstances, despite limited RCTs on safety and efficacy. Broad-spectrum micronutrients may be comparable in efficacy to conventional medications and appear safer, so first-line use is rational if the clinical presentation is not too acute. Furthermore, just as one might introduce exercise, sleep hygiene, and dietary measures in the initial phase of intervention for some individuals, broad-spectrum micronutrients might be considered in certain cases before conventional psychopharmacotherapy. Chart documentation should include a convincing statement that there is a low clinical risk to delaying established treatment.

Mechanisms of Action of Broad-Spectrum Micronutrients

Broad-spectrum micronutrients are crucially involved in many functions throughout biology, undoubtedly operating through numerous mechanisms of action.

Pervasive Upregulation of CNS Functions

In the brain, broad-spectrum micronutrients appear to have wide-ranging effects in 1) treating a variety of psychiatric symptoms, 2) enhancing a diverse range of normal brain functions, and 3) appearing to increase the potency of most CNS-active drugs. In standard pharmacological models, this broad range of effects would be difficult to explain. Broad-spectrum micronutrients appear to operate through pervasive upregulation of CNS functioning, not through mechanisms tied to particular psychiatric disorders. This is consistent with Bruce Ames' theory of a "metabolic tune-up" (Ames 2004). This theory could explain why micronutrients appear to have a "holistic effect" on brain function by supplying a broad variety of micronutrients to enhance and pervasively optimize physiological functioning.

It may seem perplexing that broad-spectrum micronutrients appear to potentiate virtually all CNS-active drugs. Speculatively, psychiatric patients might under-respond to CNS medications because their general biological functioning is not optimized. By metabolically tuning up physiological efficiency, broad-spectrum micronutrients might improve clinical response to CNS medications through enhanced pharmacodynamic responsiveness.

Possible Neurotrophic Effects

Neurotrophic effects of micronutrients could improve neuronal growth and survival, as illustrated by an animal study on micronutrient-enhanced recovery from perinatal brain damage (Halliwell et al. 2009). When rats are lesioned in the frontal or parietal cortex within a few days of birth, they grow into adults with large permanent reductions in brain tissue mass and functional performance. However, if fed chow with broad-spectrum micronutrients throughout their lives, the adult rats show more anatomic recovery (reversal of decreased brain size, increased cortical thickness, enhanced new dendritic growth, higher spine density) and more motor and cognitive functional recovery than rats on normal diets (Halliwell and Kolb 2003). This study suggests that broad-spectrum micronutrients might exert a neurotrophic effect on brain development, structure, and function following early brain injury. Speculatively, this finding could have clinical implications for children with neurobehavioral sequelae of prenatal or perinatal brain injury and for adults with traumatic brain injury.

Another type of neurotrophic effect is shown by data suggesting that broad-spectrum micronutrients have antiaging properties. As previously mentioned, Ames demonstrated in his animal model that micronutrient deficiencies can increase oxidative damage to nuclear and mitochondrial DNA, causing metabolic changes in multiple organ systems, chronic inflammation, neuronal deterioration, cancer, and accelerated aging. Dietary intake of vitamin-like substances slowed these changes (Ames 2010). In humans, as previously noted, an RCT in almost 4,500 middle-aged adults (45–50 years old) found that broad-spectrum micronutrients administered over several years produced a slowing of age-related declines in both executive functioning and verbal memory (Kesse-Guyot et al. 2011). In addition, a cross-sectional study in humans (Xu et al. 2009) found that daily users of multinutrient products have 5% longer telomeres than do nonusers ($P=0.002$). These apparent trophic effects on neurorecovery after brain damage and antiaging neuroprotection suggest further directions for research.

Risks of Narrow-Spectrum Versus Broad-Spectrum Micronutrients

Numerous studies show that treatment with only one or two micronutrients can be harmful, even at routine doses (Harvie 2014). Large-scale studies link vitamin A with increased cardiovascular deaths and lung cancer, vitamin E with colorectal cancer and prostate cancer, and beta-carotene with stomach and lung cancer. Beta-carotene, vitamin E, and vitamin A can increase all-cause mortality. Combining vitamins C and E is associated with reduced benefits of physical exercise (Ristow et al. 2009). Such single-nutrient or narrow-spectrum treatments might speculatively exert deleterious effects by inducing imbalances and relative insufficiencies among micronutrients.

Most adverse micronutrient effects have been associated with treatments involving three or fewer ingredients. The findings become more favorable with formulations of 10 or more micronutrients (Comerford 2013). This reinforces the principle that a full range of micronutrients is needed for optimal physiological functioning and for reducing potential drawbacks of narrow-spectrum approaches.

Desirable Characteristics of Broad-Spectrum Micronutrient Formulations

In selecting a commercial micronutrient formulation, the following characteristics are desirable:

- At least 10, preferably more (25 or so), minerals and vitamins
- Doses of individual micronutrients exceeding the RDA (levels 5–10 times the RDA are acceptable for some B vitamins) but below tolerable upper intake levels specified in the Dietary Reference Intake system from the Institute of Medicine (2006)
- Properly balanced ratios among ingredients (to avoid micronutrient imbalances)
- High bioavailability (which excludes many and perhaps most drugstore products)
- High quality control (to ensure appropriate contents and to exclude contaminants)
- Absence of citrus bioflavonoids and other botanicals that interact with drugs
- Availability of peer-reviewed studies on safety and efficacy using comparable formulations

Although many micronutrient commercial products are available, in the authors' opinion, two formulations stand apart from others because of their high product quality and psychiatric research examining their safety and effectiveness. These products, Daily Essential Nutrients (Hardy Nutritionals) and EMPowerplus (Truehope Nutritional Support), are available as capsules and flavored powders. The cost in 2017 was $3–$5 daily, depending on dose, and typically is not covered by health insurance.

Future Development of Broad-Spectrum Micronutrient Interventions

The entire approach of taking micronutrients in pill form might beg the question: Why not just eat more nutritious food? After all, improved dietary intake is known to contribute to better mental health (Jacka et al. 2012). An unblinded controlled study showed significant improvement in adults with MDD following a 12-week protocol involving dietary counseling, mindful eating, and motivational interviewing that encouraged adherence to a modified Mediterranean diet (Jacka et al. 2017). However, simply increasing nutrient intake may not be sufficient for everyone, in view of the diminished nutrient content of our food supply, unwise food preferences and lifestyle choices, and personal financial limitations. Even if all these factors could be ameliorated, genetic factors would probably still play a key role. Linus Pauling (1968) proposed that genes that predispose people to mental disorders might also influence brain metabolism of essential nutrients. This implies that a positive family psychiatric history might, in some cases, be associated with higher nutrient requirements than food intake alone could provide.

We know that the majority of the American population is at risk for insufficiency of at least one micronutrient. Current nutritional evaluation methods can estimate the sufficiency status of only a few micronutrients, so identification of all micronutrient insufficiencies in an individual is not yet possible. For now, it is easier and less expensive to simply supply broad-spectrum micronutrients than to characterize the specific micronutrient insufficiencies of each person.

Clearly, more research is needed (Sarris et al. 2015a, 2015b) to explore the benefits and limitations of nutrition-based therapies for developing 1) low-risk, low-stigma, health-promoting treatments for violence in prisons and conduct problems in schools; 2) nonabusable treatments for ADHD that are more likely to enhance growth than to diminish it; and 3) treatments for major depression and bipolar disorder with fewer side effects than current standard-of-care approaches. However, on the basis of current findings, it is justifiable for psychiatrists to explore the clinical effects of broad-spectrum micronutrient treatments for patients interested in these approaches.

KEY POINTS

- Single-micronutrient treatments, apart from lithium, provide modest benefits as augmentation agents (folate and perhaps vitamin D) but not as monotherapies for psychiatric symptoms.

- Evidence suggests that broad-spectrum micronutrients may aid in the treatment of aggressive behavior, conduct problems, ADHD, and mood disorders as adjunctives or, in some cases, as monotherapies.

- Broad-spectrum treatments may exert a "holistic" effect that pervasively enhances brain and physiological functioning, consistent with the "metabolic tune-up" theory, in psychiatric and nonclinical populations.

- Broad-spectrum micronutrient treatment is straightforward in individuals not using CNS-active drugs. Training and supervision are advised for treating patients taking psychiatric medications.

References

Akbaraly TN, Brunner EJ, Ferrie JE, et al: Dietary pattern and depressive symptoms in middle age. Br J Psychiatry 195(5):408–413, 2009 19880930

Almeida OP, Ford AH, Hirani V, et al: B vitamins to enhance treatment response to antidepressants in middle-aged and older adults: results from the B-VITAGE randomised, double-blind, placebo-controlled trial. Br J Psychiatry 205(6):450–457, 2014 25257064

American Psychiatric Association: Diagnostic and Statistical Manual of Mental Disorders, 5th Edition. Arlington, VA, American Psychiatric Association, 2013

Ames BN: A role for supplements in optimizing health: the metabolic tune-up. Arch Biochem Biophys 423(1):227–234, 2004 14989256

Ames BN: Optimal micronutrients delay mitochondrial decay and age-associated diseases. Mech Ageing Dev 131(7–8):473–479, 2010 20420847

Ames BN, Elson-Schwab I, Silver EA: High-dose vitamin therapy stimulates variant enzymes with decreased coenzyme binding affinity (increased K(m)): relevance to genetic disease and polymorphisms. Am J Clin Nutr 75(4):616–658, 2002 11916749

Bedson E, Bell D, Carr D, et al: Folate Augmentation of Treatment—Evaluation for Depression (FolATED): randomised trial and economic evaluation. Health Technol Assess 18(48):vii–viii, 1–159, 2014 25052890

Behzadi AH, Omrani Z, Chalian M, et al: Folic acid efficacy as an alternative drug added to sodium valproate in the treatment of acute phase of mania in bipolar disorder: a double-blind randomized controlled trial. Acta Psychiatr Scand 120(6):441–445, 2009 19392814

Bendich A: The potential for dietary supplements to reduce premenstrual syndrome (PMS) symptoms. J Am Coll Nutr 19(1):3–12, 2000 10682869

Benton D, Cook R: Selenium supplementation improves mood in a double-blind crossover trial. Psychopharmacology (Berl) 102(4):549–550, 1990 2096413

Benton D, Cook R: The impact of selenium supplementation on mood. Biol Psychiatry 29(11):1092–1098, 1991 1873372

Benton D, Griffiths R, Haller J: Thiamine supplementation mood and cognitive functioning. Psychopharmacology (Berl) 129(1):66–71, 1997 9122365

Brownley KA, Von Holle A, Hamer RM, et al: A double-blind, randomized pilot trial of chromium picolinate for binge eating disorder: results of the Binge Eating and Chromium (BEACh) study. J Psychosom Res 75(1):36–42, 2013 23751236

Centers for Disease Control and Prevention: Second National Report on Biochemical Indicators of Diet and Nutrition in the US Population 2012, Executive Summary. Atlanta, GA, Centers for Disease Control and Prevention, 2012, Available at: http://www.cdc.gov/nutritionreport/pdf/ExeSummary_Web_032612.pdf. Accessed January 1, 2017.

Comerford KB: Recent developments in multivitamin/mineral research. Adv Nutr 4(6):644–656, 2013 24228193

Coppen A, Bailey J: Enhancement of the antidepressant action of fluoxetine by folic acid: a randomised, placebo controlled trial. J Affect Disord 60(2):121–130, 2000 10967371

Davidson JR, Abraham K, Connor KM, et al: Effectiveness of chromium in atypical depression: a placebo-controlled trial. Biol Psychiatry 53(3):261–264, 2003 12559660

De Souza MC, Walker AF, Robinson PA, et al: A synergistic effect of a daily supplement for 1 month of 200 mg magnesium plus 50 mg vitamin B6 for the relief of anxiety-related premenstrual symptoms: a randomized, double-blind, crossover study. J Womens Health Gend Based Med 9(2):131–139, 2000 10746516

Docherty JP, Sack DA, Roffman M, et al: A double-blind, placebo-controlled, exploratory trial of chromium picolinate in atypical depression: effect on carbohydrate craving. J Psychiatr Pract 11(5):302–314, 2005 16184071

Eilander A, Gera T, Sachdev HS, et al: Multiple micronutrient supplementation for improving cognitive performance in children: systematic review of randomized controlled trials. Am J Clin Nutr 91(1):115–130, 2010 19889823

Facchinetti F, Borella P, Sances G, et al: Oral magnesium successfully relieves premenstrual mood changes. Obstet Gynecol 78(2):177–181, 1991 2067759

Findling RL, Maxwell K, Scotese-Wojtila L, et al: High-dose pyridoxine and magnesium administration in children with autistic disorder: an absence of salutary effects in a double-blind, placebo-controlled study. J Autism Dev Disord 27(4):467–478, 1997 9261669

Finley JS, Penland JG: Adequacy or deprivation of dietary selenium in healthy men: clinical and psychological findings. J Trace Elem Exp Med 11(1):11–27, 1998

Forbes SC, Holroyd-Leduc JM, Poulin MJ, Hogan DB: Effects of nutrients, dietary supplements and vitamins on cognition: a systematic review and meta-analysis of randomized controlled trials. Can Geriatr J 18(4):231–245, 2015 26740832

Frazier EA, Fristad MA, Arnold LE, Fristad MA: Multinutrient supplement as treatment: literature review and case report of a 12-year-old boy with bipolar disorder. J Child Adolesc Psychopharmacol 19(4):453–460, 2009 19702498

Frazier EA, Gracious B, Arnold LE, et al: Nutritional and safety outcomes from an open-label micronutrient intervention for pediatric bipolar spectrum disorders. J Child Adolesc Psychopharmacol 23(8):558–567, 2013 24138009

Gately D, Kaplan BJ: Database analysis of adults with bipolar disorder consuming a micronutrient formula. Clinical Medicine Insights: Psychiatry 4(2):3–16, 2009

Gesch CB, Hammond SM, Hampson SE, et al: Influence of supplementary vitamins, minerals and essential fatty acids on the antisocial behaviour of young adult prisoners: fandomised, placebo-controlled trial. Br J Psychiatry 181:22–28, 2002 12091259

Ghaleiha A, Davari H, Jahangard L, et al: Adjuvant thiamine improved standard treatment in patients with major depressive disorder: results from a randomized, double-blind, and placebo-controlled clinical trial. Eur Arch Psychiatry Clin Neurosci 266(8)695–702, 2016 26984349

Giannini AJ, Nakoneczie AM, Melemis SM, et al: Magnesium oxide augmentation of verapamil maintenance therapy in mania. Psychiatry Res 93(1):83–87, 2000 10699232

Godfrey PS, Toone BK, Carney MW, et al: Enhancement of recovery from psychiatric illness by methylfolate. Lancet 336(8712):392–395, 1990 1974941

Gordon HA, Rucklidge JJ, Blampied NM, Johnstone JM: Clinically significant symptom reduction in children with attention-deficit/hyperactivity disorder treated with micronutrients: an open-label reversal design study. J Child Adolesc Psychopharmacol 25(10):783–798, 2015 26682999

Grima NA, Pase MP, Macpherson H, Pipingas A: The effects of multivitamins on cognitive performance: a systematic review and meta-analysis. J Alzheimers Dis 29(3):561–569, 2012 22330823

Halliwell C, Kolb B: Vitamin/mineral supplements enhance recovery from perinatal cortical lesions in rats (abstract). Society for Neuroscience Abstracts 29:459.11, 2003

Halliwell C, Comeau W, Gibb R, et al: Factors influencing frontal cortex development and recovery from early frontal injury. Dev Neurorehabil 12(5):269–278, 2009 20477557

Hariri M, Azadbakht L: Magnesium, iron, and zinc supplementation for the treatment of attention deficit hyperactivity disorder: a systematic review on the recent literature. Int J Prev Med 6:83, 2015 26445630

Harvie M: Nutritional supplements and cancer: potential benefits and proven harms. Am Soc Clin Oncol Educ Book e478–e486, 2014 24857143

Hawkes WC, Hornbostel L: Effects of dietary selenium on mood in healthy men living in a metabolic research unit. Biol Psychiatry 39(2):121–128, 1996 8717610

Hvas AM, Juul S, Lauritzen L, et al: No effect of vitamin B-12 treatment on cognitive function and depression: a randomized placebo controlled study. J Affect Disord 81(3):269–273, 2004 15337331

Institute of Medicine: Dietary Reference Intakes: The Essential Guide to Nutrient Requirements. Edited by Otten JJ, Hellwing JP, Meyers LD. Washington, DC, National Academies Press, 2006

Jacka FN, Mykletun A, Berk M: Moving towards a population health approach to the primary prevention of common mental disorders. BMC Med 10:149, 2012 23186355

Jacka FN, O'Neil A, Opie R, et al: A randomised controlled trial of dietary improvement for adults with major depression (the 'SMILES' trial). BMC Med 15(1):23, 2017 28137247

Kaplan BJ, Fisher JE, Crawford SG, et al: Improved mood and behavior during treatment with a mineral-vitamin supplement: an open-label case series of children. J Child Adolesc Psychopharmacol 14(1):115–122, 2004 15142398

Kaplan BJ, Crawford SG, Field CJ, Simpson JS: Vitamins, minerals, and mood. Psychol Bull 133(5):747–760, 2007 17723028

Kaplan BJ, Steiger RA, Pope J, et al: Successful treatment of pill-swallowing difficulties with head posture practice. Paediatr Child Health 15:e1–e5, 2010 21532781

Kaplan BJ, Rucklidge JJ, Romijn A, McLeod K: The emerging field of nutritional mental health: inflammation, the microbiome, oxidative stress, and mitochondrial function. Clin Psychol Sci 3(6):964–980, 2015a

Kaplan BJ, Rucklidge JJ, Romijn AR, et al: A randomised trial of nutrient supplements to minimise psychological stress after a natural disaster. Psychiatry Res 228(3):373–379, 2015b 26154816

Kaplan BJ, Isaranuwatchai W, Hoch JS, et al: Hospitalization cost of conventional psychiatric care compared to broad-spectrum micronutrient treatment: literature review and case study of adult psychosis. Int J Ment Syst 11:14, 2017 28163777

Kesse-Guyot E, Fezeu L, Jeandel C, et al: French adults' cognitive performance after daily supplementation with antioxidant vitamins and minerals at nutritional doses: a post hoc analysis of the Supplementation in Vitamins and Mineral Antioxidants (SU.VI.MAX) trial. Am J Clin Nutr 94(3):892–899, 2011 21775560

Khoraminya N, Tehrani-Doost M, Jazayeri S, et al: Therapeutic effects of vitamin D as adjunctive therapy to fluoxetine in patients with major depressive disorder. Aust N Z J Psychiatry 47(3):271–275, 2013 23093054

Kjærgaard M, Waterloo K, Wang CE, et al: Effect of vitamin D supplement on depression scores in people with low levels of serum 25-hydroxyvitamin D: nest case-control study and randomised clinical trial. Br J Psychiatry 201(5):360–368, 2012

Kleijnen J, Ter Riet G, Knipschild P: Vitamin B6 in the treatment of the premenstrual syndrome—a review. Br J Obstet Gynaecol 97(9):847–852, 1990 2242373

Lawson KA, Wright ME, Subar A, et al: Multivitamin use and risk of prostate cancer in the National Institutes of Health-AARP Diet and Health Study. J Natl Cancer Inst 99(10):754–764, 2007 17505071

Li X, Huang WX, Lu JM, et al: Effects of a multivitamin/multimineral supplement on young males with physical overtraining: a placebo-controlled, randomized, double-blinded cross-over trial. Biomed Eviron Sci 26(7):599–604, 2013 23895706

Li G, Mbuagbaw L, Samaan Z, et al: Efficacy of vitamin D supplementation in depression in adults: a systematic review. J Clin Endocrinol Metab 99(3):757–767, 2014 24423304

Long SJ, Benton D: Effects of vitamin and mineral supplementation on stress, mild psychiatric symptoms, and mood in nonclinical samples: a meta-analysis. Psychosom Med 75(2):144–153, 2013 23362497

Mayer AMB: Historical changes in the mineral content of fruits and vegetables. British Food Journal 99(6):207–211, 1997

Mech AW, Farah A: Correlation of clinical response with homocysteine reduction during therapy with reduced B vitamins in patients with MDD who are positive for MTHFR C677T or A1298C polymorphism: a randomized, double-blind, placebo-controlled study. J Clin Psychiatry 77(5):668–671, 2016 27035272

Mitchell DM, Henao MP, Finkelstein JS, Burnett-Bowie SA: Prevalence and predictors of vitamin D deficiency in healthy adults. Endocr Pract 18(6):914–923, 2012 22982792

Mokhber N, Namjoo M, Tara F, et al: Effect of supplementation with selenium on postpartum depression: a randomized double-blind placebo-controlled trial. J Matern Fetal Neonatal Med 24(1):104–108, 2011 20528216

Nowak G, Siwek M, Dudek D, et al: Effect of zinc supplementation on antidepressant therapy in unipolar depression: a preliminary placebo-controlled study. Pol J Pharmacol 55(6):1143–1147, 2003 14730113

Oren DA, Teicher MH, Schwartz PJ, et al: A controlled trial of cyanocobalamin (vitamin B12) in the treatment of winter seasonal affective disorder. J Affect Disord 32(3):197–200, 1994 7852661

Pan LA, Martin P, Zimmer T, et al: Neurometabolic disorders: potentially treatable abnormalities in patients with treatment-refractory depression and suicidal behavior. Am J Psychiatry 174(1):42–50, 2017 27523499

Papakostas GI, Shelton RC, Zajecka JM, et al: L-Methylfolate as adjunctive therapy for SSRI-resistant major depression: results of two randomized, double-blind, parallel-sequential trials. Am J Psychiatry 169(12):1267–1274, 2012 23212058

Pauling L: Orthomolecular psychiatry: varying the concentrations of substances normally present in the human body may control mental disease. Science 160(3825):265–271, 1968 5641253

Pfeiffer SI, Norton J, Nelson L, et al: Efficacy of vitamin B6 and magnesium in the treatment of autism: a methodology review and summary of outcomes. J Autism Dev Disord 25(5):481–493, 1995 8567594

Popper CW: Single-micronutrient and broad-spectrum micronutrient approaches for treating mood disorders in youth and adults. Child Adolesc Psychiatr Clin N Am 23(3):591–672, 2014 24975626

Qureshi NA, Al-Bedah AM: Mood disorders and complementary and alternative medicine: a literature review. Neuropsychiatr Dis Treat 9:639–658, 2013 23700366

Rayman M, Thompson A, Warren-Perry M, et al: Impact of selenium on mood and quality of life: a randomized, controlled trial. Biol Psychiatry 59(2):147–154, 2006 16181615

Resler G, Lavie R, Campos J, et al: Effect of folic acid combined with fluoxetine in patients with major depression on plasma homocysteine and vitamin B12, and serotonin levels in lymphocytes. Neuroimmunomodulation 15(3):145–152, 2008 18716414

Ristow M, Zarse S, Oberbach A, et al: Antioxidants prevent health-promoting effects of physical exercise in humans. Proc Natl Acad Sci U. S. A. 106(21):8665–8670, 2009 19433800

Rodway M, Vance A, Watters A, et al: Efficacy and cost of micronutrient treatment of childhood psychosis. BMJ Case Rep 2012:bcr2012007213, 2012 23144350

Rucklidge JJ, Kaplan BJ: Broad-spectrum micronutrient formulas for the treatment of psychiatric symptoms: a systematic review. Expert Rev Neurother 13(1):49–73, 2013 23253391

Rucklidge JJ, Gately D, Kaplan BJ: Database analysis of children and adolescents with bipolar disorder consuming a micronutrient formula. BMC Psychiatry 10:74, 2010 20875144

Rucklidge JJ, Andridge R, Gorman B, et al: Shaken but unstirred? Effects of micronutrients on stress and trauma after an earthquake: RCT evidence comparing formulas and doses. Hum Psychopharmacol 27(5):440–454, 2012 22782571

Rucklidge JJ, Frampton CM, Gorman B, Boggis A: Vitamin-mineral treatment of attention-deficit hyperactivity disorder in adults: double-blind randomised placebo-controlled trial. Br J Psychiatry 204:306–315, 2014 24482441

Rylander M, Verhulst S: Vitamin D insufficiency in psychiatric inpatients. J Psychiatr Pract 19(4):296–300, 2013 23852104

Sánchez-Villegas A, Delgado-Rodríguez M, Alonso A, et al: Association of the Mediterranean dietary pattern with the incidence of depression: the Seguimiento Universidad de Navarra/University of Navarra follow-up (SUN) cohort. Arch Gen Psychiatry 66(10):1090–1098, 2009 19805699

Sánchez-Villegas A, Toledo E, de Irala J, et al: Fast-food and commercial baked goods consumption and the risk of depression. Public Health Nutr 15(3):424–432, 2012 21835082

Sarris J, Logan AC, Akbaraly TN, et al: International Society for Nutritional Psychiatry Research consensus position statement: nutritional medicine in modern psychiatry. World Psychiatry 14(3):370–371, 2015a 26407799

Sarris J, Logan AC, Akbaraly TN, et al: Nutritional medicine as mainstream in psychiatry. Lancet Psychiatry 2(3):271–274, 2015b 26359904

Sarris J, Murphy J, Mischoulon D, et al: Adjunctive nutraceuticals for depression: a systematic review and meta-analyses. Am J Psychiatry 173(6):575–587, 2016 27113121

Sawada T, Yokoi K: Effect of zinc supplementation on mood states in young women: a pilot study. Eur J Clin Nutr 64(3):331–333, 2010 20087376

Schoenthaler SJ, Bier ID: The effect of vitamin-mineral supplementation on juvenile delinquency among American schoolchildren: a randomized, double-blind placebo-controlled trial. J Altern Complement Med 6(1):7–17, 2000 10706231

Schoenthaler SJ, Amos S, Doraz W, et al: The effect of randomized vitamin-mineral supplementation on violent and non-violent antisocial behavior among incarcerated juveniles. J Nutr Environ Med 7(4):343–352, 1997

Sharpley AL, Hockney R, McPeake L, et al: Folic acid supplementation for prevention of mood disorders in young people at familial risk: a randomised, double blind, placebo controlled trial. J Affect Disord 167:306–311, 2014 25010374

Shelton RC, Pencina MJ, Barrentine LW, et al: Association of obesity and inflammatory marker levels on treatment outcome: results from a double-blind, randomized study of adjunctive L-methylfolate calcium in patients with MDD who are inadequate responders to SSRIs. J Clin Psychiatry 76(12):1635–1641, 2015 26613389

Shigenaga MK, Hagen TM, Ames BN: Oxidative damage and mitochondrial decay in aging. Proc Natl Acad Sci USA 91(23):10771–10778, 1994 7971961

Shor-Posner G, Lecusay R, Miguez MJ, et al: Psychological burden in the era of HAART: impact of selenium therapy. Int J Psychiatry Med 33(1):55–69, 2003 12906343

Simpson JS, Crawford SG, Goldstein ET, et al: Systematic review of safety and tolerability of a complex micronutrient formula used in mental health. BMC Psychiatry 11:62, 2011 21501484

Siwek M, Dudek D, Paul IA, et al: Zinc supplementation augments efficacy of imipramine in treatment resistant patients: a double blind, placebo-controlled study. J Affect Disord 118(1–3):187–195, 2009 19278731

Siwek M, Dudek D, Schlegel-Zawadzka M, et al: Serum zinc level in depressed patients during zinc supplementation of imipramine treatment. J Affect Disord 126(3):447–452, 2010 20493532

Smidt LJ, Cremin FM, Grivetti LE, et al: Influence of thiamin supplementation on the health and general well-being of an elderly Irish population with marginal thiamin deficiency. J Gerontol 46(1):M16–M22, 1991 1986037

Syed EU, Wasay M, Awan S: Vitamin B12 supplementation in treating major depressive disorder: a randomized controlled trial. Open Neurol J 7:44–48, 2013 24339839

Tammam JD, Steinsaltz D, Bester DW, et al: A randomised double-blind placebo-controlled trial investigating the behavioural effects of vitamin, mineral and n-3 fatty acid supplementation in typically developing adolescent schoolchildren. Br J Nutr 115(2):361–373, 2016 26573368

U.S. Department of Agriculture, Agriculture Research Service: Community Nutrition Mapping Project. Available at: http://www.ars.usda.gov/News/docs.htm?docid=15656. Accessed January 1, 2017.

Venkatasubramanian R, Kumar CN, Pandey RS: A randomized double-blind comparison of fluoxetine augmentation by high and low dosage folic acid in patients with depressive episodes. J Affect Disord 150(2):644–648, 2013 23507369

Walker AF, De Souza MC, Vickers MF, et al: Magnesium supplementation alleviates premenstrual symptoms of fluid retention. J Womens Health 7(9):1157–1165, 1998 9861593

Wyatt KM, Dimmock PW, Jones PW, et al: Efficacy of vitamin B-6 in the treatment of premenstrual syndrome: systematic review. BMJ 318(7195):1375–1381, 1999 10334745

Xu Q, Parks CG, DeRoo LA, et al: Multivitamin use and telomere length in women. Am J Clin Nutr 89(6):1857–1863, 2009 19279081

Zaalberg A, Nijman H, Bulten E, et al: Effects of nutritional supplements on aggression, rule-breaking, and psychopathology among young adult prisoners. Aggress Behav 36(2):117–126, 2010 20014286

SECTION III

Plant-Based Medicines

CHAPTER 7

Issues in Phytomedicine Related to Psychiatric Practice

Mark Blumenthal, Ph.D. (Honoris Causa)

A man may esteem himself happy
when that which is his food is also his medicine.

Henry David Thoreau

Phytomedicine, use of herbs and medicinal plants based on both traditional use and modern research, has been accepted by pharmacists, physicians, and consumers in many countries. For example, in Germany, herbs are sold primarily as government-approved nonprescription medicines and are manufactured by modern extraction and chemical standardization according to good manufacturing practices (GMPs) to produce extracts that are consistent from batch to batch. From 2000 to 2014, annual retail sales of herbal supplements in the United States rose from $4.2 billion to $6.5 billion (Smith et al. 2015). Health professionals and consumers ask: "Are herbs regulated? Are they safe? Do herbs really work? What about herb-drug interactions? Which brands can I trust?" This overview discusses the current regulation of herbal dietary supplements; the available evidence of quality, safety, and efficacy; and issues affecting the quality of research. The problems of adulteration, the limitations of DNA testing, and the need to educate professionals, media, and government oversight agencies regarding analytical testing of products are addressed. Identification of high-quality supplements and phytoequivalency are also covered.

Regulation of Herbal Dietary Supplements in the United States

One of the biggest misconceptions is that the federal government does not regulate botanical dietary supplements. Although people disagree about whether supplements are *adequately* regulated, ample evidence confirms that they *are* regulated. In 2012 a peer-reviewed assessment of herb regulation in the United States found that federal laws (e.g., the Federal Food, Drug, and Cosmetic Act as amended by the Dietary Supplement Health and Education Act of 1994 [DSHEA] and subsequent legislation) grant significant authority and responsibility to federal agencies (U.S. Food and Drug Administration [FDA] and Federal Trade Commission) to regulate herbs and other dietary supplements. Areas over which these agencies have authority include importation, storage, processing, manufacture, labeling, sales, marketing claims, and required reporting of serious adverse events (Soller et al. 2012). Regulations require marketers to send safety information about new dietary ingredients (i.e., those introduced to the United States after October 15, 1994) to the FDA for review. Many natural foods and herbs are approved under the Federal Food, Drug, and Cosmetic Act as being *generally recognized as safe* (GRAS) on the basis of scientific evidence or experience through common use in foods (www.fda.gov/Food/IngredientsPackagingLabeling/GRAS).

Some critics of the current regulatory framework advocate for herbs to be regulated in the same manner as pharmaceutical drugs, requiring premarket approval and enormous safety and efficacy research expenditures. Such requirements are not necessary for most herbal products, are not economically feasible, and would not serve the public interest because they would likely deprive consumers of access and prevent health professionals from prescribing traditionally available herbal medicines that are predominantly safe and relatively inexpensive.

The Quality of Phytomedicinal Research

Questions regarding the safety and efficacy of herbal preparations hinge on long-term traditional use, preclinical and clinical studies, postmarket surveillance, and epidemiological data. A study by a Swiss government agency concluded that the quality of design of 89 randomly selected controlled phytomedicinal clinical trials was equal, or in some cases superior, to 89 matched randomized controlled trials of conventional pharmaceuticals (Nartey et al. 2007). The matched-pair sampling method limits this study. Among herbal medicine trials, more beneficial effects were observed for preparations chemically standardized and used for indications listed in the nonofficial European Scientific Cooperative on Phytotherapy (ESCOP; http://escop.com) monographs.

The quality of a scientific "evidence base" in systematic reviews and meta-analyses is based on pooling of studies (Hung and Ernst 2010). This approach may miss identifying the true value, safety, and efficacy of phytomedicines because it was developed predominantly to assess single-chemical pharmaceuticals. Quality ratings are based not only on methodology (e.g., randomization) but also on size (number of subjects), duration, and other characteristics. The result is that quality ratings are heavily affected by the amount of available funding. It is far more expensive to study a larger group, to add control subjects, and to extend the study beyond a few weeks. Financial incentives are far greater for pharmaceutical research, whereby companies can recover their investment from the sale of patented products, than for herbal studies. One reason for this disparity in financial incentives is that it is difficult to obtain exclusive patents for herbal medicines because most have already been marketed or are in the public domain. These factors severely limit—but do not preclude—opportunities for high-quality herbal studies. In many cases, the absence of a large evidence base for herbal products does not accurately reflect their potential therapeutic value. Lack of knowledge among researchers about how to obtain high-quality extracts and ignorance regarding dosing and use of uncharacterized or poor-quality extracts in some studies can adversely affect meta-analytic outcomes. A review of herb and phytomedicine clinical trials funded by the U.S. National Institutes of Health's National Center for Complementary and Integrative Health (NCCIH) reported that most U.S.-funded trials had negative outcomes (Hopp 2015).

Bias exists in the debate about quality, safety, and efficacy of herbal dietary supplements. Bubela et al. (2008)) reported that mainstream newspapers tend toward negative bias about herbal clinical trials, often favoring news about pharmaceutical medicines. A pilot study noted that the amount of advertising for pharmaceutical drugs in 11 major medical journals was inversely proportional to the amount of coverage on dietary supplements, such as original supplement research and reviews (Kemper and Hood 2008).

Herbal Product Safety and Quality

Consumer demand for and professional use of phytomedicines are supported by clinical trials that suggest or confirm safety and efficacy. Responsible elements of the herb and supplement industry are making substantial efforts to increase compliance with GMPs as well as other means of ensuring the authenticity and purity of raw materials and extracts.

The Problem of Adulterants

One of the greatest challenges in global herbal medicine is the adulteration of botanical raw materials, extracts, and essential oils. *Adulteration* refers to the accidental or, more often, intentional substitution of an undeclared (not noted on a certificate of analysis or product label) lower-cost material or the undeclared dilution of an ingredient with a lower-cost ingredient. Intentional adulteration financially benefits the seller to the financial detriment of the buyer (Foster 2011). In addition, the buyer may experience negative health consequences from adverse reactions to adulterants or lack of expected benefits.

In 2010, to educate the herbal industry, researchers, and health professionals about adulteration problems, the nonprofit American Botanical Council, the American Herbal Pharmacopoeia, and the National Center for Natural Products Research at the University of Mississippi (ABC-AHP-NCNPR) formed the Botanical Adulterants Program, now comprising more than 175 supporters in the United Sates and internationally. The program collects data on adulteration and provides guidance to industry laboratories regarding best analytical methods for detecting adulteration and fraud. Among herbs used in psychiatric practice, adulteration is reported in ashwagandha, ginkgo (Gafner 2015), and St. John's wort in bulletins by the ABC-AHP-NCNPR Botanical Adulterants Program (http://cms.herbalgram.org/BAP/index.html; Gafner 2015).

Analytical Testing and Analytical Testing Methods in the Herbal Supplement Market

Attempts to deal with adulteration by analytical testing (e.g., genetic testing to identify botanical materials) sometimes create confusion. Consumers and many health professionals consider publicized DNA results to be credible a priori. In 2013 a *New York Times* story described an uncontrolled study at the University of Guelph in Canada in which 44 herbal supplements from 12 U.S. and Canadian companies were tested with a DNA barcode method. The results were misinterpreted as showing that many supplements were adulterated (O'Connor 2013). Mainstream media echoed the *New York Times*, decrying the state of the herbal industry. The highly flawed Canadian study was criticized by independent phytomedicinal research experts, who advised that the paper be retracted (Gafner et al. 2013). In February 2015 the *New York Times* published a front-page story about DNA-based testing of herbal supplements by a university laboratory contracted by the New York attorney general (NYAG), which indicated that 79% of seven store-labeled herbal supplements (echinacea, garlic, ginseng, ginkgo, saw palmetto, St. John's wort, and valerian) from four retail chains (GNC, Target, Walgreens, and Walmart) were misreported, containing unlisted plants or lacking herbs listed on the label (O'Connor 2015). Problems with the NYAG investigation included 1) use of only one analytical method, 2) lack of confirmation from a second laboratory, 3) nonapplicability and unreliability of the DNA barcoding method for botanical extracts, and 4) lack of knowledge about botanical identification by the NYAG office. Within weeks, the NYAG settled with retailer GNC, acknowledging that the herbal products were made in accord with state and federal regulations, were not mislabeled, and could be returned to store shelves without changes in labeling (Smith 2015).

Deficiencies in DNA Testing as the Sole Analytical Method for Determining Botanical Authenticity

The consensus of botanical analytical experts is that DNA barcode–based technologies should not be the *sole* basis for identifying botanical materials, especially for legal/regulatory investigation. DNA testing cannot differentiate among plant parts because DNA is in all parts (e.g., fruit, flower, leaf, seed, root). Conventional DNA barcode testing cannot determine the presence of DNA when botanical extraction (e.g., heat and filtration) degrades DNA or filters it out. More current methods (e.g., next-generation DNA testing) can determine the presence of certain DNA segments in extracts (Parveen et al. 2016).

Identifying High-Quality Botanical Supplements

Best-quality botanical supplements can be found in brands whose safety and efficacy have been documented in clinical trials published in peer-reviewed journals. In addition, many companies contract with accredited third-party verification programs, which audit manufacturing facilities for compliance with GMPs. If the product has been approved, the manufacturer can display a seal on the container from the accreditor (e.g., NSF International, formerly known as the National Sanitation Foundation). Updates on products from specific companies are posted on the FDA Web site www.fda.gov/Food/RecallsOutbreaksEmergencies/SafetyAlertsAdvisories/default.htm, as well as on non-peer-reviewed Web sites, such as https://supplementswatch.com and the for-profit www.consumerlab.com. The NCCIH, through its "Alerts and Advisories" (https://nccih.nih.gov/news/alerts), posts information about problems with supplements. The National Institutes of Health National Library of Medicine, through its Dietary Supplement Label Database (https://dsld.nlm.nih.gov/dsld/), provides information about more than 2,000 supplements. The Council for Responsible Nutrition and UL (Underwriters Laboratories) have initiated development of a dietary supplement registry (Supplement OWL [Online Wellness Laboratory]) wherein all information on product labels (plus additional data) will be made available to the public online. The German Commission E, which evaluated safety and efficacy of phytomedicines in German pharmacies, published authoritative, government-sponsored monographs (http://cms.herbalgram.org/commissione/index.html), but these are mostly generic rather than product specific (Blumenthal et al. 1998). The American Herbal Pharmacopoeia, which distributes authenticated botanical reference materials to industry laboratories to ensure accurate identity, publishes peer-reviewed quality control and therapeutic monographs and books on herbs and therapeutic applications (www.herbal-ahp.org/order_online.htm).

Issues of Efficacy and Phytoequivalence of Herbal Products

Conventional pharmaceuticals are usually single artificial chemicals to which the human body has never before been exposed (except for those derived from plants). In contrast, herbs and phytomedicines are chemically complex mixtures of naturally occurring plant compounds. Some have a history of traditional use, going back hundreds, or even thousands, of years. There has been a long-standing debate about the level of evidence required to assess the safety and efficacy of a traditionally used herb or phytomedicinal preparation. More conservative, critical practitioners adhere to randomized controlled clinical trials to determine efficacy. A science-based approach, called *rational phytotherapy*, includes herbs used in clinical practice and/or self-medication *only* if they have a basis in published pharmacological and/or clinical trials (Schulz et al. 2004). Alternatively, other practitioners adhere to the doctrine of *reasonable certainty*, described by the late Varro E. Tyler, professor of pharmacognosy at Purdue University and dean of the School of Pharmacy and Pharmaceutical Sciences, and used by the German Commission E to include *all* levels of evidence (Blumenthal et al. 1998). These levels of evidence include clinical trials on specific phytomedicinal products; phytomedicinal products containing clinically tested ingredients; phytomedicinal products containing ingredients that are phytoequivalent to clinically tested ingredients; phytomedicinal products containing ingredients that conform to an official compendium, such as a national or regional pharmacopoeia (e.g., European Pharmacopoeia); products and/or ingredients that have been subjected to in vivo pharmacological research studies to determine bioactivity in test animals; historical use in a system of traditional medicine (e.g., Ayurveda); and historical, folkloric use.

Phytoequivalence, the physiological equivalence of two herbal products or the applicability of data on safety of one herbal product to another, is more complex than comparisons between generic and brand pharmaceuticals. For herbs whose research data are based primarily on a single proprietary formula (e.g., ginkgo EGb 761®), generic extracts may not produce the same outcomes.

KEY POINTS

- In the United States, herbal supplements are regulated by the U.S. Food and Drug Administration and the Federal Trade Commission.

- The *quantity* of research and the *subject size* of studies on phytomedicinals are less than for conventional pharmaceuticals, primarily because of large disparities in funding.

- Governmental and professional organizations monitor and provide generally up-to-date information on botanical supplements.

References

Blumenthal M, Busse Werner R, Goldberg A, et al (eds): The Complete German Commission E Monographs: Therapeutic Guide to Herbal Medicines. Translated by Klein S, Rister RS. Austin, TX, American Botanical Council/Boston, MA, Integrative Medicine Communications, 1998

Bubela T, Boon H, Caulfield T: Herbal remedy clinical trials in the media: a comparison with the coverage of conventional pharmaceuticals. BMC Med 6:35–49, 2008 19036123

Foster S: A brief history of adulteration of herbs, spices, and botanical drugs. HerbalGram 92:42–57, 2011

Gafner S: Ginkgo extract adulteration in the global market: a brief review. HerbalGram 109:58–59, 2015

Gafner S, Blumenthal M, Reynaud DH, et al: ABC review and critique of the research article "DNA Barcoding Detects Contamination and Substitution in North American Herbal Products" by Newmaster et al. HerbalGram 10(11), 2013. Available at: http://cms.herbalgram.org/heg/volume10/11November/DNAbarcodingReviewandCritique.html?t=1383684796. Accessed June 30, 2016.

Hopp C: Past and future research at National Center for Complementary and Integrative Health with respect to botanicals. HerbalGram 107:44–51, 2015

Hung S-K, Ernst E: Herbal medicine: an overview of the literature from three decades. J Diet Suppl 7(3):217–226, 2010 22432513

Kemper KJ, Hood KL: Does pharmaceutical advertising affect journal publication about dietary supplements? BMC Complement Altern Med 8:11–19, 2008 18400092

Nartey L, Huwiler-Müntener K, Shang A, et al: Matched-pair study showed higher quality of placebo-controlled trials in Western phytotherapy than conventional medicine. J Clin Epidemiol 60(8):787–794, 2007 17606174

O'Connor A: Herbal supplements are often not what they seem. New York Times (online), November 3, 2013. Available at: www.nytimes.com/2013/11/05/science/herbal-supplements-are-often-not-what-they-seem.html. Accessed November 2014.

O'Connor A: New York attorney general targets supplements at major retailers. New York Times (online), February 3, 2015. Available at: http://well.blogs.nytimes.com/2015/02/03/new-york-attorney-general-targets-supplements-at-major-retailers/. Accessed May 12, 2015.

Parveen I, Gafner S, Techen N, et al: DNA barcoding for the identification of botanicals in herbal medicine and dietary supplements: strengths and limitations. Planta Med 82(14):1225–1235, 2016 27392246

Schulz V, Hansel R, Tyler VE, et al: Rational Phytotherapy: A Reference Guide for Physicians and Pharmacists, 5th Edition. Berlin, Springer, 2004

Smith T: The supplement saga: a review of the New York attorney general's herbal supplement investigation. HerbalGram 106:44–55, 2015

Smith T, Lynch ME, Johnson J: Herbal dietary supplement sales in US increase 6.8% in 2014. HerbalGram 107:52–59, 2015

Soller RW, Bayne HJ, Shaheen C: The regulated dietary supplement industry: myths of an unregulated industry dispelled. HerbalGram 93:42–57, 2012

CHAPTER 8

Adaptogens in Psychiatric Practice

Rhodiola rosea, Schisandra chinensis, Eleutherococcus senticosus, and *Withania somnifera*

Alexander Panossian, Ph.D., D.Sci.

Jay D. Amsterdam, M.D.

Health is the ability to adapt to one's environment.

Georges Canguilhem, Le Normal et le pathologique, *1943*

In this chapter, we review molecular mechanisms and clinical studies of four botanical adaptogens: golden root (*Rhodiola rosea* [L.], radix and rhizome), Siberian ginseng (*Eleutherococcus senticosus*), schisandra (*Schisandra chinensis* [Turcz.] Baill., fructus), and ashwagandha (*Withania somnifera* [L.] Dunal, radix). These herbs are of particular interest because they have an adequate evidence base of safety and efficacy for treating disorders commonly encountered in psychiatric practice. Used for thousands of years in traditional folk medicines, they are included as conventional therapies in several national pharmacopoeias in Asia and Europe for treatment of neuropsychiatric disorders.

Botanical adaptogens are plant extracts and constituents that increase the ability of an organism to tolerate, adapt, survive, and perform under a wide range of stressors. The term *adaptogen* was introduced in 1959 to describe substances that increase the "state of non-specific resistance" of an organism under stress, "normalize" physiological states, and mitigate the effects of environmental or emotional stress (Brekhman and Dardymov 1969). Recent definitions of adaptogen may include mechanisms of action such as upregulating expression of neuropeptide Y (NPY) and heat shock protein 70 (Hsp70; Asea et al. 2013; Panossian and Wikman 2010; Panossian et al. 1999).

Molecular Mechanisms

Adaptive stress response involves activation of intracellular and extracellular signaling pathways and increased expression of antiapoptotic proteins, neuropeptides, and antioxidant enzymes. Accordingly, botanical adaptogens have been proposed to act as mild stress "vaccines," inducing stress-protective responses. Although acute administration of an adaptogen may produce a stimulatory effect, the stress-protective effects of chronic adaptogen administration are more likely the result of adaptive changes in response to repeated stress-mimetic or booster vaccine–like effects. These may be mediated through the hypothalamic-pituitary-adrenal (HPA) axis and nitric oxide (Panossian and Wagner 2005).

Russian medical manuals recognize adaptogens as a group of synthetic and natural medications with stimulant and/or psychotropic properties, which are prescribed for psychiatric disorders such as asthenia (mental or physical fatigue), neurosis, depression, and alcoholism and as an adjuvant with conventional psychotropics (Mashkovskiy 2000; Panossian and Wikman 2008; Panossian et al. 2010). Compared with prescription stimulants such as amphetamines, adaptogens are lower in side effects, provide a better quality of arousal, have no addiction potential, cause no withdrawal syndrome, do not deplete energy, enhance performance and survival under stress, improve recovery after exhausting physical workload, and cause no loss of appetite (Panossian 2003).

Adaptogens may exert *polyvalent* (more than one direction of change) biological activity and multi-target effects on transcriptional, proteomic, and metabolomic regulation, potentially affecting signaling pathways and molecular networks with a beneficial effect on stress-induced limbic-hypothalamic–mediated responses (Panossian et al. 2012, 2013, 2014). The following molecular mechanisms have been proposed to contribute to adaptogen effects on neuroendocrine regulation of the HPA axis through mediators of stress response (see Panossian 2013 for review of molecular mechanisms): molecular chaperones Hsp70 and NPY, membrane-bound G-protein-coupled receptors (GPCRs) and G-protein-signaling pathways, regulation of cyclic adenosine monophosphate (cAMP) and protein kinase A (PKA), and G-protein-signaling phosphatidylinositol and phospholipase C pathways.

Molecular Chaperones

HEAT SHOCK PROTEIN 70

Hsp70 proteins protect cells from stress-induced damage by temporarily binding to partially denatured proteins, preventing aggregation and allowing repair of the proteins. In addition, Hsp70 participates in disposal of damaged or defective proteins and inhibits programmed cell death. In mice, ADAPT-232 (combination of *R. rosea*, *E. senticosus*, and *S. chinensis*) significantly increased stress tolerance, accompanied by a dramatic increase in serum levels of circulating Hsp70. ADAPT-232 and one active constituent, salidroside, both stimulated expression and release of Hsp70 from isolated human neuroglial cells (Panossian et al. 2012).

NEUROPEPTIDE Y

Salidroside and ADAPT-232 stimulate expression and release of NPY from isolated human brain glioblastoma T98G cells (Panossian et al. 2012). NPY is a stress-responsive hormone present throughout the central and peripheral nervous systems. NPY stimulates the HPA axis and modulates secretion of hypothalamic neuropeptides. Stressors such as strenuous exercise, cold exposure, panic disorder, and chronic fatigue syndrome (CFS) produce sympathoadrenal activation and NPY release from sympathetic nerve endings. The elevation of serum NPY in CFS patients correlates with the severity of stress, negative mood, and clinical symptoms. In healthy subjects, psychological stress elevates plasma NPY. In the periphery, sympathetic nerve–derived and platelet-derived NPY are stimulatory, potentiate stress response synergistically with glucocorticoids and catecholamines, and induce vasoconstriction. In the central nervous system, NPY paradoxically serves as an anxiolytic and inhibits sympathetic activity and cortisol production (Hirsch and Zukowska 2012). NPY can regulate immune response, that is, inhibit nitric oxide synthesis, which prevents interleukin (IL-1β) release. NPY promotes adenosine triphosphate (ATP) formation by decreasing expression of mitochondrial uncoupling protein.

Preclinical and clinical evidence suggests mood and cognitive enhancement by NPY. Elevated NPY concentration was found in soldiers who had reduced psychological distress or who belonged to elite Special Forces. In contrast, decreased NPY levels were documented in depressed patients and in brain tissues of persons who committed suicide (Panossian 2013). The release of stress hormones, NPY, and Hsp70 into the blood can be considered an innate defense response to mild stressors, such as adaptogens, which increases tolerance and adaptation to stress.

Membrane-Bound G-Protein-Coupled Receptors and G-Protein-Signaling Pathways

Genes that encode cell membrane–bound GPCRs include serotonin type 3 receptor (5-HT$_3$) and key proteins of G-protein intracellular signaling downstream pathways: cAMP and phospholipase C/phosphatidylinositol (Panossian et al. 2013). GPCRs are involved in many physiological processes related to stress tolerance:

- Binding of neurotransmitters, including serotonin, dopamine, γ-aminobutyric acid (GABA), and glutamate, that are involved in regulation of mood, behavior, and cognitive functions
- Regulation of sympathetic and parasympathetic nervous systems
- Regulation of immune system activity and inflammation
- Maintaining homeostasis in response to stressors

Many neuropsychiatric drugs either bind directly to specific GPCRs (e.g., antipsychotics) or act indirectly via GPCRs, affecting the amount of available agonist (e.g., antidepressants). Adaptogens downregulate the gene *HTR1A* encoding the 5-HT$_3$ GPCR that activates an intracellular second-messenger cascade to produce excitatory or inhibitory neurotransmission. Serotonin receptors modulate release of glutamate, GABA, dopamine, epinephrine, norepinephrine, and acetylcholine, as well as hormones, including oxytocin, prolactin, vasopressin, cortisol, corticotropin, and substance P. Serotonin receptors influence aggression, anxiety, appetite, cognition, learning, memory, mood, nausea, sleep, and thermoregulation. Downregulation of *HTR1A* by salidroside and tyrosol (active constituents of *R. rosea*) is consistent with involvement of serotonin receptors in preclinical and clinical effects of *R. rosea*, including the antidepressant effects (Panossian et al. 2014).

Regulation of Cyclic Adenosine Monophosphate and the Activity of Protein Kinase A

In brain cells, adaptogens regulate the dopamine-cAMP-PKA–ceramide transfer protein (CERT) signaling pathway (Panossian et al. 2013; Rao et al. 2007). Adaptogens downregulate expression of adenylate cyclase, which activates generation of cAMP from ATP and upregulates expression of phosphodiesterases, which activates degradation of cAMP (Panossian et al. 2013). Predicted downstream effect of *Rhodiola* and salidroside is an inhibition of PKA- and mitogen-activated protein kinase kinase (MEK)–mediated pathways followed by inhibition of cAMP response element-binding protein, a transcription factor involved in both the mechanism of action of antidepressants and the disease itself. Regulation of cAMP and PKA is a key mechanism of energy homeostasis and metabolism—the shifting between catabolic and anabolic states. Downregulation of cAMP and PKA by adaptogens decreases stress-induced catabolic transformations and is associated with stress-protective effects. Inhibition of adenylate cyclase by adaptogens can increase intracellular ATP (Abidov et al. 2003) when less of it is converted to cAMP. This contributes to the ability of adaptogens to maintain energy supplies during stress over long periods of time.

Prefrontal cortex cells contain hyperpolarization-activated channels that can open when exposed to cAMP during stress. Excess opening of these channels has been associated with impairment of higher cognitive function. It has been suggested that cAMP inhibitors may close the channels, enabling neurotransmission of information connecting neural networks, thus improving working memory, which plays a key role in such tasks as abstract thinking, planning, and organizing. This mechanism could contribute to treatment of age-related cognitive decline and cognitive dysfunctions in schizophrenia, bipolar disorder, and attention-deficit/hyperactivity disorder. It may contribute to cognitive-enhancing effects of ADAPT-232 and *R. rosea* in humans (Panossian et al. 2013, 2014).

G-Protein-Signaling Phosphatidylinositol and Phospholipase C Pathways

Adaptogens upregulate the gene *PLCB1* encoding phosphoinositide-specific phospholipase C and phosphatidylinositol 3-kinases (Panossian et al. 2013). G proteins catalyze the hydrolysis of phosphatidylinositol 4,5-bisphosphate into diacylglycerol and inositol-1,4,5-triphosphate, which is involved in cellular signaling pathways associated with depression. Phosphatidylinositol 4,5-bisphosphate is required for the long-term potentiation (long-lasting enhancement in neuronal signal transmission), which is critical for memory and learning.

Safety and Effectiveness of Adaptogens in Psychiatric Disorders

Studies of adaptogens for treatment of psychological conditions have been published since the 1940s. The methodology of most of the older studies does not meet current criteria, and diagnostic categories differ from those in use today. Nevertheless, such studies provide useful information regarding potential benefits that would be worth current investigation. Level I and II evidence (defined in Table 8–2 footnote) supports the use of *R. rosea* for fatigue, life stress, and depression; *S. chinensis* for depression; *E. senticosus* for bipolar disorder; and *W. somnifera* for bipolar disorder, anxiety, and schizophrenia (Tables 8–1 and 8–2). For insomnia, *S. chinensis* and *W. somnifera* have shown benefits. In addition, *R. rosea*, *S. chinensis*, and *E. senticosus* have been found to improve cognitive function. Tables 8–1 and 8–2 summarize research in mental disorders and potential applications; details on active constituents can be found in Figure 8–1. For a summary of clinical trials of *E. senticosus*, *R. rosea*, *S. chinensis*, and *W. somnifera* in mental disorders in tabulated form, see Panossian and Wikman (2010; available at www.mdpi.com/1424-8247/3/1/188/pdf). Table 8–3 summarizes clinical trials of *W. somnifera* in anxiety and bipolar disorders.

TABLE 8–1. *Rhodiola rosea, Eleutherococcus senticosus, Schisandra chinensis,* and *Withania somnifera*: types of evidence and applications

Herbal medicine	Type of evidence					Potential applications
	Dep	**Anx**	**Ins**	**Sch**	**Ast**	
Roseroot (*R. rosea*)	1, 2, 3	1, 2, 3	–	–	1, 2, 3	Stress-induced fatigue, cognitive impairment, depression, anxiety
Schisandra (*S. chinensis*)	1	2	2	1	1, 2, 3	Fatigue, cognitive impairment, nervous exhaustion, schizophrenia
Siberian ginseng (*E. senticosus*)	1, 2	2	–	–	1, 2, 3	Chronic fatigue, cognitive impairment, bipolar disorder
Withania (*W. somnifera*)	1, 2, 3	1, 2, 3	2, 3	1, 2	1, 2, 3	Anxiety, insomnia, bipolar disorder

Note. Anx=anxiety; Ast=asthenia, fatigue; Dep=depression; Ins=insomnia; Sch=schizophrenia. 1=human clinical data; 2=experimental preclinical evidence of activity; 3=traditional systems of medicine and pharmacopoeias endorse use.

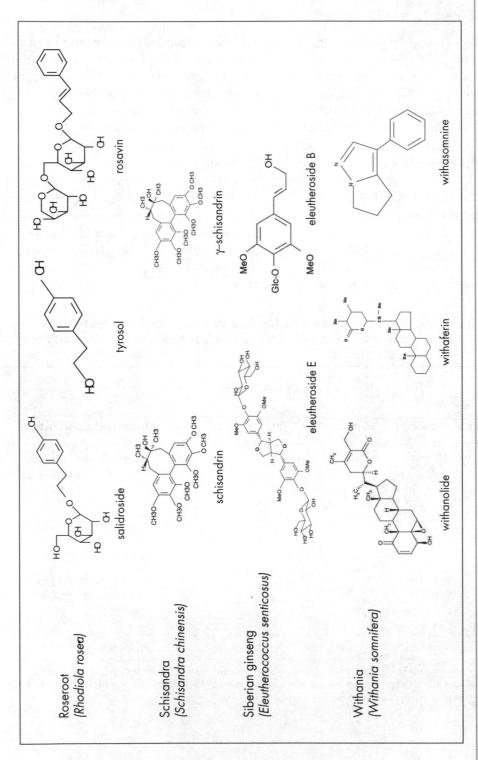

FIGURE 8–1. Major active constituents of *R. rosea, S. chinensis, E. senticosus,* and *W. somnifera.*

TABLE 8–2. Clinical trials of *Eleutherococcus senticosus*, *Rhodiola rosea*, *Schisandra chinensis*, and *Withania somnifera* in psychiatric disorders

Condition	Adaptogen	Design	Duration, weeks	Jadad score[b]	Number of subjects	Level of evidence[e]	Reference[f]
Chronic fatigue syndrome	*E. senticosus*	DBRPCT	4, 8, 16	5	96	Ib	Hartz (2004)
Fatigue syndrome (stress induced)	*R. rosea*	DBRPCT	4	5	60	Ib	Olsson et al. (2009)
Life-stress symptoms	*R. rosea*	OL	4	1	101	IIa	Edwards et al. (2012)
Diagnosis	*R. rosea*	OL	6, 12	0	120	III	Fintelmann and Gruenwald (2007)
Depression	*R. rosea*	DBRPCT	12	5	57	Ib	Mao et al. (2014, 2015)
	R. rosea	DBRPCT	6	5	91	Ib	Darbinyan et al. (2007)
	R. rosea	OL, C[a]		0	78/56[a]	IIa	Brichenko (1986)[a]
	S. chinensis	OL, UC		0	37		Staritsina (1946)
Astheno-depressive syndrome (stress-induced depression)	*R. rosea*	OL, UC	2–3	0	128		Krasik et al. (1970)d
	R. rosea	OL, UC	2–3	0	135/27		Krasik et al. (1970)d
	R. rosea	OL	8	0	58		Mikhailova (1983)
	S. chinensis	OL, UC		0	13		Zakharov (1956)
	S. chinensis	OL, UC		0	40		Leman (1952)
	S. chinensis	OL	2–6		36		Galant (1958)
	S. chinensis	OL	1.5		30		Zakharova (1948)

TABLE 8–2. Clinical trials of *Eleutherococcus senticosus*, *Rhodiola rosea*, *Schisandra chinensis*, and *Withania somnifera* in psychiatric disorders *(continued)*

Condition	Adaptogen	Design	Duration, weeks	Jadad score[b]	Number of subjects	Level of evidence[e]	Reference[f]
Neurosis (stress-induced depression)	*R. rosea*	OL	1.5	0	65		Saratikov 1965[d]
	R. rosea	SBPC		1	70/80[c]		Kaliko (1966)
	S. chinensis	OL	2–8	0	386[d]		Sudakov (1986)
	S. chinensis	OL	2–10	0	250		Rossijskij (1952)
	E. senticosus	OL, PC	3–4	2	80		Strokina (1966, 1967)
Bipolar disorder/manic depression	*W. somnifera*	DBRPCT	8	4	60	Ib	Chengappa et al. (2013)
	W. somnifera	DBRPCT	8	3	60		Gannon et al. (2014)
	E. senticosus		6	5	76	Ib	Weng et al. (2007)
Anxiety	*R. rosea*	OL	10	0	10	III	Bystritsky (2008)
	W. somnifera	DBRPCT	8.5	2	64	Ib	Chandrasekhar et al. (2012)
	W. somnifera	R, C, PC	6	1	40/41		Cooley et al. (2009)
	W. somnifera	DBRPCT	6	2	39		Andrade et al. (2000)
	W. somnifera	DBRPCT	8.5	3	30/35/35/30		Auddy et al. (2008)

TABLE 8–2. Clinical trials of *Eleutherococcus senticosus*, *Rhodiola rosea*, *Schisandra chinensis*, and *Withania somnifera* in psychiatric disorders *(continued)*

Condition	Adaptogen	Design	Duration, weeks	Jadad score[b]	Number of subjects	Level of evidence[e]	Reference[f]
Schizophrenia	*S. chinensis*	OL	?	0	79/41[d]	III	Romas (1958, 1962)
	S. chinensis	OL, C	?	0	30/20[d]		Zakharova (1948)[d]
	S. chinensis	OL	?	0	48		Lastovetskiy (1963)
	W. somnifera	DBRPCT	4.5	2	30	IIa	Agnihotri et al. (2013)

Note. C=controlled; CO=crossover; DBRPCT=double-blind, randomized placebo-controlled trial; OL=open-label; PC=placebo-controlled; R=randomized; SB=single-blind; UC=uncontrolled.

[a]The control group was treated with tricyclic antidepressants; the study group was treated with tricyclic antidepressants and *R. rosea* as adjuvant therapy.

[b]Jadad AR, Moore RA, Carroll D, et al: "Assessing the quality of reports of randomized clinical trials: is blinding necessary?" *Controlled Clinical Trials* 17:1–12, 1996.

[c]Neurotic, stress-related, and somatoform disorders (ICD-10-CM F40–F48).

[d]Mixed patient population, sick/healthy subjects.

[e]According to the World Health Organization, U.S. Food and Drug Administration, and European Medicines Evaluation Agency. Ia=meta-analyses of randomized and controlled studies; Ib=evidence from at least one randomized study with control group; IIa=evidence from at least one well-performed study with control group; IIb=evidence from at least one well-performed quasi-experimental study; III=evidence from well-performed nonexperimental descriptive studies as well as comparative studies, correlation studies, and case studies; IV=evidence from expert committee reports or appraisals and/or clinical experiences by prominent authorities.

[f]For references not listed in the reference list, see Panossian and Wikman (2010).

Grade of recommendation based on the European Medicines Agency Assessment Scale (European Medicines Agency. Committee on Medicinal Products EMEA/HMPC/104613/2005. Available at: http://www.ema.europa.eu/ema/index.jsp?curl=pages/regulation/general/general_content_000830.jsp&mid=WC0b01ac058003a9b. Accessed February 2, 2017):

- *Grade A: Evidence levels quality Ia, Ib*—Requires at least one randomized controlled trial as part of the body of literature of overall good consistency addressing the specific recommendation
- *Grade B: Evidence levels IIa, IIb, III*—Requires availability of well-conducted clinical studies but no randomized clinical trials on the topic of recommendation
- *Grade C: Evidence level IV*—Requires evidence from expert committee reports or opinions and/or clinical experience of respected authorities but indicates absence of directly applicable studies of good quality

Source. Updated and adapted from Panossian and Wikman 2010; www.mdpi.com/1424-8247/3/1/188/.pdf.

TABLE 8–3. Summary of clinical trials: *Withania somnifera* in anxiety and bipolar disorders

Author, year	Sample size	Design	Duration, weeks	Daily dose, extraction solvent, marker, trade name	Diagnosis	Primary outcomes	Adverse events (*n*)	Jadad score[b]
Gannon et al. (2014)[a]	30+30	DBRPCT	8	500 mg NS, NS, NS, Sensoril	Bipolar disorder	Serum thyroxine	NS	2
Chengappa et al. (2013)[a]	24+29	DBRPCT	8	500 mg, 250-mg capsules water, 8% withanolides, 2% withaferin Sensoril	DSM-IV bipolar disorder, YMRS, MADRS, and HARS scores	Cognitive tasks: auditory digit span, flanker test, Penn Emotional Acuity Test; social cognition test: Penn Emotional Acuity Test	26 placebo 19 *verum*	4
Chandrasekhar et al. (2012)	32+32	DBRPCT	8.5	300-mg capsules NS, 5% withanolides, KSM-66	Stress; score: <5 (WHO-5), <14 (PSS)	Serum cortisol, PSS, DASS, GHQ-28 questionnaires	6 placebo 5 *verum*	2
Cooley et al. (2009)	40+41	R, C, PC	12	300-mg pills NS, 1.5% withanolides, ISRCTN78995974	Anxiety	BAI, SF-36, FSI, MY-MOP	7+7	1
Andrade et al. (2000)	20+19	DBRPCT	6	500 mg, 250-mg tablets ethanol, NS	Generalized anxiety, mixed anxiety, depression	Hamilton anxiety score, global rating scale, SAFTEE symptom checklist	17 placebo 16 *verum*	3

TABLE 8-3. Summary of clinical trials: *Withania somnifera* in anxiety and bipolar disorders *(continued)*

Author, year	Sample size	Design	Duration, weeks	Daily dose, extraction solvent, marker, trade name	Diagnosis	Primary outcomes	Adverse events (*n*)	Jadad score[b]
Auddy et al. (2008)	30+35+ 35+30	DBRPCT	8.5	125-mg and 250-mg capsules NS, 11.9% withanolides, 1% withaferin A, Sensoril	Anxiety	Modified HARS, serum cortisol, serum C-reactive protein, pulse rate and blood pressure	0	3
Singy and Malviya (1978)	30	OL	4	40 mL fermented water extract corresponding to 12 g dry roots	Anxiety, neurosis	Anxiety: nervousness, palpitation, tremors, headache, anorexia, insomnia, lack of concentration, dyspepsia, fatigue, irritability	NS	0

[a]Two publications are related to the same study: NCT00761761.

[b]Jadad AR, Moore RA, Carroll D, et al.: "Assessing the Quality of Reports of Randomized Clinical Trials: Is Blinding Necessary?" *Controlled Clinical Trials* 17:1–12, 1996.

Note. BAI=Beck Anxiety Inventory; C=positive control, psychotherapy intervention; DASS=Depression Anxiety Stress Scales; DBRPCT=double-blind, randomized placebo-controlled trial; FSI=Fatigue Symptom Inventory; GHQ-28=28-Item General Health Questionnaire; HARS=Hamilton Anxiety Rating Scale; MADRS=Montgomery-Åsberg Depression Rating Scale; MY-MOP=Measure Yourself Medical Outcomes Profile; NS=not specified; OL=open-label; PC=placebo-controlled; PSS=Perceived Stress Scale; R=randomized; SAFTEE=Systematic Assessment for Treatment Emergent Events technique scale; SF=Short Form 36; WHO-5=WHO (Five) Well-Being Index; YMRS=Young Mania Rating Scale.

Rhodiola rosea

Rhodiola rosea is an ancient medicinal herb that grows at high altitudes in Europe and Asia. The roots and rhizomes are used to make tea, alcohol extracts, and water extracts, which are used to either promote physical fortitude or reduce mental strain during conditions of stress, including physical exertion, military training and warfare, cold stress, low oxygen, bacterial and viral infections, wound healing, mental performance, cognitive demands, cancer, athletic competition, and space travel (Cuerrier and Ampong-Nyarko 2014).

Effects of *Rhodiola rosea* on Asthenia, Fatigue, and Exhaustion

In 1969, the Pharmacological Committee of the Ministry of Health of the former Soviet Union recommended *R. rosea* extract for the treatment of neuropsychiatric disorders including "asthenic syndrome," "neurosis," "vascular dystonia," hypotension, and "schizophrenia asthenic type" (Rhizome and roots of Rhodiola rosea 1999). Asthenic syndrome, characterized by general weakness, reduced work capacity, poor concentration and memory, irritability, headache, insomnia, and anorexia, usually occurs after prolonged intensive work requiring high levels of mental exertion. *R. rosea* extract was found to improve performance and shorten recovery time in essentially healthy individuals when given during heavy physical or mental work (Krasik et al. 1970). It also protected individuals prone to asthenia from the adverse effects of intensive workloads. Other uncontrolled, open-label studies suggested that *R. rosea* extract also may be effective in reducing psychogenic and somatogenic exhaustion caused by CFS and infectious diseases. For example, individuals suffering from post-influenza fatigue showed improved mental and physical work capacity and concentration ability and a reduction in headaches after 3 days of *R. rosea* extract therapy (Krasik et al. 1970; Saratikov and Krasnov 2004).

Effects of *Rhodiola rosea* on Cognitive Function

In an early observational study, *R. rosea* extract in combination with piracetam, a synthetic *nootropic* (brain function enhancer), improved cognitive function, memory, and affect in individuals with organic amnestic disorders, such as Korsakoff syndrome, dementias, intellectual disability, and acquired organic mental syndromes (Sudakov et al. 1986). Limited studies in subjects with cognitive impairment showed improvement in cognitive deficits: forgetfulness, memory loss, and impaired concentration. Randomized controlled trials (RCTs) in healthy adults found that *R. rosea* standardized extract alone and in combination with *E. senticosus* and *S. chinensis* (ADAPT formula) improved intellectual performance on complex tasks, short-term memory, concentration, learning, and performance under stress (Aslanyan et al. 2010).

Studies of *Rhodiola rosea* for Treatment of Anxiety and Depression

In an open-label study (Bystritsky et al. 2008), *R. rosea* (Rhodax) 340 mg given daily for 10 weeks to 10 subjects with DSM-IV (American Psychiatric Association 1994) generalized anxiety disorder (Table 8–2) significantly reduced the mean Hamilton Anxiety Rating Scale score ($P=0.01$) and Hamilton Rating Scale for Depression (Ham-D) score ($P=0.001$) at endpoint.

An observational study reported that *R. rosea* used as an adjunctive treatment for depression may have enhanced antidepressant efficacy and may reduce side effects of tricyclic antidepressants in depressed patients. More recently, Darbinyan et al. (2007) conducted a randomized double-blind, placebo-controlled trial of *R. rosea* extract (SHR-5; Swedish Herbal Institute, Vallberga, Halland, Sweden) in 89 subjects ages 18–70 years with mild to moderate DSM-IV-classified major depressive disorder. Subjects received either *R. rosea* extract 340 mg daily ($n=31$), *R. rosea* extract 680 mg daily ($n=29$), or placebo ($n=29$) for 6 weeks. At endpoint, mean Ham-D score significantly declined for both doses of *R. rosea* ($P<0.0001$) versus no significant reduction in Ham-D score for placebo ($P=0.2206$). Intergroup analysis found lower mean Ham-D scores for both *R. rosea* treatment conditions versus placebo ($P<0.001$, $P<0.001$, respectively) (Panossian and Wikman 2014). However, such dramatic drug-placebo differences in an underpowered pilot study are questionable. These promising results need to be replicated in larger RCTs.

Subsequently, Mao et al. (2015) performed a 12-week RCT of *R. rosea* extract versus sertraline or placebo in 57 adults with mild to moderate major depressive disorder (DSM-IV), baseline Ham-D score≥10. Identically appearing capsules containing either pharmaceutical-grade *R. rosea* (SHR-5) powdered extract 340 mg (rosavins 3.07%, rhodioloside [salidroside] 1.95%) (Swedish Herbal Institute, Vallberga, Halland, Sweden), sertraline 50 mg HCl (North Star Pharmaceuticals, Memphis, Tennessee), or placebo (lactose monohydrate NF; Spectrum Quality Products, New Brunswick, New Jersey) were dispensed under the aegis of the U.S. Food and Drug Administration (investigational new drug 105,063). Starting with one capsule daily for 2 weeks, subjects with ≤50% reduction in Ham-D score (versus baseline) had the dose increased to two capsules daily during weeks 3 and 4 of therapy. This continued every 2 weeks up to a maximum of four capsules daily during weeks 6–12. Subjects unable to tolerate increased drug doses had their dosage reduced to a minimum of one capsule daily. Measurements were obtained at baseline and after 2, 4, 6, 8, and 12 weeks. The study was powered to detect relatively large differences between treatment conditions and to identify trends in the data that might inform future study design. There was no statistically significant difference in change over time on Ham-D among treatment groups ($P=0.79$), and the decline in Ham-D scores by week 12 was slightly greater for sertraline (−8.2; 95% confidence interval [CI] −12.7 to −3.6) versus *R. rosea* (−5.1; 95% CI −8.8 to −1.3) and placebo (−4.6; 95% CI −8.0 to −0.6). Nevertheless, there were clinically meaningful odds ratios (95% CI) of global improvement by week 12 (versus placebo) of 1.39 (0.38–5.04) for *R. rosea* and 1.90 (0.44–8.20) for sertraline, indicating that subjects taking *R. rosea* had 1.4 times the odds of improvement, and subjects taking sertraline had 1.9 times the odds of improvement versus placebo. More subjects who were taking sertraline (63.2%) versus *R. rosea* (30.0%) or placebo (16.7%) reported adverse events ($P=0.012$). Two subjects prematurely discontinued sertraline; none discontinued *R. rosea* or placebo.

Overall, these studies suggest a possible antidepressant action for *R. rosea* in adults.

Safety and Drug Interactions

In comparison with most conventional antidepressants, *R. rosea* is well tolerated in short-term studies and shows a favorable safety profile (Amsterdam and Panossian 2016). In 31 patients with schizophrenia, high doses of *R. rosea* extract (25–40 drops twice daily) for 4–6 weeks reduced neuroleptic-induced extrapyramidal side effects. A similar reduction in extrapyramidal symptoms was also observed in 9 patients with schizophrenia in whom an anticholinergic drug was ineffective (Krasik et al. 1970).

R. rosea ethanolic extract inhibits cytochrome P450 (CYP) 3A4 in isolated Caco-2 cells in vitro (Hellum et al. 2010), suggesting that it may suppress metabolic transformation of warfarin or other drugs in the liver, increasing serum concentration of such drugs. However, these effects on the activity of isolated enzymes do not appear to have clinical significance because concomitant treatment of rats with warfarin or theophylline and SHR-5 brand of *R. rosea* did not give rise to significant effects on the pharmacokinetics of warfarin or theophylline. Simultaneous administration of SHR-5 and warfarin did not alter significantly the pharmacokinetics or the anticoagulant activity of warfarin. It was concluded that interaction of *Rhodiola* with coadministered drugs is likely to be negligible (Panossian et al. 2009).

Schisandra chinensis

Schisandra chinensis, known in traditional Chinese medicine as bei wu wei zi or gomischi, is a woody vine that grows naturally in northern China, eastern Russia, Korea, and Japan. Its berries and seeds have been used for millennia to increase strength, energy, and stress resilience. Extracts of *S. chinensis* show antidepressant and anti-stress properties (for a review, see Panossian and Wikman 2008).

Effects of *Schisandra chinensis* on Asthenia

An open case study of more than 250 individuals found that taking *S. chinensis* extract for 2–10 weeks reduced symptoms of "asthenia," "exhaustion," and poor physical and mental work performance. A nonrandomized open-label comparative study of 95 subjects with "neurasthenia" syndrome reported that virtually all subjects receiving *S. chinensis* seed tincture had a substantial reduction in generalized weakness, insomnia, anorexia, irritability, and headaches versus 55% of the control group not receiving *S. chinensis*. These open-label, uncontrolled studies are subject to bias and require validation by RCTs (Panossian and Wikman 2005, 2008, 2010).

Effects of *Schisandra chinensis* on Depression and Other Neuropsychiatric Disorders

Studies using older diagnostic categories and methodologies have reported a beneficial effect of *S. chinensis* extract on "asthenic" and depressive states. For example, Leman (1952) observed that *S. chinensis* administration for up to 40 days in 40 individuals with asthenic and "psychogenic" or "somatic" depression led to improvement in mood, energy, activity, insomnia, and anorexia. *S. chinensis* was well tolerated, with a stimulatory effect less troubling than either caffeine or amphetamine. Another uncontrolled, open-label study (Galant 1957) reported better recovery from psychosis following *S. chinensis* treatment in 19 patients with schizophrenia, 6 patients with "reactive psychosis," 4 patients with "alcoholic psychosis," and 3 patients with psychotic depression. A subsequent uncontrolled, open-label study of *S. chinensis* in 41 subjects with schizophrenia and 197 subjects with chronic alcoholism (Romas 1967) showed that *S. chinensis* tincture (5–25 drops per day) helped patients become calm, sociable, active, undepressed, free of anxiety, and willing to work. These early open studies suggest a possible role for *S. chinensis* in the treatment of psychosis. Considering the adverse effects of chronic medications used to treat psychoses, these preliminary observations warrant future controlled study. Adjunctive administration of *S. chinensis* with conventional neuroleptic or antidepressant medications appeared to reduce the side-effect burden (e.g., anticholinergic effects) of synthetic drugs. None of these studies were rigorously controlled or randomized, and the results need to be validated using modern methodologies.

Safety and Adverse Reactions

Overall, *S. chinensis* has a favorable safety profile; however, it can stimulate uterine contractions and should be avoided during pregnancy. Other possible side effects include heartburn, upset stomach, decreased appetite, stomach pain, skin rash, urticaria, and itching. *S. chinensis* may affect serum levels of medications metabolized by CYP3A4 isozymes, such as warfarin. However, in vivo and human studies have not shown clinically significant effects on serum levels of medications metabolized by the same enzymes. Such discrepancies are not uncommon when herbal extracts are tested in vitro.

Eleutherococcus senticosus

Eleutherococcus (Acanthopanax) senticosus, or ben cao gang mu in traditional Chinese medicine, is a thorny shrub that is widely used in Russia and China to increase performance and quality of life and to treat respiratory infections and flu. It is sometimes called Siberian ginseng, although it does not belong to the ginseng family. Studies of extracts from *E. senticosus* roots show antistress, antiulcer, anti-irradiation, anticancer, anti-inflammatory, and hepatoprotective activity (Panossian 2003; Panossian and Wikman 2010).

Therapeutic Effect of *Eleutherococcus senticosus* in Chronic Fatigue Syndrome

Ben Cao Gang Mu (An Outline of Herbs), written by Li Shi Zhen in 1596, describes the use of *E. senticosus* root for promoting vigor, vitality, and longevity (Weng et al. 2007). In one recent study (Hartz et al. 2004), an extract of *E. senticosus* (standardized to a total of 0.12% eleutherosides B and E) 2,000 mg daily was given to subjects with CFS. The botanical preparation was effective after 2 months; however, by 4 months the efficacy was not significantly different from that of placebo. In China, standardized *E. senticosus* extracts (0.82% eleutherosides B and E) are approved for treatment of insomnia, weakness, lack of appetite, and muscle soreness—symptoms associated with depression and CFS (Weng et al. 2001). Another study found no statistically significant difference between improvements with the *E. senticosus* extract versus imipramine in subjects with moderate depression (Weng et al. 2001). In numerous studies, *E. senticosus* was examined in the combination formula, with *R. rosea* rhizome and *S. chinensis* berry extracts (ADAPT) (e.g., Aslanyan et al. 2010; Narimanian et al. 2005; Panossian et al. 2012, 2013).

Effects of *Eleutherococcus senticosus* in Bipolar Disorder

A 6-week RCT compared the safety and efficacy of *E. senticosus* extract plus lithium with fluoxetine plus lithium for bipolar depression in 76 adolescents (45 females and 31 males), ages 12–17 (Weng et al. (2007). Outcomes were assessed using the Ham-D and Young Mania Rating Scale (YMRS) at baseline and after weeks 1, 2, 4, and 6. Response was defined as >50% reduction in baseline Ham-D score, remission as Ham-D score <7, and mania as an increase in YMRS score >16 for at least 7 days at any time during treatment. Subjects were queried regarding adverse events. Response rates were comparable between adjunctive *E. senticosus* and fluoxetine (67.6% vs. 71.8%). Remission rates between groups were also similar (51.4% vs. 48.7%). During treatment, there was a significant time effect ($F=183.06$; $P<0.01$) but not a significant group effect ($F=0.99$) or effect by duration of treatment interaction ($F=0.779$). Three subjects in the fluoxetine group versus no subjects in the *E. senticosus* group experienced a manic switch episode. A greater frequency of adverse events was reported with fluoxetine versus *E. senticosus*. For adolescents with bipolar disorder, *E. senticosus* is a promising adjunctive treatment (Weng et al. 2007). Studies of *E. senticosus* with mood stabilizers other than lithium are warranted.

Safety and Adverse Reactions

E. senticosus generally produces few side effects and is usually well tolerated. The contraindication of arterial hypertension is not evidence based and should be carefully reevaluated (Schmidt et al. 2014). Safety during pregnancy or breast-feeding has not been established.

Withania somnifera

Withania somnifera (L.) Dunal (*W. somnifera*; Solanaceae), known as ashwagandha in Sanskrit and as Indian ginseng (Kulkarni and Dhir 2008), is used both in Ayurveda and Unani traditional medicinal systems for treating numerous conditions, including neurological and mental disorders. *W. somnifera* has more than 30 steroidal lactone withanolides; withaferin A is used for standardization of extracts (Lavie et al. 1965).

Other phytosterols (sitoindosides), alkaloids, saponins, flavonoids, and other phenolic compounds also contribute to the herb's broad spectrum of activities (Choudhary et al. 2013).

Withania somnifera for Stress, Anxiety, Insomnia, and Depression

Anxiolytic-like and antidepressant-like activity of the alcohol root extract and isolated glycowithanolides, sitoindosides, and withaferin A has been demonstrated in animal models of depression and anxiety (Bhattacharya and Muruganandam 2003; Bhattacharya et al. 2000; Singh et al. 1982). *W. somnifera* root extract produced sedation, reduction in locomotor activity, potentiation of thiopental-induced sleep, reduction of catecholamines and acetylcholine with an increase in histamine and serotonin in brain tissue of mice, and a delay in semicarbazide- and pentylenetetrazole-induced seizures (Day and Chatterjee 1968; Singh et al. 1979; Yidya Prabhu and Rao 1990). It is possible that GABAergic activity is the mechanism for improving GABAergic signaling dysfunctions such as in anxiety disorders and insomnia (Candelario et al. 2015).

Seven clinical studies have described *W. somnifera* as a safe and effective adaptogen for treating stress-related neuropsychiatric conditions—anxiety and bipolar disorder (Tables 8–1 and 8–3). For example, in a double-blind, randomized placebo-controlled trial, 64 adult subjects exposed to chronic stress were randomly assigned to take either one capsule twice daily of *W. somnifera* extract 300 mg or placebo for 60 days (Chandrasekhar et al. 2012). Telephone interviews assessed safety and compliance on days 15, 30, and 45 and at endpoint day 60. At study endpoint, subjects taking *W. somnifera* extract showed significantly greater reductions on all stress scales versus placebo ($P<0.0001$) and a significantly greater reduction in serum cortisol levels versus placebo ($P=0.0006$). Adverse event rates were comparable in both groups.

Table 8–3 shows anxiolytic effects of five different *Withania* preparations from five clinical studies with a total of 157 patients. Three of these were double-blind, randomized placebo-controlled trials with quality scores 2–3 out of 5. Study limitations include insufficient details regarding extract preparation, treatment administration, and randomization procedures. The best study (quality score 4), an 8-week double-blind RCT, used a water extract, 250–500 mg/day *Withania* (Sensoril), in 60 subjects with bipolar disorder (Chengappa et al. 2013). Compared with the control subjects, subjects taking *W. somnifera* had significantly better performance on three cognitive tasks: digit span backward ($P=0.035$), flanker neutral response time ($P=0.033$), and social cognition response of the Penn Emotional Acuity Test ($P=0.045$). Other cognitive tests were not significantly different between groups. Adverse events were similar in both groups. These encouraging results need confirmation in clinical trials of standardized products.

Safety, Adverse Events, and Contraindications

W. somnifera has a benign side-effect profile. Compared with other adaptogens, it is more calming. *Withania* is contraindicated in pregnancy because it may precipitate abortion. A 2010 review noted the potential for additive effects if given with sedatives

(Brinker 2010). The presence of *W. somnifera* may cause false positive readings for digoxin levels in fluorescence polarization immunoassay.

Limitations

An important limitation in assessment of herbal studies in general is variability in the composition and activity of bioactive constituents due to genetic and environmental (e.g., climate, soil characteristics, plant infections, fertilization) factors. Differences in processing raw materials, extraction, purification, and storage also affect the final composition and activity. Batch-to-batch reproducibility is not always evaluated. Heterogeneity in results among clinical studies may be due in part to the use of nonidentical herbal preparations. Of note, the dose-effect curve of adaptogens is bell-shaped in animal studies, such that excessively high doses are not more effective (Kurkin et al. 2003; Panossian and Wagner 2005; Wiegant et al. 2009). This may be due to feedback regulation of signaling systems and/or differences in threshold concentration for binding of extract constituents to receptors.

KEY POINTS

- Adaptogens demonstrate multi-target effects on the regulation of cellular responses to stress by influencing neuroendocrine, neurotransmitter, receptor, and molecular networks associated with beneficial effects on mood and cognitive function.

- Adaptogens may be better tolerated than conventional psychotropics; however, this needs confirmation in controlled comparative trials.

- Pilot clinical trials show therapeutic benefits of adaptogens for depression and anxiety, as well as cognitive and memory impairment.

- Further large-scale studies of standardized products are indicated for exploration of numerous potential clinical applications.

References

Abidov M, Crendal F, Grachev S, et al: Ziegenfuss T. Effect of extracts from Rhodiola rosea and Rhodiola crenulata (Crassulaceae) roots on ATP content in mitochondria of skeletal muscles. Bull Exp Biol Med 136(6):585–587, 2003 15500079

Agnihotri AP, Sontakke SD, Thawani VR, et al: Effects of Withania somnifera in patients of schizophrenia: a randomized, double blind, placebo controlled pilot trial study. Indian J Pharmacol 45(4):417–418, 2013 24014929

American Psychiatric Association: Diagnostic and Statistical Manual of Mental Disorders, 4th Edition. Washington, DC, American Psychiatric Association, 1994

Amsterdam JD, Panossian AG: Rhodiola rosea L. as a putative botanical antidepressant. Phytomedicine 23(7):770–783, 2016 27013349

Andrade C, Aswath A, Chaturvedi SK, et al: A double-blind, placebo-controlled evaluation of the anxiolytic efficacy of an ethanolic extract of Withania somnifera. Indian J Psychiatry 42(3):295–301, 2000 21407960

Asea A, Kaur P, Panossian A, Wikman KG: Evaluation of molecular chaperons Hsp72 and neuropeptide Y as characteristic markers of adaptogenic activity of plant extracts. Phytomedicine 20(14):1323–1329, 2013 23920279

Aslanyan G, Amroyan E, Gabrielyan E, et al: Double-blind, placebo-controlled, randomised study of single dose effects of ADAPT-232 on cognitive functions. Phytomedicine 17(7):494–499, 2010 20374974

Auddy B, Hazra J, Mitra A, et al: A standardized Withania somnifera extract significantly reduces stress related parameters in chronically stressed humans: a double blind, randomized, placebo controlled study. Journal of American Nutraceutical Association 11:50–56, 2008

Bhattacharya SK, Muruganandam AV: Adaptogenic activity of Withania somnifera: An experimental study using a rat model of chronic stress. Pharmacol Biochem Behav 75(3):547–555, 2003 12895672

Bhattacharya SK, Bhattacharya A, Sairam K, Ghosal S: Anxiolytic-antidepressant activity of Withania somnifera glycowithanolides: an experimental study. Phytomedicine 7(6):463–469, 2000 11194174

Brekhman II, Dardymov IV: New substances of plant origin which increase non-specific resistance. Ann Rev Pharmacol 9:419–430, 1969 4892434

Brinker F: Herbal Contraindications and Drug Interactions Plus Herbal Adjuncts With Medicines. Sandy, OR, Eclectic Medical Publishers, 2010

Brown RP, Gerbarg PL, Ramazanov Z, et al: A phytomedical review of Rhodiola rosea. Herbalgram 56:40–62, 2002

Bystritsky A, Kerwin L, Feusner JD: A pilot study of Rhodiola rosea (Rhodax®) for generalized anxiety disorder (GAD). J Altern Complement Med 14(2):175–180, 2008 18307390

Candelario M, Cuellar E, Reyes-Ruiz JM, et al: Direct evidence for GABAergic activity of Withania somnifera on mammalian ionotropic GABAA and GABAp receptors. J Ethnopharmacol 171:264–272, 2015 26068424

Chandrasekhar K, Kapoor J, Anishetty S: A prospective, randomized double-blind, placebo-controlled study of safety and efficacy of a high-concentration full-spectrum extract of ashwagandha root in reducing stress and anxiety in adults. Indian J Psychol Med 34(3):255–262, 2012 23439798

Chengappa KN, Bowie CR, Schlicht PJ, et al: Randomized placebo-controlled adjunctive study of an extract of Withania somnifera for cognitive dysfunction in bipolar disorder. J Clin Psychiatry 74(11):1076–1083, 2013 24330893

Choudhary MI, Yousuf S, Rahman AU: Chemistry and antitumor activity., in Natural Products. Edited by Ramawat KG, Merillon JM. Berlin, Springer-Verlag, 2013, pp 3465–3495

Cooley K, Szczurko O, Perri D, et al: Naturopathic care for anxiety: a randomized controlled trial ISRCTN78958974. PLoS One 4(8):e6628, 2009 19718255

Cuerrier A, Ampong-Nyarko K: *Rhodiola rosea* (Traditional Herbal Medicines for Modern Times). Boca Raton, FL, CRC Press, 2014, pp 203–221

Darbinyan V, Aslanyan G, Amroyan E, et al: Clinical trial of Rhodiola rosea L. extract SHR-5 in the treatment of mild to moderate depression. Nord J Psychiatry 61(5):343–348, 2007 17990195

Day PK, Chatterjee BK: Studies on the neuropharmacological properties of several Indian medicinal plants. J Res Indian Med 3(1):9–17, 1968

Edwards D, Heufelder A, Zimmermann A, et al: Therapeutic effects and safety of Rhodiola rosea extract WS® 1375 in subjects with life-stress symptoms—results of an open-label study. Phytother Res 26(8):1220–1225, 2012 22228617

Fintelmann V, Gurenwald J: Efficacy and tolerability of a Rhodiola rosea extract in adults with physical and cognitive deficiencies. Adv Ther 24(4):929–939, 2007 17901042

Galant IB, Kuznetsova AI, Suvorina NA, et al: The experience in using Schizandra chinensis in psychiatric practice, in Clinical Development and Therapy of Mental Diseases and Organisation of Psychoneurological Assistance. Moscow, State Research Institute of Psychiatry of the Ministry of Health of RSFSR, 1957, pp 112–113

Gannon JM, Forrest PE, Roy Chengappa KN: Subtle changes in thyroid indices during a placebo-controlled study of an extract of Withania somnifera in persons with bipolar disorder. J Ayurveda Integr Med 5(4):241–245, 2014 25624699

Hartz AJ, Bentler S, Noyes R, et al: Randomized controlled trial of Siberian ginseng for chronic fatigue. Psychol Med 34(1):51–61, 2004 14971626

Hirsch D, Zukowska Z: NPY and stress 30 years later: the peripheral view. Cell Mol Neurobiol 32(5):645–659, 2012 22271177

Hellum BH, Tosse A, Hoybakk K, et al: Potent in vitro inhibition of CYP3A4 and P-glycoprotein by Rhodiola rosea. Planta Med 76(4):331–338, 2010 19790032

Krasik ED, Morozova ES, Petrova KP: Therapy of asthenic conditions: clinical perspectives of applica-tion of Rhodiola rosea extract (golden root), in Proceedings Modern Problems in Psycho-pharmacology. Edited by Avrutskiy GY. Kemerovo City, USSR, Siberian Branch of Russian Academy of Sciences, 1970, pp 298–330

Kulkarni SK, Dhir A: Withania somnifera: an Indian ginseng. Prog Neuropsychopharmacol Biol Psychiatry 32(5):1093–1105, 2008 17959291

Kurkin VA, Zapesochnaya GG: Chemical composition and pharmacological properties of Rhodiola rosea. Journal of Medicinal Plants 20(10):1231–1244, 1986

Kurkin VA, Dubishchev AV, Titova IN, et al: Potent in vitro inhibition of CYP3A4 and P-glycoprotein by Rhodiola rosea. Rastit Resursi 3:115–122, 2003

Lavie D, Glotter E, Shvo Y: Constituents of Withania somnifera dun—part IV: the structure of Withaferin A. J Chem Soc 30:7517–7531, 1965

Leman MF: Treatment of reactive and asthenic states of exogenous etiology using the Far East Schizandra. Zh Nevropatol Psikhiatr Im S S Korsakova 52:67–70, 1952

Mao JJ, Lie QS, Soeller J, et al: Rhodiola rosea therapy for major depressive disorder: a study protocol for a randomized, double-blind, placebo-controlled trial. J Clin Trials 4:170, 2014 25610752

Mao JJ, Xie SX, Zee J, et al: Rhodiola rosea versus sertraline for major depressive disorder: a randomized placebo-controlled trial. Phytomedicine 22(3):394–399, 2015 25837277

Mashkovskiy MD: Extractum Eleutherococci fluidum, in Medicinal Agents (Drug Index) Manual for Doctors, Vol 1 [in Russian]. Moscow, Novaya Volna, 2000, pp 133–136

Narimanian M, Badalyan M, Panosyan V, et al: Impact of Chisan (ADAPT-232) on the quality-of-life and its efficacy as an adjuvant in the treatment of acute non-specific pneumonia. Phytomedicine 12(10):723–729, 2005 16323290

Olsson EM, von Schéele B, Panossian AG: A randomised, double-blind, placebo-controlled, parallel-group study of the standardised extract shr-5 of the roots of Rhodiola rosea in the treatment of subjects with stress-related fatigue. Planta Med 75(2):105–112, 2009 19016404

Panossian AG: Adaptogens: Tonic herbs for fatigue and stress. Alternative & Complementary Therapies 9(6):327–331, 2003

Panossian AG: Adaptogens in mental and behavioral disorders. Psychiatr Clin North Am 36(1):49–64, 2013 23538076

Panossian A, Wagner H: Stimulating effect of adaptogens: an overview with particular reference to their efficacy following single dose administration. Phytother Res 19(10):819–838, 2005 16261511

Panossian A, Wikman G: Effect of adaptogens on the central nervous system. Arq Bras Fitomed Cient 2:108–130, 2005

Panossian AG, Wikman G: Pharmacology of Schisandra chinensis Bail.: an overview of Russian research and uses in medicine. J Ethnopharmacol 118(2):183–212, 2008 18515024

Panossian A, Wikman G: Effects of adaptogens on the central nervous system and the molecular mechanisms associated with their stress-protective activity. Pharmaceuticals (Basel) 3(1):188–224, 2010

Panossian A, Wikman G: Evidence based efficacy and effectiveness of Rhodiola SHR-5 extract in treating stress- and age-associated disorders, in Rhodiola Rosea. Edited by Cuerrier C, Ampong-Nyarko K. Boca Raton, CRC Press, 2014, pp 203–221

Panossian A, Wikman G, Wagner H: Plant adaptogens: new concepts on their mode of action. Phytomedicine 6:287–300, 1999

Panossian A, Hovhannisyan A, Abrahamyan H, et al: Pharmacokinetic and pharmacodynamic study of interaction of Rhodiola rosea SHR-5 extract with warfarin and theophylline in rats. Phytother Res 23(3):351–357, 2009 18844284

Panossian A, Wikman G, Sarris J, et al: Rosenroot (Rhodiola rosea): traditional use, chemical composition, pharmacology and clinical efficacy. Phytomedicine 17(7):481–493, 2010 20378318

Panossian A, Wikman G, Kaur P, et al: Adaptogens stimulate neuropeptide Y and Hsp72 expression and release in neuroglia cells. Front Neurosci 6:6, 2012 22347152

Panossian A, Hamm R, Kadioglu O, et al: Synergy and antagonism of active constituents of ADAPT-232 on transcriptional level of metabolic regulation of isolated neuroglial cells. Front Neurosci 7:16, 2013 23430930

Panossian A, Hamm R, Wikman G, et al: Mechanism of action of Rhodiola, salidroside, tyrosol and triandrin in isolated neuroglial cells: an interactive pathway analysis of the downstream effects using RNA microarray data. Phytomedicine 21(11):1325–1348, 2014 25172797

Rao RP, Yuan C, Allegood JC, et al: Ziegenfuss T. Ceramide transfer protein function is essential for normal oxidative stress response and lifespan. Proc Natl Acad Sci USA 104(27):11,364–11,369, 2007 17592126

Rhizome and roots of Rhodiola rosea, in National Pharmacopoeia of the USSR, 11th Edition, Vol 2, Pharmacopoeia Paper 75, Update 2, Moscow, USSR Ministry of Health, 1999, pp 317–319

Romas RS: About the effect of Schizandra chinensis on higher brain structures of schizophrenia patients and chronic alcoholics. Thesis, Faculty of Medicine, Pirogov's Medical Institute, Vinnitsa, USSR, 1967

Saratikov AS, Krasnov EA: Rhodiola Rosea (Golden Root), 4th Edition. Tomsk, Russia, Tomsk State University Publishing House, 2004

Schmidt M, Thomsen M, Kelber O, et al: Myths and facts in herbal medicines: Eleutherococcus senticosus (Siberian ginseng) and its contraindication in hypertensive patients. Botanics: Targets and Therapy 4:27–32, 2014

Singh N, Nath R, Lata A, et al: Withania somnifera (Ashwagandha), a rejuvenating herbal drug which enhances survival during stress (an adaptogen). Int J Crude Drug Res 20(1):29–35, 1982

Singh RH, Malviya PC: Studies on the psychotropic effect of an indigenous rasayana drug, Asvagandha (Withania somnifera dunol) part I: (clinical studies). J Res Educ Indian Med 13(1):15–24, 1978

Singh RH, Malviya PC, Sarkar FH, et al: Studies on the psychotropic effect of an indigenous rasayana drug, Asvagandha (Withania somnifera dunol) part II: (experimental studies). J Res Educ Indian Med 14(1):49–54, 1979

Sudakov VN, Savinykh AB, Agapov YK: The role of adaptogens in the psychoprophylaxis of patients with borderline states of exogenous-organic genesis, in Modern Problems of Pharmacology and Search for New Medicines, Vol 2. Edited by Goldsberg ED. Tomsk, Russia, Tomsk State University Press, 1986, pp 298–330

Udintsev SN, Schakhov VP: Decrease of cyclophosphamide haematotoxicity by Rhodiola rosea root extract in mice with Ehrlich and Lewis transplantable tumors. Prog Neuropsychopharmacol Eur J Cancer 27(9):1182, 1991 1835634

Weng S, Cheng Z, Wang H, et al: An open-label study of capsule Acanthopanax senticosus for treatment of depression in patients. Hubei Journal of Chinese Traditional Medicine 6:8–9, 2001

Weng S, Tang J, Wang G, et al: Comparison of the addition of Siberian ginseng (Acanthopanax senticosus) versus fluoxetine to lithium for the treatment of bipolar disorder in adolescents: a randomized, double-blind trial. Curr Ther Res Clin Exp 68(4):280–290, 2007 24683218

Wiegant FAC, Surinova S, Ytsma E, et al: Plant adaptogens increase lifespan and stress resistance in C. elegans. Biogerontology 10(1):27–42, 2009 18536978

Yidya Prabhu M, Rao A: Neuropharmacological activity of Withania somnifera. Fitoterapia 66(3):237–240, 1990

CHAPTER 9

Integrating *Rhodiola rosea* in Clinical Practice

Clinical Cases

Patricia L. Gerbarg, M.D.

Richard P. Brown, M.D.

Its flower rises on twin stalks a cubit high. In color it resembles the Korykian crocus, and the root in the earth is like newly cut flesh. Like the dark moisture from an oak on the mountains, she [Medea] had gathered its sap in a Caspian shell.

Apollonius of Rhodes, third century B.C.,
Jason and the Golden Fleece

The polyvalent effects of *Rhodiola rosea* and other adaptogens create opportunities for many clinical applications. In Chapter 8, "Adaptogens in Psychiatric Practice," the biochemistry and preclinical and clinical studies of adaptogens were reviewed. In this chapter, we provide examples of clinical diagnoses and cases in which we have found *R. rosea*—which we have prescribed for more than 20 years—to be exceptionally helpful. Although skeptics could point out that the observed benefits may be attributed to a placebo effect, many of the case examples on which this chapter is based were patients who had tried many previous trials of medications and other treatments without success, suggesting that they were not placebo responders. Furthermore, placebo response is known to fade over time, unlike the improvements in these cases, which were observed to persist for years. Clinical observations have provided the impetus for scientific studies to investigate and validate many of the treatments in use today. The conditions discussed include anxiety disorders, fatigue, cognitive and memory impairment, attention-deficit/hyperactivity disorder (ADHD), and menopausal depression.

Anxiety, Posttraumatic Stress, and Phobias

Angela, a highly successful computer programmer, was constantly worried about failure, criticism, and rejection. Angela began psychotherapy twice weekly at age 31. It became evident that she had been emotionally abused by her mother and sexually molested by her stepfather between ages 6 and 10 years. She was beset by self-doubt, self-blame, and frequent thoughts of running away or shooting herself. She denied suicidal impulses or intent. This self-directed anger was addressed repeatedly in therapy sessions. Angela was extremely sensitive to medication side effects and tolerated a maximum dose of 25 mg/day of sertraline, 5 mg twice daily of buspirone, and 0.25 mg of diazepam (when needed for crossing bridges). She began R. rosea 50 mg (Rosavin by Ameriden International, 3% rosavins, 1% salidrosides) in the morning by opening a 100-mg capsule and sprinkling half the contents into her tea. The dose was gradually increased to 100 mg twice a day over several months, which reduced her anxiety and enabled her to speak up for herself more at work. Angela also learned coherent breathing at five cycles per minute. In addition to a 20-minute morning practice, she used the breath technique to stay calm whenever she felt pressured at work. She became more hopeful and self-confident, with far less frequent thoughts of running away or suicide. Over the next 7 years, she continued psychotherapy, gradually reducing her sessions to once a month.

Fatigue Due to Medical Illness or Medication Treatments

Sharon was diagnosed with breast cancer at age 51. During and after treatment with radiation and chemotherapy, she complained of severe fatigue, cognitive impairment ("chemo brain"), and radiation burns on her chest. She began taking R. rosea 360 mg (EnergyKare by Kare-N-Herbs, 4% rosavins, 2% salidrosides) in the morning. Within 1 week, her energy increased, and by the sixth week, her mental clarity and cognitive functions began to improve. She reported that the R. rosea seemed to accelerate the healing of her radiation burns. She continued R. rosea and remained cancer free at her 5-year follow-up.

Many cancer patients experience fatigue and cognitive impairment. R. rosea can rapidly relieve fatigue, usually in 1 week, followed by more gradual cognitive recovery in 6–12 weeks. These benefits are also seen in patients who have fatigue or cognitive impairment due to other medical conditions or medication side effects.

Cognitive Impairment

Traumatic Brain Injury

Morgan, a 40-year-old accountant, lost consciousness for 2 hours after a car accident. She became cognitively impaired, was unable to do mathematical calculations, lost her job, and went on disability. She complained of feeling as if she were "moving through molasses"; even simple tasks required great effort. Despite trials of selective serotonin reuptake inhibitors (SSRIs), other antidepressants, and stimulants, she made no progress in 2 years. She was started on a trial of 300 mg/day of *R. rosea* (3% rosavins, 1% salidrosides; Rosavin Plus by Ameriden International). After 4 weeks, she noticed some improvement in cognitive function, which continued over the subsequent 6 months. At that point, she was able to return to work half time and believed that her ability to think had come back to normal speed.

Attention-Deficit/Hyperactivity Disorder

Mrs. Alvarez brought her 22-year-old son, Ramon, for evaluation after he dropped out of college, moved back home, and started spending most of his time alone in his room playing video games. He had a history of ADHD, depression, and poor social functioning. A previous consultant thought that he might be developing schizophrenia. Trials of SSRIs had no effect on his symptoms. Stimulants (methylphenidate and mixed amphetamine salts) were intolerable, causing severe anxiety, jitteriness, and insomnia.

Some patients with ADHD who cannot tolerate prescription stimulants do well with the milder stimulating and cognitive-enhancing effects of *R. rosea*. When Ramon started taking 300 mg of *R. rosea* (Arctic root, SHR-5 by Swedish Herbal Institute, 4% rosavins, 2% salidrosides) every morning, he immediately noticed better mental focus, followed by greater ability to organize and follow through with activities. His depression remitted. Ramon returned to college, graduated, moved to his own apartment, and now supports himself by working.

Neurodegeneration: Parkinson's Disease

Mr. Campbell, a 78-year-old man with Parkinson's disease, had been passively sitting in a chair at home, rarely speaking or initiating any action for 5 years, despite treatment with levodopa and dopaminergic agents. He was brought for consultation by his family, who agreed to a trial of *R. rosea*. On the first day, he took 150 mg (Rosavin Plus, Ameriden). No adverse reaction occurred, so the dose was increased to 300 mg the second and third days. Two hours after taking the morning dose of *R. rosea* on the third day of treatment, Mr. Campbell rose from his chair, told his wife that it looked like a nice day to be outside, put on his hat, walked out the door, and began working in his garden. He continued talking spontaneously, gardening, doing small home repairs, and enjoying life at home with his wife until he died at age 82.

Mr. Campbell had a robust response to *R. rosea*. Obviously, not all patients will have this type of response; however, in practice, we find that most patients with cognitive, neurodegenerative, or cerebrovascular-related impairments benefit to some degree from this herb. Such cases may be examples of neuroprotective, antioxidative, anti-inflammatory, stimulating, and other adaptogenic effects.

Menopausal Depression

Women spend one-third of their lives in menopause, a time when estrogen decline is associated with diminished energy, mood, stress tolerance, cognitive function, memory, and sexual function. Simultaneously, menopausal women face increased risks for cardiovascular diseases, dementia, cancer, and osteoporosis. Selective estrogen receptor modulators (SERMs) are estrogen receptor ligands with tissue-specific agonistic or antagonistic effects. The "perfect" SERM would exert agonistic effects on estrogen receptors in bone, vascular, and brain tissues while causing antiestrogenic or no estrogenic effects in breast, endometrium, or ovaries.

Adaptogen constituents act on estrogen receptors, intracellular signaling, genomic regulation, and intercellular transmission involved in supporting the brain functions that become impaired with estrogen decline and aging (Gerberg and Brown 2015). Studies indicate that *R. rosea* could mitigate these pathophysiological processes and thereby improve many symptoms experienced by menopausal women (Gerbarg and Brown 2016; Gerbarg et al. 2015).

Studies in vitro and in animals show neuroprotection by salidrosides from *R. rosea* extracts (Chapter 8). By enabling cells to maintain energy production, *R. rosea* may help to fuel cellular repair systems, preventing the cumulative damage that contributes to brain aging. In addition, *R. rosea* provides direct antioxidant protection of cellular elements. In clinical trials, *R. rosea* improved cognitive functions and physical performance, especially under stress (Chapter 8) (Brown et al. 2009). Vascular aging accelerates during menopause, with reduced endothelial-dependent vasodilation and large artery stiffening, risk factors for cardiovascular and cerebrovascular disease. *R. rosea*–derived salidroside and estrogen provide similar protective activities. In animal studies, salidroside protected endothelium from hydrogen peroxide (H_2O_2) cytotoxicity, upregulated mitochondrial biogenesis factors, inhibited nuclear factor kappa-light-chain-enhancer of activated B cells (NF-κB), and prevented H_2O_2-induced overactivation of oxidative stress–related downstream signaling pathways (Xing et al. 2014). In vitro and in vivo studies reported that salidrosides protected endothelial functions from reactive oxygen species, preserved nitric oxide bioavailability, and protected mitochondria (Wu et al. 2009; Xing et al. 2015; Zhao et al. 2015). Thus, through these mechanisms, *R. rosea* could be used to compensate for estrogen deficiency during menopause by helping preserve endothelial-dependent vasodilation and arterial wall flexibility (Gerbarg and Brown 2015, 2016).

In contrast to hormone replacement therapy, *R. rosea* may reduce the risk of breast, ovarian, and uterine cancer. Salidrosides inhibited proliferation and induced cell cycle arrest and apoptosis in human breast cancer MDA-MB-231 (estrogen receptor–negative) and MCF-7 (estrogen receptor–positive) cells in vitro (Hu et al. 2010). Studies of human tumors transplanted into rodents showed that *R. rosea* increased the effectiveness of chemotherapies and protected stem cells in bone marrow and liver from toxic effects of chemotherapy (Brown et al. 2004, 2009). A standardized extract of *R. rosea* (3% rosavins, 1% salidrosides) was tested in ovariectomized rats, with evidence of strong estrogen receptor binding without estrogen receptor activation in vitro (Eagon et al. 2004). Ovariectomized rats fed therapeutic doses of *R. rosea* had no increase in circulating estradiol levels, no reduction of serum luteinizing hormone levels, and no increase in uterine size.

The development of *R. rosea* and other adaptogens to counteract adverse effects of estradiol decline would require further clarification of the interactions with estrogen receptors in different tissues. By interacting with cellular signaling molecules (rather than the estrogen receptors only), *R. rosea* affects a myriad of targets, genes, molecules, and downstream mechanisms that are involved in cognitive function, mood regulation, energy, cardiovascular function, and bone structuring. The following case illustrates integrative treatment with *R. rosea*.

Case Example: Anxiety, Depression, Fatigue, Cognitive Dysfunction, and Stress in a Menopausal Woman and Her Husband

Now in their early 60s, Dr. S and her husband, Dr. H, were highly regarded in their academic fields. Prolific researchers, writers, and teachers, they maintained an intense work and travel schedule until Dr. S. began to complain of fatigue, forgetfulness, and increasing ruminations that she would make a mistake or forget something vital. This snowballed into episodes of shortness of breath and feelings of terror. She became depressed and exhausted. Trials of antidepressants were discontinued because SSRIs caused rapid weight gain, bupropion exacerbated her anxiety, tricyclics caused left bundle branch block, and trazodone impaired her cognitive function. Dr. S hoped to avoid further medication reactions, so she consulted an integrative psychiatrist. Her chief complaint was fatigue because she needed energy and mental alertness to function at work. She was started on *R. rosea* 150 mg (3% rosavins, 1% salidrosides; Rosavin Plus by Ameriden International) 20 minutes before breakfast and lunch. Within 3 days, she noticed increased energy, which quickly led to improved mental focus, mood, and productivity. To reduce anxiety, Dr. S learned coherent breathing (see Chapter 21, "Breathing Techniques in Psychiatric Treatment"), which she practiced 20 minutes every morning and throughout the day whenever she felt stressed. It relaxed her body and stopped her anxious ruminations. No longer struggling to complete her work further reduced anxiety. After 3 weeks, 150 mg of *R. rosea* was added to her morning dose. Over the next month, her memory and processing speed improved. As his wife perked up and recovered her normal positive personality, Dr. H wondered if he could try the herb. Although he never talked about it, he had been feeling tired and somewhat depressed himself. Being pessimistic and critical were acceptable traits in his profession, but he was bothered by the fact that during lectures he could no longer recall all the references he previously knew by heart. He contacted his wife's psychiatrist, who prescribed increasing doses of *R. rosea* until he was taking 300 mg twice daily over a period of 2 weeks. Dr. S was delighted with the improvements in her husband's mood and energy, but Dr. H. was particularly pleased with the restoration of his reference recall.

Safety, Adverse Reactions, and Contraindications

R. rosea is generally well tolerated, even in elderly populations (Fintelmann and Gruenwald 2007). The most common side effects are due to stimulating properties, which are beneficial for patients who complain of fatigue, poor concentration, loss of motivation, or cognitive slowing. In patients with anxiety, sensitivity to stimulants, or cardiac arrhythmias, administration of activating agents such as *R. rosea* may exacerbate anxiety and insomnia or occasionally increase heart rate or frequency of irregular rhythms. Patients should avoid combining *R. rosea* with large amounts of caffeine because the stimulating effects are additive and can lead to tachycardia. As with antidepressants, there is a potential risk for triggering or exacerbating hypomanic or manic symptoms in patients with bipolar disorder, particularly when manic symptoms are not fully controlled by prescription medications.

In general, the dose of *R. rosea* extract should not exceed 800 mg/day (3% rosavins, 1% salidrosides). At higher doses, some individuals manifest increased bruising, probably as a result of an antiplatelet effect (as is seen with SSRIs). Concurrent use of anticoagulants requires monitoring and possibly dose adjustments. To our knowledge, to date, no cases of bleeding attributable to *R. rosea* have been reported. Although in vitro studies show that *R. rosea* affects cytochrome P450 (CYP) enzyme systems, in vivo and human studies show either no effects or effects that are too small to be of clinical significance. This is to be expected because, unlike the direct application of herbal extract to in vitro enzymes, orally ingested extracts undergo digestion, metabolism, and conversion to secondary metabolites, which often lack effects on CYP. Furthermore, human studies of *R. rosea* with CYP substrates would help identify any potentially significant herb-drug interactions (Hellum et al. 2010; Panossian et al. 2009).

KEY POINTS

- The polyvalent effects of *Rhodiola rosea* have therapeutic potential in a wide range of disorders.

- *R. rosea* can ameliorate fatigue, anxiety, cognitive and memory impairment, and menopausal depression.

- *R. rosea* has a high degree of safety in appropriate therapeutic doses.

References

Brown RP, Gerbarg PL, Graham B: The Rhodiola Revolution. New York, Rodale Press, 2004

Brown RP, Gerbarg PL, Muskin PR: How to Use Herbs, Nutrients, and Yoga in Mental Health Care. New York, WW Norton, 2009

Eagon PK, Elm MS, Gerbarg PL, et al: Evaluation of the medicinal botanical Rhodiola rosea for estrogenicity (abstract 2878), Proceedings of the American Association for Cancer Research 64:663, 2010

Fintelmann V, Gruenwald J: Efficacy and tolerability of a Rhodiola rosea extract in adults with physical and cognitive deficiencies. Adv Ther 24(4):929–939, 2007 17901042

Gerbarg PL, Brown RP: Therapeutic nutrients, herbs, and hormones, in Psychiatric Care of the Medical Patient, 3rd Edition. Edited by Fogel B, Greenberg D. New York, Oxford University Press, 2015, pp 545–608

Gerbarg PL, Brown RP: Pause menopause with Rhodiola rosea, a natural selective estrogen receptor modulator. Phytomedicine 23(7):763–769, 2016 26776957

Gerbarg P, Illeg P, Brown RP: Rhodiola rosea in psychiatric and medical practice, in Rhodiola Rosea (Traditional Herbal Medicines for Modern Times). Edited by Cuerrier A, Ampong-Nyarko K. New York, Taylor & Francis, 2015, pp 225–252

Hellum BH, Tosse A, Hoybakk K, et al: Potent in vitro inhibition of CYP3A4 and P-glycoprotein by Rhodiola rosea. Planta Med 76(4):331–338, 2010 19790032

Hu X, Zhang X, Qiu S, et al: Salidroside induces cell-cycle arrest and apoptosis in human breast cancer cells. Biochem Biophys Res Commun 398(1):62–67, 2010 20541529

Panossian A, Hovhannisyan A, Abrahamyan H, et al: Pharmacokinetic and pharmacodynamic study of interaction of Rhodiola rosea SHR-5 extract with warfarin and theophylline in rats. Phytother Res 23(3):351–357, 2009 18844284

Wu T, Xhou H, Jin Z, et al: Cardioprotections of slidroside from ischemia/reperfusion injury by increasing N-acetylglucosamine linkage to cellular proteins. EurJ Pharmacol 613(1–3):93–99, 2009 19376110

Xing S, Yang X, Li W, et al: Salidroside stimulates mitochondrial biogenesis and protects against H_2O_2-induced endothelial dysfunction. Oxid Med Cell Longev 2014:904834, 2014 24868319

Xing SS, Yang XY, Zheng T, et al: Salidroside improves endothelial function and alleviates atherosclerosis by activating a mitochondria-related AMPK/PI3K/Akt/eNOS pathway. Vascul Pharmacol 72:141–152, 2015 26187353

Zhao G, Shi A, Fan Z, Du Y: Salidroside inhibits the growth of human breast cancer in vitro and in vivo. Oncol Rep 33(5):2553–2560, 2015 25814002

CHAPTER 10

St. John's Wort (*Hypericum perforatum*) in the Treatment of Depression

Jerome Sarris, N.D., M.H.Sc., Ph.D.

I must gather the mystic St. John's Wort to-night;
The wonderful herb whose leaf will decide
If the coming year shall see me a bride.

Folkloric German poem

St. John's wort (*Hypericum perforatum*; SJW), traditionally used for a variety of nervous system conditions, is a popular modern-day herbal treatment for depression. Many clinical trials consistently demonstrate SJW's effectiveness in major depressive disorder (MDD); several have shown it to be equivalent to pharmaceutical antidepressants (Sarris 2013). However, because most of these studies used highly characterized, standardized SJW preparations, the findings cannot be extrapolated to all over-the-counter SJW supplements. In this chapter, I discuss the mechanisms of action of SJW, emerging pharmacogenetic data, current evidence of the efficacy of SJW in treating depression, safety and clinical considerations, and a case study.

Antidepressant Mechanisms of Action and Pharmacology

SJW contains constituents that exert antidepressant actions, including hypericin, pseudohypericin, hyperforin, and flavonoids (Butterweck and Schmidt 2007). Preclinical studies suggest several mechanisms of action, but the neurochemical effects were reported in preclinical studies that used exceedingly high doses of SJW or its isolated constituents. Considering the poor bioavailability of many constituents and the lack of penetration across the blood-brain barrier, it cannot be assumed that such effects would occur with therapeutic doses (Cott 2010). Preclinical studies have found the following:

- Nonselective inhibition of neuronal reuptake of serotonin, dopamine, and norepinephrine
- Weak inhibition of monoamine oxidase A and B
- Decreased degradation of and increased release of neurochemicals
- Sensitization of and increased binding of ligands to various receptors (e.g., γ-aminobutyric acid [GABA], glutamate, and adenosine)
- Increased dopaminergic activity in the prefrontal cortex
- Neuroendocrine modulation (Butterweck 2003)

Preclinical pharmacogenetic studies show a range of the epigenetic effects of SJW. A rodent study analyzing hypothalamic and hippocampal tissue genes found that genes involved with inflammatory processes and oxidative stress were upregulated by both SJW and fluoxetine (Jungke et al. 2011). A proteomic animal model study found that SJW differentially affected expression of 64 proteins involving energy metabolism and axonal outgrowth and regeneration (Pennington et al. 2009). Wong et al. (2004) found that gene expression was differentially regulated in 66 genes (concerning synaptic and energy metabolism functions). Finally, a cross-sectional study showed that SJW use was associated with higher serum levels of brain-derived neurotrophic factor in depressed patients compared with nonmedicated control subjects (Molendijk et al. 2011).

Evidence of Efficacy as an Antidepressant

More than 40 clinical trials of varying methodological quality have assessed the efficacy of SJW in treating depression. A Cochrane review and meta-analysis by Linde et al. (2008) reported that 18 combined randomized controlled trials (RCTs) showed a significantly greater relative risk (ratio of the portion of responders) of 1.48 with SJW compared with placebo and an effect equivalent to that of selective serotonin reuptake inhibitors (SSRIs). Although most studies tend to last 6–12 weeks, a longer-term RCT involving 426 clinical responders to 6 weeks of SJW extract WS 5570 (Dr. Willmar Schwabe Pharmaceuticals, Karlsruhe, Germany) found that after continuation of SJW or matching placebo for up to 26 weeks, SJW completers had a relapse rate of 18% compared with 25.7% for placebo (Kasper et al. 2008).

For more severe depression, SJW is not considered a first-line treatment. A 6-week RCT in 251 subjects with moderate to severe depression (Hamilton Rating Scale for Depression [Ham-D] score≥22) found that SJW extract WS 5570 showed a slightly superior reduction in Ham-D score compared with paroxetine (and placebo) (Szegedi et al. 2005). However, not all studies support SJW for treatment of MDD. The widely publicized 2002 National Institute of Mental Health–funded Hypericum Depression Trial Study Group (2002) three-arm RCT ($n=340$) was a failed trial in which neither SJW nor sertraline was significantly different from placebo in reducing Ham-D score at week 8. Reanalysis of the Ham-D score at week 26 follow-up found no significant difference among treatments and a pronounced placebo effect (Sarris et al. 2012).

Efficacy of SJW has not been established for use in antepartum, peripartum, or postpartum depression. Currently, no RCT has assessed its use for depression in menopausal transition. No firm evidence supports the efficacy and safety of SJW in adolescents with MDD; however, two 8-week open-label trials involving SJW in small samples of adolescents ages 6–17 years have been completed (Findling et al. 2003; Simeon et al. 2005). The results of these trials indicated modest response rates for SJW, but the studies were limited by the lack of placebo groups. In addition, the trials had a high percentage of dropouts because of continuing depression or noncompliance.

Safety, Side Effects, and Drug Interactions

Compared with prescription antidepressant medications, SJW has a sound safety profile. A review of 16 postmarketing surveillance studies ($N=34,834$) found that SJW was tenfold safer than synthetic antidepressants (Knüppel and Linde 2004). A meta-analysis also showed a significant difference in favor of SJW over conventional antidepressants for discontinuation due to adverse events (Rahimi et al. 2009). Aside from rare idiosyncratic reactions, most adverse effects involve reversible dermatological (phototoxic rash) and gastrointestinal (nausea, heartburn, loose stools) symptoms. At higher doses, SJW may cause side effects similar to but milder than those of SSRIs, including gastrointestinal symptoms, sexual dysfunction, bruxism (teeth clenching), and restless legs syndrome. Several case reports of serotonin syndrome, documented by drug surveillance agencies, are attributable to the use of high-dose SJW and concomitant use of synthetic antidepressants (Sarris 2013). SJW can augment response to tricyclic antidepressants, bupropion, venlafaxine, and *S*-adenosylmethionine but should not be combined with monoamine oxidase inhibitors. Although many of the reported cases of mania in patients taking SJW involved concomitant use of other medications and/or recreational drugs, as well as a background of cyclothymia, a clear temporal association appears to exist between SJW use and induction of hypomania or mania. Therefore, as with conventional antidepressants, caution is advised in people with a personal or family history of bipolar disorder. The use of SJW in combination with other serotonergic antidepressants (SSRIs, serotonin-norepinephrine reuptake inhibitors) also may increase the risk of serotonin syndrome. Nevertheless, there may be a role for low-dose SJW when a patient is withdrawing from an antidepressant under clinical supervision, as the following case illustrates.

> A 46-year-old woman was taking 150 mg per day of Zoloft (sertraline) for more than 10 years for what began as a postpartum depressive episode. Her life was generally stable and her mood was good. She wished to stop taking the medication because she was worried about long-term side effects. Two previous attempts to discontinue antidepressants resulted in recurrence of depression. Fearful that her depression might return, she

wanted to try a "natural option." She was taking no other medications and had no significant medical conditions other than mild arthritis in her knees.

In this case the psychiatrist considered whether SJW would be appropriate and how best to reduce the dose of sertraline while initiating and increasing SJW. Because antidepressant medication and SJW should not be used together at higher doses, clinical judgment determines when the antidepressant is at a sufficiently low dose before introduction of SJW. In addition, the half-life of the antidepressant needs to be considered. This patient was taking an average dose of sertraline, which has a half-life of about 26 hours. To avoid discontinuation syndrome, sertraline should be titrated down over several weeks. When the sertraline is reduced to 100 mg per day, SJW could be started at a minimum standard dose (300 mg per day) and increased by 300 mg every 7 days until response occurs, usually at 300 mg three times daily. The sertraline dose may need to be reduced more gradually to avoid recurrence of depression. If depression recurs, it may be necessary to temporarily increase sertraline. Although serotonin syndrome is highly unlikely with this regime, the patient should be monitored using criteria such as Sternbach or Hunter criteria (Dunkley et al. 2003).

Although concerns have been raised over potential interactions with pharmaceuticals, this is more likely to occur with SJW extracts containing higher amounts of hyperforin, a constituent known to induce cytochrome P450 (CYP) pathways and the P-glycoprotein drug efflux pump, thereby reducing drug serum levels (Izzo 2004). Case reports and human studies indicate that SJW can interfere with absorption, metabolism, and effectiveness of medications, including alprazolam, amitriptyline, anticoagulants, clonazepam, cyclosporine, digoxin, HIV protease inhibitors, dextromethorphan, indinavir, oral contraceptives, reverse transcriptase inhibitors, simvastatin, tacrolimus, theophylline, and warfarin (Knüppel and Linde 2004; Van Strater and Bogers 2012). SJW constituents hypericin, hyperforin, and flavones are used for standardization. Studies indicate that high-dose hyperforin extracts (≥ 10 mg/day) induce CYP3A4; low-dose hyperforin extracts (≤ 4 mg/day) showed no significant effects on CYP3A4 (Sarris 2013). Therefore, for patients taking other medications, it is advisable to prescribe only low-hyperforin SJW. However, low-hyperforin SJW may be potentially less effective in treating depression because it is the major constituent found to cross the blood-brain barrier (Cott 2010).

The safety of SJW during pregnancy and lactation has not been established. A prospective study compared 54 SJW-exposed pregnant women with a matched group of pregnant women taking other pharmacological medicines for depression and a third matched group of healthy women (not exposed to any known teratogens) (Moretti et al. 2009). Follow-up information indicated that the rates of major malformations were similar across the three groups and at 3%–5% risk, the same as expected in the general population. However, such a small study without long-term follow-up is insufficient to establish safety during pregnancy.

Clinical Considerations

Caution is advised when combining SJW with other antidepressants because of the potential for serotonin syndrome. SJW also has been reported to cause "switching" in bipolar disorder. An overarching consideration is the marked difference in quality and standardization among SJW products. The results of high-quality European pharmaceutical-grade extracts cannot be generalized to inferior extracts. Therefore, clinicians are advised to use standardized SJW products that have proved to be effective in clinical trials. The common daily dosage of SJW is between 900-mg and 1,800-mg tablets standardized to 0.3% of hypericin and/or 1%–5% of hyperforin, given in two to three doses. Standardization to less than 2% hyperforin reduces the risk of CYP3A4 induction. SJW is not recommended as a first-line intervention in cases of severe mental illness or when significant suicidal ideation is present. It has not yet been studied in treatment-resistant depression. SJW has shown benefits in mild depression, wintertime seasonal affective disorder (Cott and Fugh-Berman 1998; Hänsgen et al. 1994; Wheatley 1999), and somatoform disorder (Volz et al. 2002).

KEY POINTS

- Studies showing well-characterized, standardized St. John's wort (SJW) preparations to be as effective as standard antidepressants for treatment of major depressive disorder cannot be extrapolated to all over-the-counter SJW supplements.

- SJW products standardized for lower amounts of hyperforin and higher levels of hypericin and flavonoids are less likely to induce cytochrome P450 pathways but may be less effective clinically.

- Combining high doses of SJW and serotonergic prescription antidepressants increases the risk of serotonin syndrome.

References

Butterweck V: Mechanism of action of St John's wort in depression: what is known? CNS Drugs 17(8):539–562, 2003 12775192

Butterweck V, Schmidt M: St. John's wort: role of active compounds for its mechanism of action and efficacy. Wien Med Wochenschr 157(13–14):356–361, 2007 17704987

Cott J: St John's Wort, 2nd Edition. Informacare, 2010

Cott JM, Fugh-Berman A: Is St. John's wort (Hypericum perforatum) an effective antidepressant? J Nerv Ment Dis 186(8):500–501, 1998 9717868

Dunkley EJ, Isbister GK, Sibbritt D, et al: The Hunter Serotonin Toxicity Criteria: simple and accurate diagnostic decision rules for serotonin toxicity. QJM 96(9):635–642, 2003 12925718

Findling RL, McNamara NK, O'Riordan MA, et al: An open-label pilot study of St. John's wort in juvenile depression. J Am Acad Child Adolesc Psychiatry 42(8):908–914, 2003 12874492

Hänsgen KD, Vesper J, Ploch M: Multicenter double-blind study examining the antidepressant effectiveness of the Hypericum extract LI 160. J Geriatr Psychiatry Neurol 7(1 suppl 1):S15–S18, 1994 7857501

Hypericum Depression Trial Study Group: Effect of Hypericum perforatum (St John's wort) in major depressive disorder: a randomized controlled trial. JAMA 287(14):1807–1814, 2002 11939866

Izzo AA: Drug interactions with St. John's wort (Hypericum perforatum): a review of the clinical evidence. Int J Clin Pharmacol Ther 42(3):139–148, 2004 15049433

Jungke P, Ostrow G, Li JL, et al: Profiling of hypothalamic and hippocampal gene expression in chronically stressed rats treated with St. John's wort extract (STW 3-VI) and fluoxetine. Psychopharmacology (Berl) 213(4):757–772, 2011 20924750

Kasper S, Volz HP, Möller HJ, et al: Continuation and long-term maintenance treatment with Hypericum extract WS 5570 after recovery from an acute episode of moderate depression—a double-blind, randomized, placebo controlled long-term trial. Eur Neuropsychopharmacol 18(11):803–813, 2008 18694635

Knüppel L, Linde K: Adverse effects of St. John's wort: a systematic review. J Clin Psychiatry 65(11):1470–1479, 2004 15554758

Linde K, Berner MM, Kriston L: St John's wort for major depression. Cochrane Database Syst Rev 4(4):CD000448, 2008 18843608

Molendijk ML, Bus BA, Spinhoven P, et al: Serum levels of brain-derived neurotrophic factor in major depressive disorder: state-trait issues, clinical features and pharmacological treatment. Mol Psychiatry 16(11):1088–1095, 2011 20856249

Moretti ME, Maxson A, Hanna F, et al: Evaluating the safety of St. John's wort in human pregnancy. Reprod Toxicol 28(1):96–99, 2009 19491000

Pennington K, Föcking M, McManus CA, et al: A proteomic investigation of similarities between conventional and herbal antidepressant treatments. J Psychopharmacol 23(5):520–530, 2009 18562437

Rahimi R, Nikfar S, Abdollahi M: Efficacy and tolerability of Hypericum perforatum in major depressive disorder in comparison with selective serotonin reuptake inhibitors: a meta-analysis. Prog Neuropsychopharmacol Biol Psychiatry 33(1):118–127, 2009 19028540

Sarris J: St. John's wort for the treatment of psychiatric disorders. Psychiatr Clin North Am 36(1):65–72, 2013 23538077

Sarris J, Fava M, Schweitzer I, et al: St John's wort (Hypericum perforatum) versus sertraline and placebo in major depressive disorder: continuation data from a 26-week RCT. Pharmacopsychiatry 45(7):275–278, 2012 22592504

Simeon J, Nixon MK, Milin R, et al: Open-label pilot study of St. John's wort in adolescent depression. J Child Adolesc Psychopharmacol 15(2):293–301, 2005 15910213

Szegedi A, Kohnen R, Dienel A, et al: Acute treatment of moderate to severe depression with hypericum extract WS 5570 (St John's wort): randomised controlled double blind non-inferiority trial versus paroxetine. BMJ 330(7490):503, 2005 15708844

Van Strater AC, Bogers JP: Interaction of St John's wort (Hypericum perforatum) with clozapine. Int Clin Psychopharmacol 27(2):121–124, 2012 22113252

Volz HP, Murck H, Kasper S, et al: St John's wort extract (LI 160) in somatoform disorders: results of a placebo-controlled trial. Psychopharmacology (Berl) 164(3):294–300, 2002 12424553

Wheatley D: Hypericum in seasonal affective disorder (SAD). Curr Med Res Opin 15(1):33–37, 1999 10216809

Wong ML, O'Kirwan F, Hannestad JP, et al: St John's wort and imipramine-induced gene expression profiles identify cellular functions relevant to antidepressant action and novel pharmacogenetic candidates for the phenotype of antidepressant treatment response. Mol Psychiatry 9(3):237–251, 2004 14743185

CHAPTER 11

Ginkgo biloba

Psychiatric Indications, Mechanisms, and Safety

Bruce J. Diamond, Ph.D., M.Ed.

Ashley Mondragon, B.A.

> Like a dancing phoenix, its trunk soars to the clouds, like a coiled dragon perching on a cliff, its invisible qi.
>
> *Wang Chunwu*, A Chronicle of Mt. Qingcheng (Qingcheng Shan Zhi)

The maidenhair tree, *Ginkgo biloba*, known in China as the silver almond tree (yinxing), has grown on Earth for 300 million years. The ginkgo tree, last living species of the Ginkgoaceae family, once thought to be extinct, was rediscovered in a Japanese garden in the seventeenth century and has since been widely cultivated. Traditional Chinese medicine used the seeds for asthma, phlegm, and cough and applied the circulatory effects of the leaves to heart and brain conditions. Medicinal properties of ginkgo were described nearly 5,000 years ago by Chen Noung (2767–2687 B.C.) in the first pharmacopoeia, the *Chen Noung Pen T'sao*. Primary clinical indications for ginkgo leaf extracts are cerebrovascular, peripheral vascular, and ischemic tissue damage. Most randomized controlled trials (RCTs) use the *G. biloba* special extract EGb 761, known commercially as Tebonin, Tanakan, and Rökan. Ginkgold, ginkgo biloba (Vitanica, VI3), Ginkgoforte (Blackmores), and Lichtwer's LI1370 extract also contain standardized flavone glycoside and terpene lactone fractions. Products containing one of the scientifically tested standardized forms of ginkgo are more likely to be effective.

The authors wish to recognize Ashley Bujalski and Alana Summers-Plotno for their editorial support for this chapter.

In this chapter, the term *ginkgo* refers to special extract EGb 761, unless otherwise specified. EGb 761 is manufactured to pharmaceutical standards and is standardized to contain 24% ginkgo-flavone glycosides; 6% terpenoids; and other major constituents (>0.1%) (e.g., quercetin 3-0-glucoside, quercetin 3-0-rhamnoside, bilobalide, ginkgolide A, ginkgolide B, ginkgolide C, ginkgolide J) (Diamond and Bailey 2013). When evaluating ginkgo in clinical practice and research, it is advisable to compare qualitative and quantitative characteristics of products with EGb 761.

Clinical Indications for Neurological and Neuropsychiatric Symptoms: Overview

The German Commission E (equivalent to the U.S. Food and Drug Administration) approved *G. biloba* for treating impairments in memory, concentration, attention, and mood; vertigo; and vascular tinnitus (Valli and Giardina 2002). Randomized placebo-controlled trials suggest that ginkgo exerts neuroprotective and cognitive-enhancing properties, supporting a role in neuropsychiatric and cognitive dysfunctions (e.g., memory, information processing, attention, psychomotor, mood, fatigue, and functional activities) (Diamond et al. 2000; Ponto and Schultz 2003).

Alzheimer's, Mixed, and Vascular Dementia: Cognitive and Neuropsychiatric Symptoms

A growing number of controlled trials suggest that ginkgo can be a beneficial adjunctive therapy for dementias and, in some cases, a primary treatment for cognitive, neuropsychiatric, and functional sequelae when acetylcholinesterase inhibitors (AChEIs) are ineffective or contraindicated. One study rated the quality of evidence for ginkgo's use in treating dementia as low compared with AChEIs (Laver et al. 2016). However, of four methodologically sound trials with 1,294 patients with dementia, three reported that ginkgo was more effective than placebo. In the fourth trial (Ihl 2013), ginkgo was equivalent to donepezil, with animal data suggesting that combination ginkgo and donepezil therapy may be more effective than either alone (Stein et al. 2015).

Schizophrenia

In a meta-analysis of eight double-blind, randomized placebo-controlled trials of 1,033 patients with schizophrenia taking antipsychotic medications, those given *G. biloba* ($n=571$) had significantly reduced total and negative symptoms compared with those given placebo ($n=462$) (Chen et al. 2015).

Attention-Deficit/Hyperactivity Disorder

An open pilot study in which EGb 761 was given to 20 children with attention-deficit/hyperactivity disorder (ADHD) for 3–5 weeks (maximum dosage=240 mg/day) suggested that ginkgo may be beneficial (Uebel-von Sandersleben et al. 2014). Ginkgo T.D. (Tolid Daru, Iran) was compared with methylphenidate in patients with ADHD in a 6-week double-blind RCT. Improvement in the ginkgo group was about 50% of that found in the methylphenidate group. However, methylphenidate caused more insomnia, headaches, and decreased appetite (Salehi et al. 2010). In clinical practice, Richard P. Brown, M.D., coeditor of this book, finds the combination of ginkgo and American ginseng to be particularly beneficial (see Chapter 13, "*Panax ginseng* and American Ginseng in Psychiatric Practice"). American ginseng can improve working memory, which is often impaired in ADHD. Controlled studies of ginkgo plus American ginseng are needed.

Multiple Sclerosis

A review of complementary and alternative medicine in multiple sclerosis suggested that clinicians should counsel patients that ginkgo is ineffective for cognition and possibly effective for fatigue, according to available pilot studies (Yadav and Narayanaswami 2014).

> Mrs. M, a 48-year-old married woman, was diagnosed with definite multiple sclerosis (relapsing-remitting type of 10 years' duration) by a board-certified neurologist. She was fully ambulatory but with moderate disability. Mrs. M was one subject in a larger double-blind, randomized placebo-controlled trial. Mrs. M was administered 240 mg/day (60-mg tablets four times per day) of ginkgo for 4 weeks. At study conclusion, she showed improvement in fatigue, symptom severity, and functional performance.

This case suggests that ginkgo may help ameliorate fatigue and symptom severity in multiple sclerosis, with possible application to other disorders in which fatigue figures prominently.

Healthy Participants

In a randomized placebo-controlled trial, 132 healthy young adults were randomly assigned to daily doses of 480 mg EGb 761, 240 mg EGb 761, or placebo for 4 weeks. Both treatment groups had improved scores on the Hamilton Anxiety Scale (Ham-A) and secondary outcome measures (Woelk et al. 2007). A meta-analysis of 13 studies involving 1,145 healthy individuals reported that 120–240 mg/day EGb 761 for durations of 1 week to 4 months showed no measurable effects on memory, attention, or executive function (Laws et al. 2012). However, in a double-blind crossover study, a single 600-mg dose of ginkgo improved memory and scanning speed 1 hour later (Shi et al. 2010).

Dose-Dependent Effects, Dosage, and Treatment Duration

Dose-dependent benefits of ginkgo have been documented in cerebrovascular insufficiency, cognitive impairment, aging, hypoxia, tinnitus, and vestibular disorders

(Diamond et al. 2000). Significant dose-dependent decreases in P300 event–related potential latencies were reported after daily doses of 80 mg and 160 mg in 15 young participants (mean age=29) (Diamond et al. 2000). Electroencephalogram alpha power also changed in a dose-dependent manner (greater at 600 vs. 240 vs. 120 mg/day) in frontal and occipital regions, accompanied by enhanced alertness (Diamond et al. 2000). A meta-analysis of seven RCTs involving 2,684 patients diagnosed with Alzheimer's disease, vascular dementia, and mixed dementia reported that EGb 761 at doses between 120 and 240 mg/day for 22–26 weeks improved cognition. The 240-mg/day dose was more effective than the 120-mg/day dose (Gauthier and Schlaefke 2014).

The German Commission E recommends 120–240 mg/day ginkgo extract in two to three divided doses for cerebral vascular insufficiency (Valli and Giardina 2002). Doses up to 720 mg/day have been used in trials for dementia, memory, and circulatory disorders. Improvement on one or more measures has been associated with doses ranging from 120 to 300 mg/day for 3–12 weeks (Bressler 2005). In a multicenter double-blind, randomized placebo-controlled trial involving 410 outpatients with mild to moderate dementia, a single daily dose of 240 mg EGb 761 for 24 weeks was safe, showing a significant advantage over placebo for apathy or indifference, sleep and nighttime behavior, irritability or lability, depression, dysphoria, and aberrant motor behavior (Bachinskaya et al. 2011). Overall, studies indicated that 4–6 weeks are needed for positive effects on memory, mood, or physiological function with studies of 4–52 weeks (80–720 mg/day). Doses between 120 and 240 mg taken two or three times per day are considered optimal in most cases.

Drug Interactions

Patients taking ginkgo must be monitored for possible drug interactions.

Antiplatelet Drugs

Inhibition of platelet-activating factor (PAF) by ginkgolide B led to cautions regarding concomitant use of ginkgo with drugs that affect platelet function and coagulation, such as aspirin, ibuprofen, nonsteroidal anti-inflammatory drugs, rofecoxib, anticoagulants, and warfarin (Ponto and Schultz 2003). Case reports described intracerebral hemorrhage in a patient taking ginkgo and warfarin and blurred vision and spontaneous bleeding from the iris into the eye's anterior chamber in a patient taking aspirin, with cessation of bleeding when ginkgo was discontinued (Williamson 2003). Recent trials have not confirmed these effects. Systematic reviews of case reports and RCTs do not support causal relations between ginkgo and bleeding or changes in blood coagulation parameters (Izzo and Ernst 2009).

Calcium Channel Antagonists and Monoamine Oxidase Inhibitors

In an animal model (doses exceeding recommendation for humans), ginkgo attenuated the hypotensive effect of nicardipine via induction of cytochrome P450 (CYP)

3A2 and other liver metabolizing enzymes (Shinozuka et al. 2002). Although this finding is not substantiated, caution is advised when long-term, high-dose ginkgo extract is used with calcium channel antagonists metabolized by CYP3A2 (Williamson 2003). Ginkgo administered for 1 month (120 mg/day) showed no inhibitory effects on brain monoamine oxidase A or B on positron emission tomography (Ponto and Schultz 2003).

Depression, Herbs, and Surgery

Trazodone, which is used to treat depression in the elderly, purportedly interacted with ginkgo in a patient with Alzheimer's disease, resulting in a coma (Galluzzi et al. 2000). However, little support exists for a causal relation between ginkgo and coma (Williamson 2003). Although interactions between herbal supplements and anesthetics have not been well established, the American Society of Anesthesiologists recommends that herbal supplements be stopped 2–3 weeks before elective surgery, with ginkgo specifically identified because of anti-PAF activity.

Mechanisms of Action

Flavone, ginkgolide B, and bilobalide components exert concentration-dependent antioxidant, metabolic, antiplatelet, and neurotransmitter regulatory effects that modulate cerebrovasculature, receptor/transmitter activity, glucose metabolism, and electroencephalographic activity (Diamond and Bailey 2013).

Effects of Flavonol Constituents on Dopamine and Acetylcholine Release

EGb 761 and its flavonol constituents increased dopamine and acetylcholine release in rat medial prefrontal cortex, with acylated flavonol glycosides quercetin and kaempferol as the putative constituents contributing to these effects (Kehr et al. 2012).

Cerebral Blood Flow, Metabolism, Antioxidation, and Anti-inflammatory Properties

Flavonoids act as free radical scavengers, and terpene lactones (ginkgolides) inhibit PAF, thereby facilitating blood flow. Pretreatment with high-dose ginkgo can benefit cerebrovascular disease and vascular dementia by reducing ischemia reperfusion injury, enhancing cerebral blood flow, and inhibiting platelets (Valli and Giardina 2002). Determining whether ginkgo's beneficial effects on age-related cognitive decline are mediated by altering cerebral blood flow, metabolic rate, or cerebral vascular reserve awaits more definitive studies. Hypothesized neuroprotective mechanisms in Alzheimer's disease include nitric oxide toxicity; antiapoptosis (via intracellular signaling pathways, flavonoids, and terpenes); anti-inflammation; protection against mitochondrial dysfunction, amyloidogenesis, and Aβ aggregation; ion homeostasis; modulation of tau protein phosphorylation; and possibly induction of growth factors (Shi et al. 2010).

Electroencephalographic and Event-Related Potential–Mediated Mechanisms

Ginkgo-induced changes in P300 latency and increases in the power of higher-frequency electroencephalogram components are consistent with enhanced processing efficiency and memory updating (Diamond and Bailey 2013; Diamond et al. 2000).

Tolerability and Safety

A meta-analysis of 75 clinical trials involving 7,115 patients with Alzheimer's disease, peripheral arterial disease, autism spectrum disorder, ischemic stroke, macular degeneration, cancer, and tinnitus taking EGb 761 at 60–1,000 mg/day for 2 days to 20 years found EGb 761 to be well tolerated with no adverse events (Heinonen and Gaus 2015). In trials in which 240 mg/day was administered for 24 weeks to patients with Alzheimer's disease or vascular dementia (Ihl et al. 2011) and in a meta-analysis with patients who mostly had mild to moderate dementia of vascular and nonvascular origin (Kellermann and Kloft 2011), ginkgo was safe, with no increased risk of bleeding. Moreover, in comparison with patients taking other substances, such as AChEIs, similar proportions of patients discontinued treatment because of side effects (Kurz and Van Baelen 2004).

KEY POINTS

- Standardized *Ginkgo biloba* extracts, manufactured to pharmaceutical standards, contain the following active ingredients: 24% ginkgo-flavone glycosides and 6% terpenoids.

- Mechanisms of action include modulation of cholinergic and monoamine pathways, antioxidant or anti-inflammatory activities and anti-platelet-activating factor, metabolic and neurotransmitter regulation, and increased nitric oxide activity.

- Sufficient evidence supports ginkgo as an adjunctive treatment for cognitive and neuropsychiatric symptoms associated with Alzheimer's disease, vascular dementia, normal aging, cerebral insufficiency, and tinnitus.

- In general, effective doses of ginkgo are about 120–480 mg/day for 4–12 weeks.

- Ginkgo has a long history of safety in traditional medicine and controlled clinical trials. Nevertheless, monitoring for herb-drug interactions is advised.

References

Bachinskaya N, Hoerr R, Ihl R: Alleviating neuropsychiatric symptoms in dementia: the effects of Ginkgo biloba extract EGb 761: findings from a randomized controlled trial. Neuropsychiatr Dis Treat 7(1):209–215, 2011 21573082

Bressler R: Herb-drug interactions: interactions between Ginkgo biloba and prescription medications. Geriatrics 60(4):30–33, 2005 15823059

Chen X, Hong Y, Zheng P: Efficacy and safety of extract of Ginkgo biloba as an adjunct therapy in chronic schizophrenia: a systematic review of randomized, double-blind, placebo-controlled studies with meta-analysis. Psychiatry Res 228(1):121–127, 2015 25980333

Diamond BJ, Bailey MR: Ginkgo biloba: indications, mechanisms, and safety. Psychiatr Clin North Am 36(1):73–83, 2013 23538078

Diamond BJ, Shiflett SC, Feiwel N, et al: Ginkgo biloba extract: mechanisms and clinical indications. Arch Phys Med Rehabil 81(5):668–678, 2000 10807109

Galluzzi S, Zanetti O, Binetti F, et al: Coma in a patient with Alzheimer's disease taking low-dose trazodone and Ginkgo biloba. J Neurol Neurosurg Psychiatry 68(5):679–680, 2000 10836866

Gauthier S, Schlaefke S: Efficacy and tolerability of Ginkgo biloba extract EGb 761® in dementia: a systematic review and meta-analysis of randomized placebo-controlled trials. Clin Interv Aging 9:2065–2077, 2014 25506211

Heinonen T, Gaus W: Cross matching observations on toxicological and clinical data for the assessment of tolerability and safety of Ginkgo biloba leaf extract. Toxicology 327:95–115, 2015 25446328

Ihl R: Effects of Ginkgo biloba extract EGb 761 ® in dementia with neuropsychiatric features: review of recently completed randomised, controlled trials. Int J Psychiatry Clin Pract 17 (suppl 1):8–14, 2013 23808613

Ihl R, Bachinskaya N, Korczyn AD, et al: Efficacy and safety of a once-daily formulation of Ginkgo biloba extract EGb 761 in dementia with neuropsychiatric features: a randomized controlled trial. Int J Geriatr Psychiatry 26(11):1186–1194, 2011 21140383

Izzo AA, Ernst E: Interactions between herbal medicines and prescribed drugs: an updated systematic review. Drugs 69(13):1777–1798, 2009 19719333

Kehr J, Yoshitake S, Ijiri S, et al: Ginkgo biloba leaf extract (EGb 761®) and its specific acylated flavonol constituents increase dopamine and acetylcholine levels in the rat medial prefrontal cortex: possible implications for the cognitive enhancing properties of EGb 761®. Int Psychogeriatr 24 (suppl 1):S25–S34, 2012 22784425

Kellermann AJ, Kloft C: Is there a risk of bleeding associated with standardized Ginkgo biloba extract therapy? A systematic review and meta-analysis. Pharmacotherapy 31(5):490–502, 2011 21923430

Kurz A, Van Baelen B: Ginkgo biloba compared with cholinesterase inhibitors in the treatment of dementia: a review based on meta-analyses by the Cochrane collaboration. Dement Geriatr Cogn Disord 18(2):217–226, 2004 15237280

Laver K, Dyer S, Whitehead C, et al: Interventions to delay functional decline in people with dementia: a systematic review of systematic reviews. BMJ Open 6(4):27, 2016

Laws KR, Sweetnam H, Kondel TK: Is Ginkgo biloba a cognitive enhancer in healthy individuals? A meta-analysis. Hum Psychopharmacol 27(6):527–533, 2012 23001963

Ponto LLB, Schultz SK: Ginkgo biloba extract: review of CNS effects. Ann Clin Psychiatry 15(2):109–119, 2003 12938868

Salehi B, Imani R, Mohammadi MR, et al: Ginkgo biloba for attention-deficit/hyperactivity disorder in children and adolescents: a double blind, randomized controlled trial. Prog Neuropsychopharmacol Biol Psychiatry 34(1):76–80, 2010 19815048

Shi C, Liu J, Wu F, et al: Ginkgo biloba extract in Alzheimer's disease: from action mechanisms to medical practice. Int J Mol Sci 11(1):107–123, 2010 20162004

Shinozuka K, Umegaki K, Kubota Y, et al: Feeding of Ginkgo biloba extract (GBE) enhances gene expression hepatic cytochrome P-450 and attenuates the hypotensive effects of nicardipine in rats. Life Sci 70(23):2783–2792, 2002 12269382

Stein C, Hopfeld J, Lau H, et al: Effects of Ginkgo biloba extract EGb 761, donepezil and their combination on central cholinergic function in aged rats. J Pharm Pharm Sci 18(4):634–646, 2015 26626253

Uebel-von Sandersleben H, Rothenberger A, Albrecht B, et al: Ginkgo biloba extract EGb 761® in children with ADHD. Z Kinder Jugendpsychiatr Psychother 42(5):337–347, 2014 25163996

Valli G, Giardina EG: Benefits, adverse effects and drug interactions of herbal therapies with cardiovascular effects. J Am Coll Cardiol 39(7):1083–1095, 2002 11923030

Williamson EM: Drug interactions between herbal and prescription medicines. Drug Saf 26(15):1075–1092, 2003 14640772

Woelk H, Arnoldt KH, Kieser M, et al: Ginkgo biloba special extract EGb 761 in generalized anxiety disorder and adjustment disorder with anxious mood: a randomized, double-blind, placebo-controlled trial. J Psychiatr Res 41(6):472–480, 2007 16808927

Yadav V, Narayanaswami P: Complementary and alternative medical therapies in multiple sclerosis—the American Academy of Neurology guidelines: a commentary. Clin Ther 36(12):1972–1978, 2014 25467189

CHAPTER 12

Kava (*Piper methysticum*) in the Treatment of Anxiety

Jerome Sarris, N.D., M.H.Sc., Ph.D.

When a child is born, kava is presented and for a lot of Pacifica people, they believe that if you fail to do that, the child's life is cursed.

Apo Aporosa

Kava (*Piper methysticum*) has been popularized in recent decades in Western countries, with dozens of kava products (of varying quality) being sold for anxiety and sleep disorders. Although compelling evidence supports the use of kava in the treatment of anxiety (Pittler and Ernst 2003), concerns about hepatotoxicity have led to its withdrawal or restriction in many countries since 2002 (Clouatre 2004). These concerns led to recent research on water-soluble extracts that use "noble" peeled rootstock (Savage et al. 2015). In this chapter, I discuss current evidence of kava's psychopharmacological activity, efficacy, safety issues, and clinical considerations and provide a case study.

Pharmacology and Anxiolytic Mechanisms of Action

The pharmacodynamic mechanism for kava's anxiolytic action is thought to be due to kavalactones, lipophilic constituents that are concentrated mainly in the rhizomes, roots, and root stems (Bilia et al. 2002; Raduege et al. 2004; Singh and Singh 2002). Collectively, 96% of the total pharmacological activity is attributed to six kavalactones: methysticin, dihydromethysticin, kavain, dihydrokavain, desmethoxyyangonin, and yangonin (Lebot and Lévesque 1989; Singh and Singh 2002). Preclinical studies document a wide spectrum of pharmacological effects, including anxiolytic (Kinzler et al. 1991), hypnotic (Wheatley 2001), anticonvulsant (Gleitz et al. 1996), antistress (Kinzler et al. 1991), muscle relaxant (Singh 1983), neuroprotective (Gleitz et al. 1996), sedative (Gleitz et al. 1996), and analgesic (Jamieson and Duffield 1990). Possible mechanisms mediating the actions of kava extract and specific kavalactones include blockade of voltage-gated sodium ion channels, reduced excitatory neurotransmitter release resulting from blockade of calcium ion channels, enhanced ligand binding to γ-aminobutyric acid (GABA) type A receptors, reversible inhibition of monoamine oxidase B, and reduced neuronal reuptake of norepinephrine and dopamine (Sarris et al. 2011a).

Evidence of Efficacy as an Anxiolytic

A Cochrane review of 11 rigorous randomized controlled trials (RCTs) that used kava (60–280 mg of kavalactones) for anxiety concluded that kava's anxiolytic activity exceeded that of placebo in all but one trial (Pittler and Ernst 2003). A meta-analysis contained in that review found that 7 of the RCTs showed that kava reduced anxiety significantly ($P=0.01$) more than placebo on the Hamilton Anxiety Scale (Ham-A), with a strong clinical effect. There were moderate differences in the type of extract, dosages, and types of anxiety conditions.

In a 6-week double-blind RCT (1-week placebo run-in, 1-week placebo run-out) of 75 patients with generalized anxiety disorder (58 randomly assigned to 120 mg/day of kavalactones, titrated to 240 mg for nonresponse), those given kava had significantly greater reduction in Ham-A scores ($P=0.046$; Cohen $d=0.62$) compared with placebo (Sarris et al. 2013a). Participants with moderate to severe DSM-IV-rated anxiety (American Psychiatric Association 1994) had greater treatment effect ($P=0.02$; $d=0.82$). No significant between-group differences were found for liver function tests, withdrawal, or perceived addiction; no significant adverse reactions occurred in the kava group (Sarris et al. 2013b). Interestingly, kava significantly increased female sexual drive compared with placebo on a subdomain of the Arizona Sexual Experience Scale (ASEX), with no negative effects in males. A highly significant correlation was seen between ASEX score reduction (improved sexual function and performance) and Ham-A score reduction in the whole sample ($P=0.009$). Of note, two GABA transporter polymorphisms were significantly ($P=0.021$; $P=0.046$) associated with reductions in Ham-A scores only in the kava group, suggesting that individual genetic differences may moderate anxiolytic effects of kava.

Safety, Side Effects, and Drug Interactions

Kava has not been noted to cause liver problems in traditional cultures where it is used only ceremonially. In 2002, kava was withdrawn from the market by the European Union in response to dozens of reported cases of kava-associated liver toxicity. In many reports, it was unclear whether kava was responsible for the toxic effects on the liver, particularly because many cases involved concomitant ingestion of other compounds with potential hepatotoxicity, and in some cases, a higher-than-recommended dose was used (Coulter and World Health Organization 2007). In most cases, formulations that included nontraditional acetone or ethanol extracts were ingested. Potential factors responsible for hepatotoxic effects include hepatic insufficiency for metabolizing kavalactones, preparations low in glutathione, use of aerial parts or root peelings (higher in alkaloids), acetonic or ethanolic extraction, poor storage or manufacture, or incorrect cultivar (specific cultivated variety; medicinal, tudei, or wichmanni varieties) (Sarris et al. 2011b). In vitro studies of kava extract and kavalactones found significant inhibition of cytochrome P450 (CYP) enzymes (CYP1A2, CYP2C9, CYP2C19, CYP2E1, CYP2D6, CYP3A4, and CYP4A9/11) involved in metabolism of many drugs, but this has not been confirmed in human trials (Gerbarg and Brown 2015). Taking kava with alcohol, benzodiazepines, or muscle relaxants can result in coma (Almeida and Grimsley 1996). Caution should be used in patients taking any medications.

Clinical Considerations

Because quality can affect efficacy and safety, it is critical to prescribe standardized kava formulations containing traditional water-soluble rhizome extracts of a "noble" cultivar (i.e., higher in kavain and lower in dihydromethysticin). The usual dose for standardized (10%–15% kavalactones per dry weight) preparations is between 60 and 120 mg kavalactones twice per day (Sarris et al. 2011a). Pharmaceutical-grade products are strongly recommended (although they may sometimes be challenging to identify). For long-term use, periodic liver function tests are recommended to assess potential liver inflammation. Liver dysfunction or chronic alcohol use contraindicates the use of kava.

Kava is most commonly used as an anxiolytic. It can also be helpful in managing benzodiazepam withdrawal, as the following case illustrates.

> A 28-year-old man who had chronic anxiety for several years was diagnosed with generalized anxiety disorder; medical causes were ruled out. Previously, he was nonadherent to antidepressant medication because of side effects. Over the past 6 months, his anxiety was treated with alprazolam (1 mg) as needed (usually twice per day). Recent work stress was causing insomnia. Although his anxiety was manageable, he complained of feeling tired from alprazolam and reported impaired mental function (poor memory, reduced concentration, and occasional feelings of confusion). Consequently, he wanted to stop taking alprazolam and try a natural option. He stated that he would consider psychological therapy if this failed but preferred taking tablets.

The initial goal is to reduce anxiety as quickly as possible and gradually taper off benzodiazepines. This can be achieved by combining an anxiolytic herbal or nutrient with lifestyle changes, ideally in concert with psychological therapy. GABAergic effects of kava can reduce anxiety and may reduce symptoms of benzodiazepine withdrawal. In a double-blind RCT of 40 patients during benzodiazepine taper, kava extract WS 1490 reduced Ham-A score ($P<0.01$) and withdrawal symptoms ($P<0.002$)

significantly more than did placebo (Malsch and Kieser 2001). Insomnia, common in anxiety disorders, may adversely affect neuroendocrine balance and exacerbate anxiety. Treating insomnia should lessen anxiety; treating anxiety can improve sleep. 5-Hydroxytryptophan (5-HTP, a serotonin precursor) and melatonin (see Chapter 19, "Melatonin and Melatonin Analogs for Psychiatric Disorders") can ameliorate insomnia. Although it may not be possible to alleviate work stress, meditation, mindfulness, and psychological treatment can help modify work stress response.

Lifestyle advice to reduce perceived stress and anxiety should focus on balancing meaningful work, adequate rest and sleep, appropriate exercise, positive social interactions, and pleasurable hobbies (Sarris et al. 2012). Although not rigorously evaluated, dietary programs emphasizing a low glycemic index diet, rich in protein and low in refined carbohydrates, may stabilize blood sugar levels, which may reduce fight-or-flight responses. Caffeine should be decreased or eliminated to reduce anxiety and insomnia (Broderick and Benjamin 2004). Sleep hygiene is advised (Stepanski and Wyatt 2003): sleep restriction, reduction of light exposure prior to sleep and increased morning sunlight, and avoidance of daytime naps and of stimulation before sleep (smoking, caffeine, stimulating technology).

In the case example, the patient's anxiety may "rebound" in the short term as benzodiazepines are withdrawn. Kava is expected to mitigate this, but benzodiazepines must be gradually tapered over weeks, possibly months (e.g., reducing the dose by 15% every 2 weeks), to avoid severe rebound anxiety. After 2 weeks of kava, if benefit is minimal, other plant-based medicines and psychological interventions may help manage external triggers of the anxiety. Although insomnia may worsen during medication withdrawal, sleep hygiene techniques, kava, 5-HTP, or melatonin may be helpful.

KEY POINTS

- The anxiolytic effects of kava have been attributed to kavalactones.

- The use of high-quality, preferably pharmaceutical-quality, kava potentially reduces risks of adverse reactions.

- Kava is contraindicated in patients with abnormal liver function, chronic alcohol use, or concomitant use of benzodiazepines.

- Kava can be beneficial for anxiety, insomnia, and benzodiazepine withdrawal.

References

Almeida JC, Grimsley EW: Coma from the health food store: interaction between kava and alprazolam. Ann Intern Med 125(11):940–941, 1996 8967683

American Psychiatric Association: Diagnostic and Statistical Manual of Mental Disorders, 4th Edition. Washington, DC, American Psychiatric Association, 1994

Bilia AR, Gallon S, Vincieri FF: Kava-kava and anxiety: growing knowledge about the efficacy and safety. Life Sci 70(22):2581–2597, 2002 12269386

Broderick P, Benjamin AB: Caffeine and psychiatric symptoms: a review. J Okla State Med Assoc 97(12):538–542, 2004 15732884

Clouatre DL: Kava kava: examining new reports of toxicity. Toxicol Lett 150(1):85–96, 2004 15068826

Coulter DL; World Health Organization: Assessment of the Risk of Hepatotoxicity With Kava Products. Geneva, Switzerland, World Health Organization, 2007

Gerbarg PL, Brown RP: Therapeutic nutrients, herbs, and hormones, in Psychiatric Care of the Medical Patient, 3rd Edition. Edited by Fogel B, Greenberg D. New York, Oxford University Press, 2015, pp 545–608

Gleitz J, Tosch C, Beile A, et al: The protective action of tetrodotoxin and (+/–)-kavain on anaerobic glycolysis, ATP content and intracellular Na+ and Ca2+ of anoxic brain vesicles. Neuropharmacology 35(12):1743–1752, 1996 9076753

Jamieson DD, Duffield PH: The antinociceptive actions of kava components in mice. Clin Exp Pharmacol Physiol 17(7):495–507, 1990 2401103

Kinzler E, Krömer J, Lehmann E: Effect of a special kava extract in patients with anxiety-, tension-, and excitation states of non-psychotic genesis: double blind study with placebos over 4 weeks [in German]. Arzneimittelforschung 41(6):584–588, 1991 1930344

Lebot V, Lévesque J: The origin and distribution of kava (Piper methysticum Forst. f. and Piper wichmannii C. DC., Piperaceae): a phytochemical approach. Allertonia 5(2):223–280, 1989

Malsch U, Kieser M: Efficacy of kava-kava in the treatment of non-psychotic anxiety, following pretreatment with benzodiazepines. Psychopharmacology (Berl) 157(3):277–283, 2001 11605083

Pittler MH, Ernst E: Kava extract for treating anxiety. Cochrane Database Syst Rev (1):CD003383, 2003 12535473

Raduege KM, Kleshinski JF, Ryckman JV, et al: Anesthetic considerations of the herbal, kava. J Clin Anesth 16(4):305–311, 2004 15261327

Sarris J, LaPorte E, Schweitzer I: Kava: a comprehensive review of efficacy, safety, and psychopharmacology. Aust N Z J Psychiatry 45(1):27–35, 2011a 21073405

Sarris J, Teschke R, Stough C, et al: Re-introduction of kava (Piper methysticum) to the EU: is there a way forward? Planta Med 77(2):107–110, 2011b 20814850

Sarris J, Moylan S, Camfield DA, et al: Complementary medicine, exercise, meditation, diet, and lifestyle modification for anxiety disorders: a review of current evidence. Evid Based Complement Alternat Med 2012:809653, 2012 22969831

Sarris J, Stough C, Bousman CA, et al: Kava in the treatment of generalized anxiety disorder: a double-blind, randomized, placebo-controlled study. J Clin Psychopharmacol 33(5):643–648, 2013a 23635869

Sarris J, Stough C, Teschke R, et al: Kava for the treatment of generalized anxiety disorder RCT: analysis of adverse reactions, liver function, addiction, and sexual effects. Phytother Res 27(11):1723–1728, 2013b 23348842

Savage KM, Stough CK, Byrne GJ, et al: Kava for the treatment of generalised anxiety disorder (K-GAD): study protocol for a randomised controlled trial. Trials 16(1):493, 2015 26527536

Singh YN: Effects of kava on neuromuscular transmission and muscle contractility. J Ethnopharmacol 7(3):267–276, 1983 6308355

Singh YN, Singh NN: Therapeutic potential of kava in the treatment of anxiety disorders. CNS Drugs 16(11):731–743, 2002 12383029

Stepanski EJ, Wyatt JK: Use of sleep hygiene in the treatment of insomnia. Sleep Med Rev 7(3):215–225, 2003 12927121

Wheatley D: Stress-induced insomnia treated with kava and valerian: singly and in combination. Hum Psychopharmacol 16(4):353–356, 2001 12404572

CHAPTER 13

Panax ginseng and American Ginseng in Psychiatric Practice

Lila Massoumi, M.D., ABIHM

Panax ginseng

Properties of *Panax ginseng*

Panax ginseng (Asian ginseng, Korean ginseng, true ginseng) has been used in traditional Chinese medicine for thousands of years as an adaptogen to increase resistance to physical or mental stress, illness, and aging. *Panax* derives from Greek (*pan*—all, *axos*—cure), meaning "all-healing." *Ginseng* translates from the Chinese ren shen, which means "man root." Literally translated, *Panax ginseng* means "all-healing man root." Among the species of *Panax* genus, five are used medicinally, *P. ginseng* being the most common and American ginseng (*Panax quinquefolius*) the second most common (see Table 13–1). Other invigorating herbs colloquially called "ginsengs" that are not within the *Panax* genus are ashwagandha, Indian ginseng; tongkat ali, Malaysian ginseng; maca, Peruvian ginseng; Southern ginseng; suma, Brazilian ginseng; Kerala ginseng; Thai ginseng; Nam ginseng; and Siberian ginseng.

The bioactive molecules unique to ginseng species are ginsenosides (triterpene saponins). Some ginsenosides are shared by several *Panax* species, whereas others are unique to a specific species. Heat-treated *P. ginseng* contains unique bioactives (e.g., ginsenosides Rh2 and Rg3) and is called Korean red ginseng because heating turns the white powder red.

TABLE 13–1.   Medicinal plants within the *Panax* genus

Common name	Botanical name	Chinese (Pinyin) name
Panax ginseng, true ginseng, Asian ginseng, Korean ginseng, Chinese ginseng, mountain ginseng, red ginseng (heated), white ginseng (sun-dried)	*Panax ginseng*	Ren shen
American ginseng	*Panax quinquefolius*	Xi yang shen
Vietnamese ginseng	*Panax vietnamensis*	Yue nan ren shen, ou mei san qi
Japanese ginseng	*Panax japonicus*	Da ye san qi, ri ben ren shen, zhu jie shen, xia ye zhu jie shen, xia ye jia ren shen
Pseudoginseng	*Panax notoginseng*	San qi

The highest concentration of ginsenosides is in the main rhizome root, which is ground into a medicinal powder. Plants intended for medicinal use must be grown for more than 4 years to increase ginsenoside potency (Smith et al. 2014). As with all herbal preparations, the concentrations of bioactives within a species can vary between batches because of genetic variations, environmental conditions, time of harvest, and processing techniques. Some manufacturers produce standardized products similar to pharmaceutical quality, such as G115, a *P. ginseng* extract marketed as Ginsana (Pharmaton SA, Bioggio, Switzerland) containing 4% ginsenosides. Despite a long medicinal history and the veneration for *P. ginseng*, most research has been on animal models and in vitro. Clinical trials focus mainly on acute dosing, and some use daily doses for up to 3 months. A 2009 Cochrane review of ginseng for cognition in healthy adults and those with mild cognitive impairment or dementia concluded that the clinical and preclinical studies taken together suggest that a single 200–400 mg dose of *P. ginseng* improves at least one cognitive domain (e.g., quality of memory, secondary memory, speed of attention), although no single aspect of cognition has been improved consistently across studies (Geng et al. 2010).

In an 8-week double-blind, randomized placebo-controlled trial (DBRPCT) of 70 drug-free children ages 6–15 years with mild to moderate attention-deficit/hyperactivity disorder and evidence of chronic stress (morning cortisol<10 ng/mL), the treatment group who received 1 g of concentrated Korean red ginseng extract showed improvements in attention and hyperactivity, as well as a decrease in the theta-to-beta ratio on electroencephalogram (i.e., increased beta waves for increased concentration) (Ko et al. 2014). The effect size was medium. No adverse events and no change in cortisol or dehydroepiandrosterone levels occurred.

P. ginseng may have a greater effect size, or greater chance of an effect, in patients who are older or have greater infirmity. For example, some clinical evidence shows that *P. ginseng* improves cognition in healthy middle-aged people but not in healthy young adults (Forgo et al. 1981; Reay et al. 2005, 2006, 2010; Sorensen and Sonne 1996). In more neurologically compromised states (e.g., Alzheimer's disease, Parkinson's disease, ischemic stroke), the beneficial effects may be achieved through disease-modifying pathways that indirectly affect cognition—for example, reducing inflammation or neurotoxicity—and therefore may not translate into cognitive benefits in healthy subjects. Another mechanism attributed to ginseng is increased endothelial nitric oxide (via decreased nitric oxide degradation), which dilates blood vessel walls, increasing brain perfusion.

Similarly, for physical energy and fatigue, *P. ginseng* has a greater effect size or chance of effect in patients who are older or have greater infirmity. Five DBRPCTs on healthy athletes showed that a single 200-mg dose of *P. ginseng* taken 1 hour prior to performance, or daily for up to 8 weeks, did not improve aerobic performance (Allen et al. 1998; Engels and Wirth 1997; Engels et al. 2003; Kulaputana et al. 2007; Oh et al. 2010). However, in a 4-week DBRPCT of 90 adults with idiopathic chronic fatigue, those who took *P. ginseng* 1 g twice a day for 4 weeks had a reduction in some symptoms of fatigue, with a small effect size (Kim et al. 2013). In a 3-month DBRPCT of 52 female patients with fatigue from relapsing-remitting multiple sclerosis, those taking *P. ginseng* 250 mg twice a day for 3 months had a 75% decrease in mental fatigue and reported improved quality of life, with an overall medium effect size (Etemadifar et al. 2013). In cancer-related fatigue, an open-label study showed that *P. ginseng* taken daily for 4 weeks improved energy, quality of life, appetite, and nighttime sleep (Yennurajalingam et al. 2015). Proposed mechanisms included hypothalamic-pituitary-adrenal (HPA) axis regulation and modulation of inflammatory cytokines.

Increased endothelial nitric oxide (via decreased nitric oxide degradation) with vasodilation also has been linked to enhanced tumescence and improved erectile function. A meta-analysis of six DBRPCTs evaluating *P. ginseng* for erectile dysfunction (total $N=349$) concluded that taking *P. ginseng* (untreated or in the heated Korean red ginseng form) 1,000–1,350 mg twice a day for 8 weeks improved sexual function in men with erectile dysfunction ($P<0.001$), with a medium to large effect size (Jang et al. 2008). Subgroup analyses found beneficial effects for psychogenic erectile dysfunction ($N=135$; $P=0.001$).

Korean red ginseng may improve sexual function in menopausal women. In a crossover DBRPCT, 32 menopausal women ages 40–60 years who had no menses for 1 year were randomly assigned to receive placebo or Korean red ginseng 1,000 mg three times a day for 8 weeks (Oh et al. 2010). After a 2-week washout period, patients were switched to the other treatment arm for an additional 8 weeks. Compared with placebo, 28 of the 32 women reported improved sexual arousal while taking ginseng (Female Sexual Function Index score, $P=0.006$; Global Assessment Questionnaire, $P=0.046$). Two cases of vaginal bleeding were associated with ginseng use, possibly as a result of estrogenic effects.

Panax ginseng in Clinical Practice

P. ginseng should be given in divided doses (two or three times a day) for a daily total of 2–3 g of the dried plant or 300–800 mg of a supplement extract standardized to 4%–7% ginsenosides (Yennurajalingam et al. 2015). The half-life of many ginsenosides in pharmacokinetic studies is short (0.2–18 hours), and bioavailability is low (Smith et al. 2014). A limitation in the clinical studies is that durations were generally no longer than 3 months, and thus, the safety of long-term use of *P. ginseng* beyond 3 months has not been established. In traditional Chinese and modern-day use, it is not uncommon for people to take ginseng over many years.

In a 2012 review of 40 studies, no serious adverse events were reported (Shergis et al. 2013). Infrequent side effects included insomnia, palpitations, headache, nausea, and vertigo. There have been reports of high doses causing agitation, irritability, or high blood pressure. *P. ginseng* may have estrogenic effects, but the evidence is conflicting. A few case reports of breast tenderness, postmenopausal vaginal bleeding, and menstrual abnormalities have been associated with *P. ginseng*. Some adolescent boys and others who took megadoses to build strength and endurance experienced estrogen-like effects, such as painful swelling of the breasts. Women with hormone-sensitive conditions (e.g., endometriosis; fibroids; cancer of the breast, uterus, or ovaries) should avoid taking *Panax* (Lee et al. 2003). Safety has not been established during pregnancy or breast-feeding, but in Asia, the use of this herb in traditional Chinese medicine formulas is common throughout pregnancy and lactation (Lakshmi et al. 2011). *P. ginseng* does not appear to interact with warfarin. However, it lowers alcohol levels by 35% in people who are drinking alcohol, possibly by increasing activity of alcohol and aldehyde dehydrogenase.

American Ginseng

Properties of American Ginseng

American ginseng (*Panax quinquefolius*; xi yang shen) grows mainly in North America, with much of it produced in Ontario, Canada. Wild American ginseng is so extensively sought that it has been declared an endangered species in some states in the United States. Compared with *P. ginseng*, American ginseng is gentler, less stimulating, and less likely to cause agitation or headaches. In traditional Chinese medicine, American ginseng is used to promote "yin" energy (feminine, mild, and cold), whereas *P. ginseng* is used to increase "yang" energy (masculine, strong, and hot). The two species share some ginsenosides, but American ginseng has only 19 ginsenoside types compared with 38 in *P. ginseng*. Patented extracts of American ginseng include Cereboost (Naturex, Avignon, France; standardized to 10.65% ginsenosides) and CNT 2000 (Chai-Na-Ta Corp., Langley, British Columbia, Canada).

As with *P. ginseng*, single-dose American ginseng may improve cognition. In a crossover DBRPCT of 32 healthy young adults ages 18–40 years, participants given a single dose of 100, 200, or 400 mg American ginseng (Cereboost, standardized to 10.65% ginsenosides) 1–6 hours prior to cognitive testing had significantly improved working memory at all doses ($P<0.05$) (Scholey et al. 2010). In a crossover DBRPCT of 52 healthy middle-aged adults ages 40–60 years, participants given a single 200-mg dose of Cereboost had improved working memory (Cognitive Drug Research battery; $P<0.05$) after 3 hours (Ossoukhova et al. 2015).

In a 4-week DBRPCT, daily 100-mg doses of American ginseng (HT-1001, Afexa Life Sciences, Edmonton, Alberta, Canada) were given to 64 patients with schizophrenia who were stable (defined as no change in symptoms over the previous 3 months)

(Chen and Hui 2012). The treatment group showed significant improvement in visual working memory ($P<0.006$) but not in other cognitive domains. One important finding was that the treatment group showed significant reduction in medication-induced extrapyramidal side effects, whereas the placebo group did not.

American Ginseng in Clinical Practice

American ginseng has few side effects. Some animal and in vitro studies suggest possible estrogenic activity, but the clinical significance in humans is unclear. As with other adaptogens, American ginseng has mild hypoglycemic effects. Also, it decreases international normalized ratio and reduces the effectiveness of warfarin.

KEY POINTS

- *Panax ginseng* used daily (up to 3 months) can reduce fatigue and improve physical energy in patients who are older or infirm.

- Single-dose *P. ginseng* may improve cognition, although no single aspect of cognition has consistently improved across studies.

- *P. ginseng* (untreated or heated) can improve sexual function in men, and the heated form may improve sexual function in postmenopausal women.

- The safety of *P. ginseng* use beyond 3 months has not been established.

- American ginseng is gentler and less stimulating than *P. ginseng*.

- Like *P. ginseng*, single-dose American ginseng may improve cognition.

References

Allen JD, McLung J, Nelson AG, Welsch M: Ginseng supplementation does not enhance healthy young adults' peak aerobic exercise performance. J Am Coll Nutr 17(5):462–466, 1998 9791844

Chen EY, Hui CL: HT1001, a proprietary North American ginseng extract, improves working memory in schizophrenia: a double-blind, placebo-controlled study. Phytother Res 26(8):1166–1172, 2012 22213250

Engels HJ, Wirth JC: No ergogenic effects of ginseng (Panax ginseng C.A. Meyer) during graded maximal aerobic exercise. J Am Diet Assoc 97(10):1110–1115, 1997 9336557

Engels HJ, Fahlman MM, Wirth JC: Effects of ginseng on secretory IgA, performance, and recovery from interval exercise. Med Sci Sports Exerc 35(4):690–696, 2003 12673155

Etemadifar M, Sayahi F, Abtahi SH, et al: Ginseng in the treatment of fatigue in multiple sclerosis: a randomized, placebo-controlled, double-blind pilot study. Int J Neurosci 123(7):480–486, 2014 23301896

Forgo I, Kayasseh L, Staub JJ: Effect of a standardized ginseng extract on general well-being, reaction time, lung function and gonadal hormones [in German]. Med Welt 32(19):751–756, 1981 7231139

Geng J, Dong J, Ni H, et al: Ginseng for cognition. Cochrane Database of Systematic Reviews 2014 Issue 12. Art. No.: CD007769. DOI: 10.1002/14651858.CD007769.pub2

Jang DJ, Lee MS, Shin BC, et al: Red ginseng for treating erectile dysfunction: a systematic review. Br J Clin Pharmacol 66(4):444–450, 2008 18754850

Kim HG, Cho JH, Yoo SR, et al: Ginseng in the treatment of fatigue in multiple sclerosis: a randomized, placebo-controlled, double-blind pilot study. Int J Neurosci 123(7):480–486, 2014 23301896

Ko HJ, Kim I, Kim JB, et al: Antifatigue effects of Panax ginseng C.A. Meyer: a randomised, double-blind, placebo-controlled trial. PLoS One 8(4):e61271, 2013 23613825

Kulaputana O, Thanakomsirichot S, Anomasiri W: Single doses of Panax ginseng (G115) reduce blood glucose levels and improve cognitive performance during sustained mental activity. J Med Assoc Thai 90(6):1172–1179, 2007 17624213

Lakshmi T, Roy A, Geetha RV: Panax ginseng—a universal panacea in the herbal medicine with diverse pharmacological spectrum—a review. Asian J Pharm Clin Res 4:14–18, 2011

Lee YJ, Jin YR, Lim WC, et al: Ginsenoside-Rb1 acts as a weak phytoestrogen in MCF-7 human breast cancer cells. Arch Pharm Res 26(1):58–63, 2003 12568360

Oh KJ, Chae MJ, Lee HS, et al: Effects of Korean red ginseng on sexual arousal in menopausal women: placebo-controlled, double-blind crossover clinical study. J Sex Med 7(4 Pt 1):1469–1477, 2010 20141583

Ossoukhova A, Owen L, Savage K, et al: Improved working memory performance following administration of a single dose of American ginseng (Panax quinquefolius L.) to healthy middle-age adults. Hum Psychopharmacol 30(2):108–122, 2015 25778987

Ping FW, Keong CC, Bandyopadhyay A: Effects of acute supplementation of Panax ginseng on endurance running in a hot and humid environment. J Hum Ergol (Tokyo) 40(1–2):63–72, 2011 25665208

Reay JL, Kennedy DO, Scholey AB: Single doses of Panax ginseng (G115) reduce blood glucose levels and improve cognitive performance during sustained mental activity. J Psychopharmacol 19(4):357–365, 2005 15982290

Reay JL, Kennedy DO, Scholey AB: Effects of Panax ginseng, consumed with and without glucose, on blood glucose levels and cognitive performance during sustained 'mentally demanding' tasks. J Psychopharmacol 20(6):771–781, 2006 16401645

Reay JL, Kennedy DO, Scholey AB: Panax ginseng (G115) improves aspects of working memory performance and subjective ratings of calmness in healthy young adults. Hum Psychopharmacol 25(6):462–471, 2010 20737519

Scholey A, Ossoukhova A, Owen L, et al: Effects of American ginseng (Panax quinquefolius) on neurocognitive function: an acute, randomised, double-blind, placebo-controlled, crossover study. Psychopharmacology (Berl) 212(3):345–356, 2010 20676609

Shergis JL, Zhang AL, Zhou W, Xue CC: Panax ginseng in randomised controlled trials: a systematic review. Phytother Res 27(7):949–965, 2013 22969004

Smith I, Williamson EM, Putnam S, et al: Effects and mechanisms of ginseng and ginsenosides on cognition. Nutr Rev 72(5):319–333, 2014 24666107

Sorensen H, Sonne J: A double-masked study of the effects of ginseng on cognitive functions. Curr Ther Res 57:959–968, 1996

Yennurajalingam S, Reddy A, Tannir NM, et al: High-dose Asian ginseng (Panax ginseng) for cancer-related fatigue: a preliminary report. Integr Cancer Ther 14(5):419–427, 2015 25873296

CHAPTER 14

Theanine, Lavender, Lemon Balm, and Chamomile

Lila Massoumi, M.D., ABIHM

Patricia L. Gerbarg, M.D.

I judge that the flowers of lavender quilted in a cappe and dayly worn are good for all diseases of the head that come of a cold cause and that they comfort the braine very well.

William Turner, M.A., "Herbal," 1551

L-Theanine

L-Theanine is a non-protein-forming, nonessential amino acid found almost exclusively in the tea plant *Camellia sinensis*. A well-standardized form of L-theanine supplementation used in many studies is Suntheanine (Taiyo International, Tokyo, Japan). In healthy subjects already in a relaxed state, L-theanine attenuates sympathetic nervous system activation, reduces heart rate, reduces salivary immunoglobulin A, and increases alpha brain waves, while having no effect on theta or delta waves (Nobre et al. 2008). L-Theanine, a nonsedating anxiolytic, is well suited for daytime use.

Despite the absence of sedative effects per se, L-theanine has been shown to improve sleep quality in individuals *not* experiencing insomnia, presumably through anxiolysis. In a 10-week double-blind, randomized placebo-controlled trial (DBRPCT) of 93 boys with attention-deficit/hyperactivity disorder (27 of whom were taking stimulants), those who took L-theanine (as Suntheanine) 200 mg twice per day showed significantly improved sleep quality by actigraphic watch data compared with those in the placebo group ($P<0.05$) (Lyon et al. 2011).

In an 8-week DBRPCT of 60 patients with schizophrenia or schizoaffective disorder, L-theanine 200 mg twice per day augmented antipsychotic therapy by decreasing anxiety and activation, with modest to moderate effect size (ES; 0.09–0.39) (Cohen's *d*), starting at week 2 and continuing to study's end (Ritsner et al. 2011).

L-Theanine taken orally results in peak serum levels in 30 minutes to 2 hours, with duration of effect of 5–8 hours. In clinical practice, it can be started at 200 mg one to three times per day, up to a maximum of 1,200 mg total daily. No adverse effects from L-theanine were reported in any of the studies. Animal research indicates that L-theanine is remarkably safe, even at very high doses, and shows no carcinogenicity (negative Ames test) (Rao et al. 2015).

English Lavender (*Lavandula angustifolia*)

Lavender (*Lavandula angustifolia*), from Latin *lavare* (meaning "to wash"), was used in ancient Greece, Rome, and Persia as soap or perfume. Lavender essential oil can be taken by mouth, by inhalation, or transdermally. Essential oil, the volatile or fragrant component of the plant, is extracted by steam distillation (without chemical solvents). Essential oils contain bioactive compounds that vary depending on numerous factors, including plant subspecies, season of harvest, and soil and weather conditions. Despite these variations, some manufacturers produce standardized essential oils similar to pharmaceutical quality, such as Silexan (Lasea, Dr. Willmar Schwabe GmbH & Co KG, Karlsruhe, Germany), which contains 80 mg of lavender essential oil per capsule (standardized 20%–45% linalool and 25%–46% linalyl acetate). Preliminary evidence suggests that lavender helps anxiety. In a DBRPCT, 539 adults with generalized anxiety disorder received Silexan 80 mg, Silexan 160 mg, paroxetine 20 mg, or placebo once daily for 10 weeks (Kasper et al. 2014). Silexan 160 mg and 80 mg were superior to placebo in reducing scores on the Hamilton Anxiety Scale (Ham-A; $P<0.01$), whereas paroxetine was not ($P=0.10$). Silexan was better tolerated than paroxetine and did not differ from placebo in adverse events. In a double-blind, randomized controlled trial, 170 patients with anxiety-related restlessness and disturbed sleep (Ham-A score≥18) received Silexan 80 mg or placebo once daily for 10 weeks (Kasper et al. 2015). Silexan reduced scores on the Ham-A more than did placebo ($P=0.04$).

Most studies on lavender have examined its effects when administered as aromatherapy, applied directly to the patient's skin or clothing or via a nearby diffuser. However, the term *aromatherapy* may be a misnomer because evidence suggests that lavender oil applied topically (Jäger et al. 1992) or via inhalation (Jäger et al. 1996) results in systemic absorption. Additionally, a study in mice with laboratory-induced anosmia showed that inhaled lavender oil resulted in anxiolysis, suggesting that olfactory stimulation may be unnecessary (Chioca et al. 2013). The quality of studies on aromatherapy is inferior because study participants with intact olfaction detect aromas and therefore cannot be blinded. Lavender aromatherapy has been studied for agitation in dementia, but conflicting results preclude any firm conclusions.

Lavender aromatherapy in open-label and case-control studies has been shown to improve sleep in the nonpsychiatric population. However, a review and meta-analysis of 12 Korean studies of lavender (alone or in combination with other essential oils) found the effect size of aromatherapy on sleep (ES=0.372; 95% confidence interval=0.054–0.175; $P<0.001$) to be less than that of music therapy for sleep (ES=0.424) (Hwang and Shin 2015). Moreover, lavender aromatherapy was less effective for sleep than it was for anxiety (ES=0.603) and stress (ES=0.529). Lavender's helpfulness in sleep is presumably through anxiolysis because lavender does not appear to be sedating (Kasper et al. 2015).

The most common side effects of Silexan are nausea and dyspepsia. Silexan does not cause dependency or withdrawal (Woelk and Schläfke 2010). Skin contact with lavender oil (either fresh oil or auto-oxidized constituents that develop on prolonged air exposure) can cause dermatitis. No clinically relevant effects on cytochrome P450 (CYP) 1A2, CYP2C9, CYP2C19, CYP2D6, or CYP3A4 enzymes were found in a crossover drug interaction study of Silexan 160 mg or placebo administered once daily for 11 days to 16 participants (Doroshyenko et al. 2013).

Lemon Balm (*Melissa officinalis*)

Lemon balm (*Melissa officinalis*), a lemon-scented herb native to southern Europe, was used in ancient Greece and Rome for calmness and to improve cognitive functioning. Like lavender, it is taken either orally or as aromatherapy. As monotherapy, lemon balm's greatest utility in the psychiatric population may be for behavioral disturbances of dementia, such as pacing, restlessness, wandering, irritability, or aggression. No safe and effective medications for agitation in dementia are currently available: benzodiazepines and antihistamines can exacerbate confusion and delirium, and antipsychotics increase risks of cerebrovascular events, diabetes, and tardive dyskinesia. Additionally, neuroleptic treatment of agitation of dementia is associated with increased social withdrawal and decreased engagement in constructive activities.

In a single-blind, placebo-controlled trial in 72 patients with severe dementia, the addition of lemon balm (G. Baldwin & Co., London, UK) aromatherapy, applied to arms and face twice daily, to patients' standard medications resulted in a 30% or greater reduction of agitation in 60% of the treatment group compared with 14% of the placebo (sunflower oil) group (Ballard et al. 2002). In addition, the treatment group had a significant reduction in time spent socially withdrawn ($P=0.005$) and a significant increase in time engaged in constructive activities ($P=0.001$). In a DBRPCT, 42 patients with mild to moderate Alzheimer's disease were taken off their psychotropic medications and given an oral lemon balm extract (in 45% alcohol, standardized to at least 500 µg citral/mL) or placebo over a 4-month period (Akhondzadeh et al. 2003). Subjects given lemon balm showed significant improvements in cognitive function (Alzheimer's Disease Assessment Scale: $F_1=6.93$; $P=0.01$; Clinical Dementia Rating Scale: $F_1=16.87$; $P<0.001$) compared with placebo. The treatment group also experienced significantly less agitation ($P=0.03$).

All studies of lemon balm in dementia showed adverse effects to be equivalent to those of placebo. Therefore, lemon balm may be considered as a treatment for agitation in dementia, particularly because aromatherapy is easier for geriatric patients who may have difficulty swallowing pills. Patients with alcohol use–related disorders should not be given an herbal tincture in alcohol because it could trigger a relapse to alcohol abuse.

Most studies of lemon balm have used it in combination with other calming herbs. Herbs administered together may confer synergistic effects. For example, an in vitro study of rat cortical cultures found that a 50:50 mixture of lemon balm and lavender oil inhibited flunitrazepam binding, whereas the individual oils had no significant effect (Huang et al. 2008). In a 2-week DBRPCT of 182 patients with somatoform disorder (somatization disorder or undifferentiated somatoform disorder), a fixed herbal formulation of lemon balm, valerian, passionflower, and butterbur (Ze 185; Relaxane, Max Zeller Söhne AG, Romanshorn, Switzerland) decreased anxiety (Visual Analog Scale) by 50% or more in 71% of the treatment group, compared with 17% of the placebo group (P=0.001), and reduced depression (Beck Depression Inventory) by 50% or more in 60% of the treatment group, compared with 13% of the placebo group (P=0.001) (Melzer et al. 2009).

Chamomile (*Matricaria recutita*)

Chamomile generally refers to German chamomile (*Matricaria recutita*). Used for millennia as a sleep aid, chamomile is now the most widely used herb for insomnia (Sánchez-Ortuño et al. 2009). As of this writing, the only high-quality human double-blind, randomized controlled trial evaluating chamomile for sleep did not find it helpful (Zick et al. 2011). One double-blind, randomized controlled trial found chamomile (standardized to 1.2% apigenin) mildly helpful for generalized anxiety disorder (Amsterdam et al. 2009). As a member of the ragweed family, chamomile can cause allergic reactions in anyone with ragweed allergy (as much as 20% of the population). Considering the limited research on chamomile, its utility in psychiatric patients is uncertain.

KEY POINTS

- L-Theanine 200 mg once or twice per day has a mild relaxing effect and is suitable for daytime use. It may improve sleep quality via anxiolysis.

- Lavender oil 80 mg taken orally once or twice per day is moderately helpful for anxiety, such as generalized anxiety disorder. Lavender aromatherapy is modestly helpful for sleep.

- Lemon balm taken orally or as aromatherapy is a reasonable treatment for agitation of dementia, with fewer adverse effects compared with current medications.

- The common use of chamomile for sleep far exceeds the evidence base.

References

Akhondzadeh S, Noroozian M, Mohammadi M, et al: Melissa officinalis extract in the treatment of patients with mild to moderate Alzheimer's disease: a double blind, randomised, placebo controlled trial. J Neurol Neurosurg Psychiatry 74(7):863–866, 2003 12810768

Amsterdam JD, Li Y, Soeller I, et al: A randomized, double-blind, placebo-controlled trial of oral Matricaria recutita (chamomile) extract therapy for generalized anxiety disorder. J Clin Psychopharmacol 29(4):378–382, 2009 19593179

Ballard CG, O'Brien JT, Reichelt K, et al: Aromatherapy as a safe and effective treatment for the management of agitation in severe dementia: the results of a double-blind, placebo-controlled trial with Melissa. J Clin Psychiatry 63(7):553–558, 2002 12143909

Chioca LR, Antunes VD, Ferro MM, et al: Anosmia does not impair the anxiolytic-like effect of lavender essential oil inhalation in mice. Life Sci 92(20–21):971–975, 2013 23567808

Doroshyenko O, Rokitta D, Zadoyan G, et al: Drug cocktail interaction study on the effect of the orally administered lavender oil preparation Silexan on cytochrome P450 enzymes in healthy volunteers. Drug Metab Dispos 41(5):987–993, 2013 23401474

Huang L, Abuhamdah S, Howes MJ, et al: Pharmacological profile of essential oils derived from Lavandula angustifolia and Melissa officinalis with anti-agitation properties: focus on ligand-gated channels. J Pharm Pharmacol 60(11):1515–1522, 2008 18957173

Hwang E, Shin S: The effects of aromatherapy on sleep improvement: a systematic literature review and meta-analysis. J Altern Complement Med 21(2):61–68, 2015 25584799

Jäger W, Buchbauer G, Jirovetz L, et al: Percutaneous absorption of lavender oil from a massage oil. J Soc Cosmet Chem 43(1):49–54, 1992

Jäger W, Našel B, Našel C, et al: Pharmacokinetic studies of the fragrance compound 1, 8-cineol in humans during inhalation. Chem Senses 21(4):477–480, 1996 8866111

Kasper S, Gastpar M, Müller WE, et al: Lavender oil preparation Silexan is effective in generalized anxiety disorder—a randomized, double-blind comparison to placebo and paroxetine. Int J Neuropsychopharmacol 17(6):859–869, 2014 24456909

Kasper S, Anghelescu I, Dienel A: Efficacy of orally administered Silexan in patients with anxiety-related restlessness and disturbed sleep—a randomized, placebo-controlled trial. Eur Neuropsychopharmacol 25(11):1960–1967, 2015 26293583

Lyon MR, Kapoor MP, Juneja LR: The effects of L-theanine (Suntheanine) on objective sleep quality in boys with attention deficit hyperactivity disorder (ADHD): a randomized, double-blind, placebo-controlled clinical trial. Altern Med Rev 16(4):348–354, 2011 22214254

Melzer J, Schrader E, Brattström A, et al: Fixed herbal drug combination with and without butterbur (Ze 185) for the treatment of patients with somatoform disorders: randomized, placebo-controlled pharmaco-clinical trial. Phytother Res 23(9):1303–1308, 2009 19274698

Nobre AC, Rao A, Owen GN: L-Theanine, a natural constituent in tea, and its effect on mental state. Asia Pac J Clin Nutr 17 (suppl 1):167–168, 2008 18296328

Rao TP, Ozeki M, Juneja LR: In search of a safe natural sleep aid. J Am Coll Nutr 34(5):436–447, 2015 25759004

Ritsner MS, Miodownik C, Ratner Y, et al: L-Theanine relieves positive, activation, and anxiety symptoms in patients with schizophrenia and schizoaffective disorder: an 8-week, randomized, double-blind, placebo-controlled, 2-center study. J Clin Psychiatry 72(1):34–42, 2011 21208586

Sánchez-Ortuño MM, Bélanger L, Ivers H, et al: The use of natural products for sleep: a common practice? Sleep Med 10(9):982–987, 2009 19427262

Woelk H, Schläfke S: A multi-center, double-blind, randomised study of the lavender oil preparation Silexan in comparison to lorazepam for generalized anxiety disorder. Phytomedicine 17(2):94–99, 2010 19962288

Zick SM, Wright BD, Sen A, Arnedt JT: Preliminary examination of the efficacy and safety of a standardized chamomile extract for chronic primary insomnia: a randomized placebo-controlled pilot study. BMC Complement Altern Med 11(1):78, 2011 21939549

CHAPTER 15

Saffron, Passionflower, Valerian, and Sage for Mental Health

Shahin Akhondzadeh, Ph.D., F.B.Ph.S.
Ladan Kashani, M.D.

Love fell like rainy cloud and saffron and tulip grew.

Jalaedin Mohammad Balkhi Molana, Rumi

Saffron, passionflower, valerian, and sage, used by traditional healers and physicians for thousands of years, are being probed by researchers hoping to unlock their full therapeutic potential. We have much to learn about biochemical and clinical effects of individual constituents in petals, stigmas, leaves, roots, seeds, and fruits of plants. Less than 200 years ago, the major pharmacopoeias of the world were dominated by herbal medicines. In this chapter, we discuss the quality of evidence for clinical effects of four phytomedicines in psychiatric and neurological disorders: *Crocus sativus*, *Passiflora incarnata*, *Valeriana officinalis*, and *Salvia officinalis*.

Saffron (*Crocus sativus*)

Saffron, the world's most expensive spice, comes from the flower of *C. sativus*, which grows up to 30 cm in height, bearing up to four flowers, each with three vivid crimson stigmas. This Persian herb has a history as long as that of the Persian Empire. Iran, the world's largest producer, is researching saffron's medicinal potential. The therapeutic dose of saffron as a psychotropic agent is much higher than the amount used for cooking.

Depression

It has been reported that more patients with mental disorders sought herbal treatments for somatic problems than for psychological symptoms, particularly somatic symptoms of depression (Akhondzadeh 2007). Saffron is used for depression in Persian traditional medicine (Akhondzadeh et al. 2004). Seven randomized controlled trials (RCTs) documented benefits of saffron in depression. The first RCT found saffron to be as effective as imipramine in short-term treatment (6 weeks) of mild to moderate depression in adults (n=30) (Akhondzadeh et al. 2004). Saffron was more tolerable than imipramine (which can cause anticholinergic side effects). Subsequently, in a 6-week RCT of 40 adult patients with mild to moderate depression, saffron resulted in about a 12-point reduction on the Hamilton Rating Scale for Depression (Ham-D) compared with 5 points with placebo (P=0.001). Tolerability of saffron was similar to that of placebo (Akhondzadeh et al. 2005). Both petals and stigma of C. *sativus* show benefits for treating depression (Akhondzadeh et al. 2004; Hosseinzadeh et al. 2007). Shahmansouri et al. (2014) reported in a 6-week double-blind RCT that saffron capsules twice per day (SaffroMood, IMPIRAN, Tehran, Iran; 15 mg dried hydroalcoholic extract of saffron per capsule) had antidepressant efficacy comparable to that of fluoxetine 40 mg/day in 40 depressed patients with a history of percutaneous coronary intervention (stent placements). Although not absolutely interpretable from this short-term study, the current evidence indicates that saffron is likely to show lower rates of adverse events compared with fluoxetine. Although the mechanisms underlying antidepressant effects of saffron are not fully explicated, reuptake inhibition of monoamines, N-methyl-D-aspartate (NMDA) antagonism, and possibly improved brain-derived neurotrophic factor signaling are implicated (Shimizu et al. 2011).

In a 6-week RCT of outpatients ages 20–65 years with a history of percutaneous coronary intervention in the last 6 months who met the DSM-IV-TR (American Psychiatric Association 2000) criteria for major depressive disorder, those who were given 20 mg of saffron extracts twice daily (standardized to 1.65–1.75 mg crocin) had significantly improved symptoms of mild to moderate depression compared with placebo (P<0.01) (Akhondzadeh Basti et al. 2007). Long-term studies comparing relapse rates are needed.

Reproductive Issues and Sexual Dysfunction

The only RCT for premenstrual syndrome found that saffron 15 mg twice daily for two menstrual cycles improved depression and premenstrual symptoms significantly more than did placebo (P=0.001) (Agha-Hosseini et al. 2008). In an open-label study, saffron aromatherapy reduced cortisol levels and anxiety and increased estrogen levels in follicular and luteal phases (Fukui et al. 2011). A trial compared the effect of placebo, mefenamic acid (a nonsteroidal anti-inflammatory drug), and an herbal compound (saffron, celery seed, and anise) on primary dysmenorrhea in young women. After two or three cycles, patients in the herbal group had significantly lower pain scores (P<0.001) than did those in the comparator groups (Nahid et al. 2009).

Traditionally, saffron has been used to improve sexual function. Studies in male rats found that *C. sativus* and its constituents improved all components of sexual function (Hosseinzadeh et al. 2008). Traditional wisdom was validated in an open trial in which high-dose saffron (200 mg/day) given for 10 days to 20 men with erectile dysfunction significantly improved nocturnal penile tumescence and scores on the International Index of Erectile Function (Shamsa et al. 2009). An RCT used saffron 15 mg twice daily to treat fluoxetine-induced sexual dysfunction in men ages 18–45 who met DSM-IV (American Psychiatric Association 1994) criteria for major depressive disorder. Significant improvement occurred in the erectile function and intercourse satisfaction ($P<0.05$) (but in neither desire nor orgasmic function) domains of the International Index of Erectile Function in the saffron group. Of the patients in the saffron group, 60% achieved normal erectile function by the end of the study compared with 7% in the placebo group (Modabbernia et al. 2012). Nine incidents of side effects, including decreased appetite and dry mouth, were recorded. Frequency of side effects did not differ between groups. All adverse events were mild and did not result in leaving the study. In a parallel safety study of the same patients, saffron did not affect liver, kidney, or blood tests (complete blood count, biochemical profiles) (Mansoori et al. 2011). In a study of women with fluoxetine-associated sexual dysfunction, saffron improved arousal, pain, and lubrication domains but not satisfaction, orgasm, or desire (Kashani et al. 2013).

Alzheimer's Disease

Constituents of saffron, including safranal, crocin, crocetin, and carotenoids, show neuroprotective properties in animal models of ischemic, oxidative, traumatic, and inflammatory brain injury (Papandreou et al. 2011; Yamauchi et al. 2011). Among these, crocin showed the highest neuroprotective activity in one study (Papandreou et al. 2011). Its neuroprotection is probably due to enhanced glutathione synthesis via increasing expression of glutamate cysteine ligase. In a hemi-parkinsonian mouse model, crocin pretreatment preserved levels of glutathione, dopamine, and antioxidant enzyme activity and protected substantia nigra neurons (Ahmad et al. 2005).

C. sativus is being studied as a memory enhancer. In a 16-week randomized placebo-controlled trial of 46 patients with mild to moderate Alzheimer's disease, those given saffron 15 mg twice daily showed significantly better cognitive function than did those given placebo ($P<0.01$) (Akhondzadeh et al. 2010a). In a 22-week RCT, saffron 15 mg twice daily was as effective as donepezil 5 mg twice daily but had a lower frequency of side effects than donepezil (Akhondzadeh et al. 2010b). The same group showed that 1 year of daily saffron given to patients with moderate to severe Alzheimer's disease was comparable to memantine in reducing cognitive decline (Farokhnia et al. 2014).

Adverse Effects and Toxicity

In a 1-week double-blind, randomized placebo-controlled trial, healthy volunteers received 200 or 400 mg/day of saffron tablets or placebo. High-dose saffron (400 mg/day) significantly reduced systolic blood pressure and mean arterial pressure. Although saffron slightly decreased some hematological parameters (e.g., red blood cells, hemoglobin, hematocrit, platelets) and increased sodium, serum urea nitrogen, and creatinine, none of the changes were clinically significant (Modaghegh et al. 2008). Occasional adverse effects included nausea, vomiting, and headache. In a mouse study, intraperitoneal saffron stigma and petal extract median lethal dose values were 1.6 and 6 g/kg, respectively (Modaghegh et al. 2008).

Passionflower (*Passiflora incarnata*)

Passionflower, a woody, hairy climbing vine, is widely used as a sedative and anxiolytic.

Anxiety

Several *Passiflora* species have antianxiety effects, *P. incarnata* being the most studied. Chrysin, a *Passiflora* extract, decreased anxiety-like behaviors in rats (Brown et al. 2007; Grundmann et al. 2009). In a double-blind RCT of 36 patients with generalized anxiety disorder, *P. incarnata* extract (45 drops/day) and oxazepam (30 mg/day) were equally effective in reducing anxiety on the Hamilton Anxiety Scale (Ham-A). *P. incarnata* had delayed onset of action compared with oxazepam, whereas greater impairment in job performance occurred with oxazepam (Akhondzadeh et al. 2001b). Evidence indicates that *P. incarnata* acts on the γ-aminobutyric acid (GABA)–ergic system. For example, *P. incarnata* extract prevented [(3)H]-GABA uptake into rat cortical synaptosomes without affecting GABA release or transamination. The extract modulated both $GABA_A$ and $GABA_B$ receptors without interacting with either ethanol– or benzodiazepine–$GABA_A$ receptor binding sites (Appel et al. 2011).

Symptoms of Substance Withdrawal

P. incarnata may alleviate anxiety associated with drug and alcohol withdrawal. In an RCT of 65 patients with opioid addiction, patients taking a clonidine plus *P. incarnata* extract (60 drops/day) had significantly greater improvement in mental symptoms compared with those taking clonidine (maximum=0.8 mg/day) plus placebo (Akhondzadeh et al. 2001a). A benzoflavone moiety of *P. incarnata* has been useful in treating withdrawal symptoms in mice addicted to morphine, cannabinoids, alcohol, or nicotine (Dhawan et al. 2001, 2003).

Adverse Effects and Toxicity

P. incarnata is generally well tolerated, with few side effects. In one report, gastrointestinal symptoms, drowsiness, prolonged QTc interval, and episodes of ventricular tachycardia followed self-administered therapeutic doses of *P. incarnata* in a young female (Fisher et al. 2000). Occasional side effects include dizziness, confusion, incoordination, nausea, altered consciousness, vomiting, drowsiness, and vascular inflammation. Passionflower may have additive sedative effects with benzodiazepines, sedative/hypnotics, or barbiturates. It should be used with caution in patients taking anticoagulants and should not be taken with monoamine oxidase inhibitors.

Valerian (*Valeriana officinalis*)

Valerian, an herbal sedative, is a hardy perennial flowering plant with sweetly scented pink or white flowers that bloom during the summer.

Sleep

In comparison with benzodiazepines, valerian has moderate sedative activity without hangover effect (Dorn 2000; Schmitz and Jäckel 1998). Single or multiple doses of valerian root extract did not affect alertness, reaction time, or concentration the morning after intake (Kuhlmann et al. 1999). In male mice, 1,000 mg/kg valerian extract and constituents (12 mg/kg linarin or 1.5 mg/kg apigenin) showed mild short-term sedative properties. In contrast to substantial preclinical evidence of sleep enhancement, human studies yielded mixed or modest effects. A large (N=391) three-arm Internet-based double-blind RCT did not show any beneficial effects of valerian or kava for concomitant anxiety and insomnia (Jacobs et al. 2005). A systematic review of RCTs of herbs for insomnia found only weak, unsupportive evidence for valerian (Sarris and Byrne 2011).

Anxiety

A 4-week double-blind RCT compared placebo, valerian extract (mean dose=81.3 mg/day), and diazepam (6.5 mg/day) in 36 patients with generalized anxiety disorder (each group, n=12). No significant difference was found among groups in the change in Ham-A score or State-Trait Anxiety Inventory Trait subscale score. Patients given valerian or diazepam were significantly more improved on the Ham-A psychic factor, suggesting modest benefit for anxiety (Andreatini et al. 2002).

Adverse Effects and Toxicity

Two cases of valerian-induced hepatotoxicity have been reported to date (Cohen and Del Toro 2008; Vassiliadis et al. 2009). Valerian markedly inhibits cytochrome P450 (CYP) enzymes 3A4, 2D6, and 2C19 (Lefebvre et al. 2004). Up to 65 times the human dose of valerian extract did not cause adverse reproductive outcomes in animals (Yao et al. 2007). In one report, a young patient developed hand tremor, dizziness, throbbing, and fatigue following self-administration of *V. officinalis* and *P. incarnata* while taking lorazepam (Carrasco et al. 2009). Although valerian is generally low in side effects, it can occasionally cause headache, excitability, uneasiness, or morning-after sluggishness and may have additive sedating effects with alcohol or sedative drugs, particularly benzodiazepines and central nervous system depressants. It may affect serum levels of medications metabolized by CYP3A4.

Sage (*Salvia officinalis*)

S. officinalis is an evergreen perennial subshrub with grayish leaves, woody stems, and blue to purplish flowers. Native to the Mediterranean region, it naturalized throughout the world.

Dementia

Sage inhibits cholinesterase, exerts anti-inflammatory and antioxidative effects, and improves mood and cognition in animals and healthy human subjects (Akhondzadeh and Abbasi 2006; Eidi et al. 2006; Kennedy et al. 2006b; Rodrigues et al. 2012; Scholey et al. 2008). In a 4-month double-blind, randomized placebo-controlled trial in patients with mild to moderate Alzheimer's disease, patients given 60 drops/day of sage extract (1:1 in alcohol 45%: 1 kg dried herb [leaf] to 1 L of alcohol) showed significantly better cognitive performance and less agitation than did the placebo group ($P<0.01$) (Akhondzadeh et al. 2003). Further trials are needed to validate these encouraging findings.

Adverse Effects and Toxicity

For short- and medium-term use, sage is generally well tolerated. However, like other aromatic plants, sage contains thujone, which in excess doses can cause severe adverse reactions, such as convulsion and hallucination. Therefore, limiting daily intake of thujone to no more than 0.11 mg/kg body weight (2–20 cups of sage tea) is advised (Lachenmeier and Uebelacker 2010). Tonic-clonic seizure following accidental ingestion of sage oil was reported in children (Halicioglu et al. 2011). One case of allergic contact dermatitis caused by *S. officinalis* extract was reported (Mayer et al. 2011).

KEY POINTS

- Saffron shows beneficial effects for mild to moderate depression and mild to severe Alzheimer's disease.

- Saffron is probably beneficial for sexual dysfunction and premenstrual syndrome.

- Studies of passionflower for insomnia, anxiety disorders, and substance withdrawal are promising.

- Valerian offers modest benefit for treatment of anxiety and sleep disorders.

- Sage improved symptoms of dementia in one study, which needs replication.

References

Agha-Hosseini M, Kashani L, Aleyaseen A, et al: Crocus sativus L. (saffron) in the treatment of premenstrual syndrome: a double-blind, randomised and placebo-controlled trial. BJOG 115(4):515–519, 2008 18271889

Ahmad AS, Ansari MA, Ahmad M, et al: Neuroprotection by crocetin in a hemi-parkinsonian rat model. Pharmacol Biochem Behav 81(4):805–813, 2005 16005057

Akhondzadeh S: Herbal medicine in the treatment of psychiatric and neurological disorders, in Low-Cost Approaches to Promote Physical and Mental Health: Theory, Research and Practice. Edited by L'Abate L. New York, Springer, 2007, pp 119–138

Akhondzadeh S, Abbasi SH: Herbal medicine in the treatment of Alzheimer's disease. Am J Alzheimers Dis Other Demen 21(2):113–118, 2006 16634467

Akhondzadeh S, Kashani L, Mobaseri M, et al: Passionflower in the treatment of opiates withdrawal: a double-blind randomized controlled trial. J Clin Pharm Ther 26(5):369–373, 2001a 11679027

Akhondzadeh S, Naghavi HR, Vazirian M, et al: Passionflower in the treatment of generalized anxiety: a pilot double-blind randomized controlled trial with oxazepam. J Clin Pharm Ther 26(5):363–367, 2001b 11679026

Akhondzadeh S, Noroozian M, Mohammadi M, et al: Salvia officinalis extract in the treatment of patients with mild to moderate Alzheimer's disease: a double blind, randomized and placebo-controlled trial. J Clin Pharm Ther 28(1):53–59, 2003 12605619

Akhondzadeh S, Fallah-Pour H, Afkham K, et al: Comparison of Crocus sativus L. and imipramine in the treatment of mild to moderate depression: a pilot double-blind randomized trial [ISRCTN45683816]. BMC Complement Altern Med 4:12, 2004 15341662

Akhondzadeh S, Tahmacebi-Pour N, Noorbala AA, et al: Crocus sativus L. in the treatment of mild to moderate depression: a double-blind, randomized and placebo-controlled trial. Phytother Res 19(2):148–151, 2005 15852492

Akhondzadeh S, Sabet MS, Harirchian MH, et al: Saffron in the treatment of patients with mild to moderate Alzheimer's disease: a 16-week, randomized and placebo-controlled trial. J Clin Pharm Ther 35(5):581–588, 2010a 20831681

Akhondzadeh S, Shafiee Sabet M, Harirchian MH, et al: A 22-week, multicenter, randomized, double-blind controlled trial of Crocus sativus in the treatment of mild-to-moderate Alzheimer's disease. Psychopharmacology (Berl) 207(4):637–643, 2010b 19838862

Akhondzadeh Basti A, Moshiri E, Noorbala AA, et al: Comparison of petal of Crocus sativus L. and fluoxetine in the treatment of depressed outpatients: a pilot double-blind randomized trial. Prog Neuropsychopharmacol Biol Psychiatry 31(2):439–442, 2007 17174460

American Psychiatric Association: Diagnostic and Statistical Manual of Mental Disorders, 4th Edition. Washington, DC, American Psychiatric Association, 1994

American Psychiatric Association: Diagnostic and Statistical Manual of Mental Disorders, 4th Edition, Text Revision. Washington, DC, American Psychiatric Association, 2000

Andreatini R, Sartori VA, Seabra ML, et al: Effect of valepotriates (valerian extract) in generalized anxiety disorder: a randomized placebo-controlled pilot study. Phytother Res 16(7):650–654, 2002 12410546

Appel K, Rose T, Fiebich B, et al: Modulation of the gamma-aminobutyric acid (GABA) system by Passiflora incarnata L. Phytother Res 25(6):838–843, 2011 21089181

Brown E, Hurd NS, McCall S, et al: Evaluation of the anxiolytic effects of chrysin, a Passiflora incarnata extract, in the laboratory rat. AANA J 75(5):333–337, 2007 17966676

Carrasco MC, Vallejo JR, Pardo-de-Santayana M, et al: Interactions of Valeriana officinalis L. and Passiflora incarnata L. in a patient treated with lorazepam. Phytother Res 23(12):1795–1796, 2009 19441067

Cohen DL, Del Toro Y: A case of valerian-associated hepatotoxicity. J Clin Gastroenterol 42(8):961–962, 2008 18431248

Dhawan K, Kumar R, Kumar S, et al: Correct identification of Passiflora incarnata Linn., a promising herbal anxiolytic and sedative. J Med Food 4(3):137–144, 2001 12639407

Dhawan K, Dhawan S, Chhabra S: Attenuation of benzodiazepine dependence in mice by a tri-substituted benzoflavone moiety of Passiflora incarnata Linneaus: a non-habit forming anxiolytic. J Pharm Pharm Sci 6(2):215–222, 2003 12935433

Dorn M: Efficacy and tolerability of Baldrian versus oxazepam in non-organic and non-psychiatric insomniacs: a randomised, double-blind, clinical, comparative study [in German]. Forsch Komplementarmed Klass Naturheilkd 7(2):79–84, 2000 10899744

Eidi M, Eidi A, Bahar M: Effects of Salvia officinalis L. (sage) leaves on memory retention and its interaction with the cholinergic system in rats. Nutrition 22(3):321–326, 2006 16500558

Farokhnia M, Shafiee Sabet M, Iranpour N, et al: Comparing the efficacy and safety of Crocus sativus L. with memantine in patients with moderate to severe Alzheimer's disease: a double-blind randomized clinical trial. Hum Psychopharmacol 29(4):351–359, 2014 25163440

Fisher AA, Purcell P, Le Couteur DG: Toxicity of Passiflora incarnata L. J Toxicol Clin Toxicol 38(1):63–66, 2000 10696928

Fukui H, Toyoshima K, Komaki R: Psychological and neuroendocrinological effects of odor of saffron (Crocus sativus). Phytomedicine 18(8–9):726–730, 2011 21242071

Grundmann O, Wähling C, Staiger C, et al: Anxiolytic effects of a passion flower (Passiflora incarnata L.) extract in the elevated plus maze in mice. Pharmazie 64(1):63–64, 2009 19216234

Halicioglu O, Astarcioglu G, Yaprak I, et al: Toxicity of Salvia officinalis in a newborn and a child: an alarming report. Pediatr Neurol 45(4):259–260, 2011 21907890

Hosseinzadeh H, Motamedshariaty V, Hadizadeh F, et al: Antidepressant effect of kaempferol, a constituent of saffron (Crocus sativus) petal, in mice and rats. Pharmacologyonline 2:367–370, 2007

Hosseinzadeh H, Ziaee T, Sadeghi A: The effect of saffron, Crocus sativus stigma, extract and its constituents, safranal and crocin on sexual behaviors in normal male rats. Phytomedicine 15(6–7):491–495, 2008 17962007

Jacobs BP, Bent S, Tice JA, et al: An Internet-based randomized, placebo-controlled trial of kava and valerian for anxiety and insomnia. Medicine (Baltimore) 84(4):197–207, 2005 16010204

Kashani L, Raisi F, Saroukhani S, et al: Saffron for treatment of fluoxetine-induced sexual dysfunction in women: randomized double-blind placebo-controlled study. Hum Psychopharmacol 28(1):54–60, 2013 23280545

Kennedy DO, Pace S, Haskell C, et al: Effects of cholinesterase inhibiting sage (Salvia officinalis) on mood, anxiety and performance on a psychological stressor battery. Neuropsychopharmacology 31(4):845–852, 2006b 16205785

Kuhlmann J, Berger W, Podzuweit H, et al: The influence of valerian treatment on "reaction time, alertness and concentration" in volunteers. Pharmacopsychiatry 32(6):235–241, 1999 10599933

Lachenmeier DW, Uebelacker M: Risk assessment of thujone in foods and medicines containing sage and wormwood—evidence for a need of regulatory changes? Regul Toxicol Pharmacol 58(3):437–443, 2010 20727933

Lefebvre T, Foster BC, Drouin CE, et al: In vitro activity of commercial valerian root extracts against human cytochrome P450 3A4. J Pharm Pharm Sci 7(2):265–273, 2004 15367385

Mansoori P, Akhondzadeh A, Raisi F, et al: A randomized, double-blind, placebo-controlled study of safety of the adjunctive saffron on sexual dysfunction induced by a selective serotonin reuptake inhibitor. Journal of Medicinal Plants 1(37):121–130, 2011

Mayer E, Gescheidt-Shoshany H, Weltfriend S: Allergic contact dermatitis caused by Salvia officinalis extract. Contact Dermatitis 64(4):237–238, 2011 21392032

Modabbernia A, Sohrabi H, Nasehi AA, et al: Effect of saffron on fluoxetine-induced sexual impairment in men: randomized double-blind placebo-controlled trial. Psychopharmacology (Berl) 223(4):381–388, 2012 22552758

Modaghegh MH, Shahabian M, Esmaeili HA, et al: Safety evaluation of saffron (Crocus sativus) tablets in healthy volunteers. Phytomedicine 15(12):1032–1037, 2008 18693099

Nahid K, Fariborz M, Ataolah G, et al: The effect of an Iranian herbal drug on primary dysmenorrhea: a clinical controlled trial. J Midwifery Womens Health 54(5):401–404, 2009 19720342

Papandreou MA, Tsachaki M, Efthimiopoulos S, et al: Memory enhancing effects of saffron in aged mice are correlated with antioxidant protection. Behav Brain Res 219(2):197–204, 2011 21238492

Rodrigues MR, Kanazawa LK, das Neves TL, et al: Antinociceptive and anti-inflammatory potential of extract and isolated compounds from the leaves of Salvia officinalis in mice. J Ethnopharmacol 139(2):519–526, 2012 22154965

Sarris J, Byrne GJ: A systematic review of insomnia and complementary medicine. Sleep Med Rev 15(2):99–106, 2011 20965131

Schmitz M, Jäckel M: Comparative study for assessing quality of life of patients with exogenous sleep disorders (temporary sleep onset and sleep interruption disorders) treated with a hops-valerian preparation and a benzodiazepine drug [in German]. Wien Med Wochenschr 148(13):291–298, 1998 9757514

Scholey AB, Tildesley NT, Ballard CG, et al: An extract of Salvia (sage) with anticholinesterase properties improves memory and attention in healthy older volunteers. Psychopharmacology (Berl) 198(1):127–139, 2008 18350281

Shahmansouri N, Farokhnia M, Abbasi SH, et al: A randomized, double-blind, clinical trial comparing the efficacy and safety of Crocus sativus L. with fluoxetine for improving mild to moderate depression in post percutaneous coronary intervention patients. J Affect Disord 155:216–222, 2014 24289892

Shamsa A, Hosseinzadeh H, Molaei M, et al: Evaluation of Crocus sativus L. (saffron) on male erectile dysfunction: a pilot study. Phytomedicine 16(8):690–693, 2009 19427775

Shimizu Y, Inoue E, Motegi J, et al: Pharmacological studies of Noukassei, a crude drug containing red ginseng, polygala root, saffron, antelope horn and agarwood—antidepressant-like effect in the mouse forced swimming test. Japanese Pharmacology and Therapeutics 39(6):587–594, 2011

Vassiliadis T, Anagnostis P, Patsiaoura K, et al: Valeriana hepatotoxicity. Sleep Med 10(8):935, 2009 19138557

Yamauchi M, Tsuruma K, Imai S, et al: Crocetin prevents retinal degeneration induced by oxidative and endoplasmic reticulum stresses via inhibition of caspase activity. Eur J Pharmacol 650(1):110–119, 2011 20951131

Yao M, Ritchie HE, Brown-Woodman PD: A developmental toxicity-screening test of valerian. J Ethnopharmacol 113(2):204–209, 2007 17611059

CHAPTER 16

Traditional Chinese Medicine

Treatments for Depression, Anxiety, and Insomnia

Wing-Fai Yeung, Ph.D., B.C.M.

Ka-Fai Chung, M.B.B.S., M.R.C.Psych.

恬淡虛無, 真氣從之; 精神內守, 病安從來—《黃帝內經·上古天真論》

One should remain calm and avoid excessive desires…. When internal energies are able to circulate, and the energy of the mind is focused, illness can be avoided.

The Yellow Emperor's Classic of Medicine,
Translated by Maoshing Ni

Traditional Chinese medicine (TCM) uses numerous modalities, including herbs, mind-body practices, and acupuncture. Only a minority of practitioners of Western medicine undertake rigorous training in TCM. Nevertheless, practitioners may be interested in learning about a few key Chinese formulas that can be readily used in treating psychological symptoms frequently seen in psychiatric and medical practice (Table 16–1). It is important to note that individuals of Asian descent may be less able to tolerate Western psychotropics because of differences in pharmacokinetics, pharmacodynamics, and pharmacogenetics (Lin 2001). Moreover, Asian patients may be more comfortable using Chinese herbal medicines that are familiar to them. In this chapter, we highlight a few key Chinese herbals that can be easily integrated with Western treatments.

TABLE 16–1. Chinese herbal formulas: composition, indications, evidence, and adverse reactions

Formula	Composition	Indications	Evidence base	Common adverse reactions
Jia wei xiao yao powder	Chai hu (radix Bupleuri), dang gui (radix Angelicae sinensis), bai shao (radix Paeoniae alba), bai zhu (rhizoma Atractylodis macrocephalae), fu ling (*Poria cocos*), sheng jiang (rhizoma Zingiberis recens), gan cao (radix Glycyrrhizae), bo he (herba Menthae), mu dan pi (*Paeonia suffruticosa*; cortex Moutan), zhi zi (fructus Gardeniae)	Depression, anxiety	++, –	Dyspepsia, diarrhea, dizziness, headache, fatigue, somnolence, dry mouth, bloating, constipation
Free and Easy Wanderer Plus	Similar to jia wei xiao yao powder plus bai he (lily bulb, *Lilium brownii*), sheng di huang (*Rehmannia glutinosa*; radix Rehmanniae), dan shen (red sage; *Salvia miltiorrhiza*); but no mu dan pi (*P. suffruticosa*; cortex Moutan), zhi zi (fructus Gardeniae)	Depression	++++	Dyspepsia, dizziness, headache, diarrhea, somnolence, dry mouth, bloating, constipation
Chaihu shugan powder	Chai hu (*Bupleurum chinensis* DC.), chen pi (pericarpium Citri reticulatae), bai shao (radix Paeoniae alba) zhi qiao (fructus Aurantii), xiang fu (rhizoma Cyperi), chuan xiong (*Ligusticum chuanxiong* Hort.), gan cao (*Glycyrrhiza uralensis* Fisch.)	Depression	++	Nausea, dry mouth, drowsiness
Gan mai da zao decoction	Gan cao (*Glycyrrhiza uralensis* Fisch.), fu xiao mai (*Triticum aestivum* L.), da zao (*Ziziphus jujuba* Mill.)	Depression	++	Dry mouth, constipation, melancholia, insomnia, irritability

TABLE 16–1. Chinese herbal formulas: composition, indications, evidence, and adverse reactions *(continued)*

Formula	Composition	Indications	Evidence base	Common adverse reactions
Suan zao ren decoction	Suan zao ren (*Ziziphus jujuba* var. *spinosa* [Bunge] Hu ex H.F. Chow), gan cao (*Glycyrrhiza uralensis* Fisch.), zhi mu (*Anemarrhena asphodeloides* Bge.), fu ling (*Poria cocos* [Schw.] Wolf), chuan xiong (*Ligusticum striatum* DC.)	Insomnia	++	Lethargy, diarrhea, dizziness
Gui pi decoction	Bai zhu (*Atractylodes macrocephala* Koidz.), fu shen (*Poria cocos* [Schw.] Wolf), huang qi (*Astragalus membranaceus* [Fisch.] Bunge), long yan rou (*Dimocarpus longan* Lour.), fried suan zao ren (*Ziziphus jujuba* Mill. var. *spinosa* [Bunge] Hu ex H.F. Chou), ren shen (*Panax ginseng* C.A. Mey.), mu xiang (*Aucklandia lappa* DC.), honey-toasted gan cao (*Glycyrrhiza uralensis* Fisch.), sheng jiang (rhizoma Zingiberis recens), da zao (*Ziziphus jujuba* Mill.), dang gui (*Angelica sinensis* [Oliv.] Diels), honey-toasted yuan zhi (*Polygala tenuifolia* Willd.)	Insomnia	+/−	NA

Note. +++=more than one good quality randomized controlled trial with positive results; ++=more than one positive study; +/−=study results mixed; −=single study with negative result; NA=data not available.

Depression

Chinese herbal formulas widely used in Chinese societies for treating depression (Hsu et al. 2008) include jia wei xiao yao powder (Free and Easy Wanderer Plus), chaihu shugan powder, and gan mai da zao decoction. Single herbs, such as bai shao (*Paeonia lactiflora* Pall.) and chai hu (*Bupleurum chinensis* DC.), are commonly used in formulas for depression.

Jia Wei Xiao Yao Powder (and Free and Easy Wanderer Plus)

Jia wei xiao yao powder increased plasma tumor necrosis factor α and decreased serum corticosterone levels in depressed rats (Oh et al. 2007). A systematic review including 26 randomized controlled trials (RCTs) in 1,837 patients with depression (ages 17–80 years) concluded that jia wei xiao yao powder in combination with antidepressants was more effective than antidepressants alone because of a weighted mean difference in Hamilton Rating Scale for Depression (Ham-D) score (−0.69; $P=0.02$) and self-rating depression scale score (−3.6; $P<0.001$). No significant differences were detected between jia wei xiao yao powder alone and placebo (Y. Zhang et al. 2012). Jia wei xiao yao powder may be useful as an adjunct to antidepressant medications. This review omitted double-blind, placebo-controlled trials that used the formula's English name, Free and Easy Wanderer Plus (FEWP), which contains most of the herbs in traditional jia wei xiao yao plus additional herbs to enhance effectiveness. In a 12-week double-blind RCT, 87 patients with unipolar major depression and 62 patients with bipolar depression were randomly assigned to either 36 g/day of FEWP enhanced with Baikal skullcap (*Scutellaria baicalensis*) or placebo (Zhang et al. 2006). All participants had baseline scores of 18 or higher on the 17-item Ham-D. Participants given FEWP had significantly greater improvements ($P<0.05$ on all measures) compared with placebo on Ham-D, Montgomery-Åsberg Depression Rating Scale, and Clinical Global Impression Scale–Severity. A higher clinical response rate (≥50% improvement on Ham-D) occurred with FEWP (74%) than with placebo (42%).

In an 8-week study, 150 poststroke patients (<6 weeks after a single ischemic or hemorrhagic stroke) with moderate to severe depression (>20 on Ham-D) were randomly assigned to the following groups: FEWP ($n=60$), fluoxetine ($n=60$), and placebo ($n=30$) (Li et al. 2008). Patients received either 18 g of FEWP twice daily, fluoxetine (starting at 20 mg/day, increasing to 40 mg/day, depending on response), or placebo. The FEWP formula contained *Lilium brownii*, known for antidepressant effects. Response rates were significantly higher with FEWP and fluoxetine compared with placebo (60% and 65% vs. 21.4%; $P<0.05$). FEWP had a faster onset of action (2 weeks) and led to greater improvements in activities of daily living compared with fluoxetine ($P<0.01$).

In a study comparing carbamazepine plus FEWP with carbamazepine plus placebo, 188 patients with bipolar disorder (99 with depression and 89 with mania) had no differences on measures of depression or mania after 26 weeks (Zhang et al. 2006). However, patients with bipolar depression responded better to FEWP than to placebo. In addition, 36 g/day of FEWP (in three divided doses) plus carbamazepine had a significantly lower discontinuation rate (31%) than did FEWP plus placebo (51%). Serum carbamazepine levels in those taking FEWP were 43% of the levels in those taking carbamazepine plus placebo, indicating an herb-drug interaction. This may be the result of herbal induction of the cytochrome P450 (CYP) 3A metabolizing enzyme (known to metabolize carbamazepine) as well as other pharmacokinetic actions. Interestingly, when carbamazepine levels were lowered, FEWP reduced side effects and medication discontinuation without reducing efficacy.

Common side effects of jia wei xiao yao or FEWP include diarrhea, dizziness, headache, somnolence, dry mouth, bloating, and constipation. These formulas may affect serum levels of pharmaceuticals metabolized by CYP3A4 enzymes. In such cases, medication serum levels should be monitored and dose adjustments made.

Chaihu Shugan Powder

The mechanisms of chaihu shugan powder may be due to its effect on extracellular signal-regulated kinase, which regulates neuronal plasticity, participates in stress response, and is correlated with stress-induced depressive-like behaviors (Wang et al. 2014). It also affects c-Jun amino-terminal kinase, which plays a key role in apoptosis of nerve cells and is closely correlated with depression (Li et al. 2014). A recent systematic review of 10 RCTs involving 835 patients with depression (ages 29–68 years) showed that chaihu shugan powder in combination with antidepressants for 4–13 weeks was more effective than antidepressants alone (weighted mean difference=−3.56; $P<0.001$) in improving Ham-D scores (Wang et al. 2012). The results suggested potential benefits of chaihu shugan powder as an adjunct to antidepressants, but all 10 studies had low methodological quality (Jadad score<3); hence, better-quality trials are needed. Common adverse events included nausea, dry mouth, and drowsiness, but the incidence was lower than that associated with antidepressants. No serious adverse events were reported.

Gan Mai Da Zao Decoction

Gan mai da zao decoction may downregulate the hypothalamic-pituitary-adrenal axis and enhance nitric oxide and brain-derived neurotrophic factor production (C. Zhang et al. 2012). A systematic review of 10 RCTs (968 subjects with depression, ages 15–85 years) found gan mai da zao decoction significantly more effective than antidepressants alone, and gan mai da zao plus antidepressants fared better than antidepressants alone (weighted mean difference=−4.25; $P<0.001$) (Yeung et al. 2014). However, methodological quality of all reviewed trials was low. Side effects included dry mouth, constipation, melancholia, insomnia, and irritability, and adverse events were more common with antidepressants than with gan mai da zao decoction. Long-term safety, effects of overdose, and effects of use in pregnancy and during lactation are unknown.

Clinical Considerations

According to the principles of TCM, practitioners should prescribe herbal formulas on the basis of the patient's signs, symptoms, and pulse and tongue features. For example, gan mai da zao decoction is believed to be effective for depression caused by heart deficiency, which is characterized by low mood, tendency to cry, possession-like behavior, and frequent yawning; jia wei xiao yao powder is for liver stagnation and spleen deficiency; and chaihu shugan powder is for liver-qi stagnation, a result of anger and distress repression.

Anxiety

Jia wei xiao yao powder (best known in the West as FEWP) is widely used for anxiety, but there has been no systematic review of FEWP for anxiety. In a double-blind RCT of 147 patients with generalized anxiety disorder, jia wei xiao yao was no more effective than placebo (Park et al. 2014). However, those given the Chinese formula showed greater improvements in quality of life ($P=0.02$) and in depressive ($P=0.02$), obsessive-compulsive ($P=0.04$), and somatic ($P=0.003$) symptoms. Common adverse events (dyspepsia, diarrhea, and fatigue) were self-limiting. No patients dropped out because of adverse events.

Insomnia

Chinese herbs for sleep were documented more than 2,000 years ago in *Huangdi Neijing* (*The Yellow Emperor's Inner Classic*, 206 B.C. to 220 A.D.) (Wang 2000). Two ancient formulas still in use are suan zao ren decoction and gui pi decoction. Single herbs found in formulas for insomnia are suan zao ren (semen Ziziphi spinosae), fu ling (*Poria cocos*), ye jiao teng (caulis Polygoni multiflori), gan cao (radix Glycyrrhizae), and bai shao (radix Paeoniae alba) (Yeung et al. 2012b). A systematic review of 217 studies found overall promising results, with Chinese herbal medicine superior to benzodiazepines and placebo (Yeung et al. 2012a). However, only eight studies were rated as having moderate methodological quality; meta-analyses found that Chinese herbal medicine was not significantly different from benzodiazepine hypnotics (three studies, 222 subjects) and placebo (three studies, 449 subjects). Further studies are needed to verify effectiveness of Chinese phytomedicines for insomnia. The incidence of adverse events was similar between Chinese herbals and placebo, but combining Chinese and Western medicine was associated with fewer adverse events than Western medicine alone.

Suan Zao Ren Decoction

Suan zao ren decoction was first recorded in *Jin Gui Yao Lue* (*Synopsis of Prescriptions of the Golden Chamber*, 150–219 A.D.) (Jiang and Huang 2007). Mechanisms of action involve stimulation of γ-aminobutyric acid (GABA) type A, 5-hydroxytryptamine-1A (5-HT$_{1A}$), 5-HT$_2$, and 5-HT$_3$ receptors (Yi et al. 2007a, 2007b). In a 4-week double-blind RCT, suan zao ren decoction produced statistically significant improvement in Pittsburgh Sleep Quality Index score ($P=0.007$) and average sleep efficiency ($P=0.017$) during methadone therapy for opiate withdrawal ($n=90$) (Chan et al. 2015).

Adverse events included mild, infrequent lethargy; diarrhea; and dizziness. No subjects withdrew because of adverse events.

Gui Pi Decoction

Gui pi decoction was first documented in *Ji Sheng-Fang* (*Life Helping Formulae*, 1253 A.D.) (Yan 1956). The mechanism of action involves serotonin, dopamine, norepinephrine, 5-hydroxyindoleacetic acid, and somatostatin (Deng and Li 2012; Qian et al. 2008). Previous studies on this formula found it to be more effective than estazolam (Jia 2013; Li 2013) without significant adverse events; however, the poor quality of these studies precludes conclusions regarding efficacy and safety.

Case Example: Insomnia With Depression

Mr. A, a 58-year-old teacher, complained of insomnia and depressed mood since his wife died 1 year ago. Because he had only 4–5 hours of interrupted sleep per night, daytime tiredness affected his concentration and work performance. He was uncharacteristically irritable and argumentative and avoided social activities.

After 6 months, Mr. A was evaluated by a psychiatrist, who diagnosed mild depression. Because Mr. A did not want antidepressant medication, he was prescribed zolpidem for sleep. Worried about developing zolpidem dependence and wanting an herbal sedative instead, he consulted a TCM practitioner, who noted characteristic signs (liver dysfunction leading to depressed mood and vice versa, leading to fire symptoms) of liver-qi stagnation transforming into fire: dry, reddish eyes; red and whitish tongue with thick fur; yellowish urine; and string-like pulse. The practitioner prescribed jia wei xiao yao powder (4 g in granule form), suan zao ren decoction (6 g in granule form), and single herbs he huan pi (cortex Albiziae) and yu jin (radix Curcumae) (2 g/granule, equal to 10 g raw herb). Jia wei xiao yao powder and yu jin were used to soothe the liver, and suan zao ren decoction and he huan pi were used to calm the *shen* (spirit).

After taking these formulas and individual herbs twice a day for 1 week, Mr. A reported deeper sleep, fewer awakenings, feeling refreshed after sleep, and no side effects, but he still needed zolpidem 2–3 nights per week. Over the next 6 weeks, addition of suan zao ren (*Ziziphus jujuba* var. *spinosa* [Bunge] Hu ex H.F. Chow; 2 g/granule, equal to 10 g raw herb) and shi chang pu (rhizoma Acori Tatarinowii; 1 g/granule, equal to 5 g raw herb) further improved sleep, mood, and irritability while Mr. A was tapered off zolpidem.

Risks, Contraindications, and Precautions

The available data on Chinese herbs are limited regarding long-term safety, effects of overdose, potential herb-drug interactions, and use during pregnancy and breastfeeding. According to the *2015 Pharmacopoeia of the People's Republic of China*, there are no absolute contraindications to jia wei xiao yao powder, chaihu shugan powder, gan mai da zao decoction, suan zao ren decoction, or gui pi decoction, but there is a relative contraindication to jia wei xiao yao powder, which may contain mu dan pi (cortex Moutan), during pregnancy because it may induce miscarriage (Chinese Pharmacopoeia Commission 2015). Case reports have indicated hepatic and renal toxicity due to overdose of bo he (herba Menthae) and chai hu (radix Bupleuri) (Feng 2009), which are used in jia wei xiao yao powder. Allergic reactions have been reported in case studies. Caution is advised if Chinese herbal formulas are taken with alcohol or Western medicine. However, combining jia wei xiao yao powder, chaihu shugan powder, or gan mai da zao decoction with antidepressants has not caused adverse reactions in multiple studies. In general, Chinese herbals have not been adequately tested for effects on CYP metabolizing enzymes. Therefore, careful monitoring is advisable when these formulas are used with medications that have a narrow margin of safety or a critical level for therapeutic effect.

Guidelines for the Safe and Effective Use of Chinese Herbal Medicine

Jia wei xiao yao powder, chaihu shugan powder, gan mai da zao decoction, suan zao ren decoction, and gui pi decoction are generally safe, but the dosage and composition of Chinese medicinals vary among companies. To minimize the chance of false labeling or product contamination, it is preferable to use products with a Good Manufacturing Practices certificate. Clinicians and patients can consult qualified TCM practitioners for advice on which formulas would best suit their needs. Alternatively, Western clinicians who become knowledgeable about key formulas may prescribe them as part of an integrative treatment. Clinicians find Crane Herb Company (www.craneherb.com) to be a reliable source of advice on formula selection and high-quality products. Crane Herb Company requires online prescriptions.

KEY POINTS

- Chinese herbal formulas for depression, anxiety, and insomnia are especially helpful in patients who are sensitive to side effects of Western psychotropics, particularly individuals of Asian ethnicity.

- Some Chinese herbals have been shown to be effective as solo treatments, but others are better used to augment psychotropics or reduce side effects.

- It is important to identify herbal formulas with high-quality manufacturing standards that are free of contaminants.

References

Chan YY, Chen YH, Yang SN, et al: Clinical efficacy of traditional Chinese medicine, suan zao ren tang, for sleep disturbance during methadone maintenance: a randomized, double-blind, placebo-controlled trial. Evid Based Complement Alternat Med 2015:710895, 2015 26346534

Chinese Pharmacopoeia Commission: Pharmacopoeia of the People's Republic of China 2015. Beijing, China Medical Science and Technologoy Press, 2015

Deng M, Li T: Influence of guipi decoction on the sedative-hypnotic effect and memory consolidation obstacles of the mice [in Chinese]. China Journal of Chinese Medicine 27:438–440, 2012

Feng YB: Basic and Clinical Toxicology of Chinese Medicines. Hong Kong, Commercial Press (HK) Limited, 2009

Hsu MC, Creedy D, Moyle W, et al: Use of complementary and alternative medicine among adult patients for depression in Taiwan. J Affect Disord 111(2–3):360–365, 2008 18442859

Jia QZ: Observation on modified guipi decoction on insomnia with dual deficiency of the heart and spleen. Chinese Journal of Clinical Rational Drug Use 6:60–61, 2013

Jiang D, Huang Y: Jin Gui Yao Lue. Beijing, Beijing Scientific Publishers, 2007

Li LT, Wang SH, Ge HY, et al: The beneficial effects of the herbal medi-cine Free and Easy Wanderer Plus (FEWP) and fluoxetine on post-stroke depression. J Altern Complement Med 14(7):841–846, 2008 18721085

Li YH, Zhang CH, Qiu J, et al: Antidepressant-like effects of Chaihu-Shugan-San via SAPK/JNK signal transduction in rat models of depression. Pharmacogn Mag 10(39):271–277, 2014 25210314

Li YX: Clinical observation on modified guipi decoction in treating severe insomnia. Asia-Pacific Traditional Medicine 9:140–141, 2013

Lin KM: Biological differences in depression and anxiety across races and ethnic groups. J Clin Psychiatry 62 (suppl 13):13–19, discussion 20–21, 2001 11434414

Oh JK, Kim YS, Park HJ, et al: Antidepressant effects of Soyo-san on immobilization stress in ovariectomized female rats. Biol Pharm Bull 30(8):1422–1426, 2007 17666797

Park DM, Kim SH, Park YC, et al: The comparative clinical study of efficacy of gamisoyo-san (jiaweixiaoyaosan) on generalized anxiety disorder according to differently manufactured preparations: multicenter, randomized, double blind, placebo controlled trial. J Ethnopharmacol 158 (Pt A):11–17, 2014 25456420

Qian HN, Wang L, Shen LB, et al: Guipi decoction effects on brain somatostatin levels and receptor mRNA expression in rats with spleen deficiency. Neural Regen Res 3(2):200–203, 2008

Wang B: Huangdi Nei Jing Su Wen. Shanghai, Shanghai Scientific and Technical Publishers, 2000

Wang S, Hu S, Zhang C, et al: Antidepressant-like activity of Chaihu-Shugan-San aqueous extract in rats and its possible mechanism. Pharmacogn Mag 10 (Suppl 1):S50–S56, 2014 24914308

Wang Y, Fan R, Huang X: Meta-analysis of the clinical effectiveness of traditional Chinese medicine formula chaihu-shugan-san in depression. J Ethnopharmacol 141(2):571–577, 2012 21933701

Yan Y: Ji Sheng Fang. Beijing, People's Republic Health Publisher, 1956

Yeung WF, Chung KF, Poon MM, et al: Chinese herbal medicine for insomnia: a systematic review of randomized controlled trials. Sleep Med Rev 16(6):497–507, 2012a 22440393

Yeung WF, Chung KF, Poon MM, et al: Prescription of Chinese herbal medicine and selection of acupoints in pattern-based traditional Chinese medicine treatment for insomnia: a systematic review. Evid Based Complement Alternat Med 2012:902578, 2012b 23259001

Yeung WF, Chung KF, Ng KY, et al: A meta-analysis of the efficacy and safety of traditional Chinese medicine formula ganmai dazao decoction for depression. J Ethnopharmacol 153(2):309–317, 2014 24632021

Yi PL, Lin CP, Tsai CJ, et al: The involvement of serotonin receptors in suan zao ren tang-induced sleep alteration. J Biomed Sci 14:829–840, 2007a

Yi PL, Tsai CH, Chen YC, Chang FC: Gamma-aminobutyric acid (GABA) receptor mediates suanzaoren-tang, a traditional Chinese herb remedy, -induced sleep alteration. J Biomed Sci 14:285–298, 2007b

Zhang C, Wei W, Zhang XL, et al: The effect of Ganmai Dazao decoction on the regulation of HPA-axis of depression rats. Chin J Gerontol 32:5450–5452, 2012

Zhang Y, Han M, Liu Z, et al: Chinese herbal formula xiao yao san for treatment of depression: a systematic review of randomized controlled trials. Evid Based Complement Alternat Med 2012:931636, 2012 21869903

Zhang ZJ, Kang WH, Li Q, Tan QR: The beneficial effects of the herbal medicine Free and Easy Wanderer Plus (FEWP) for mood disorders: double-blind, placebo-controlled studies. J Psychiatr Res 41(10):828–836, 2012 17010995

CHAPTER 17

Sceletium tortuosum

Olga Gericke, M.D., F.C.Psych.

Nigel Gericke, B.Sc. (Hons), M.B.B.Ch.

Dan J. Stein, Ph.D., FRCPC

They look upon it as the greatest Cheerer of the Spirits, and the noblest Restorative in the World

Peter Kolben, The Present State of the Cape of Good-Hope, *1731*

Sceletium tortuosum (L.) N.E.Br., a succulent South African medicinal plant belonging to the subfamily Mesembryanthemoideae, is commonly known as *Sceletium* or by its indigenous name, Kanna. The plant has been used for millennia as a masticatory and an infusion by indigenous San hunter-gatherers and Nama pastoralists for coping with the physical and mental stress of subsisting in the arid Namaqualand and Karoo regions in South Africa. In this chapter, we outline emerging scientific knowledge on *Sceletium* and how it is used in a clinical setting.

Chemistry and Pharmacology

The key compounds of *Sceletium* that act on the central nervous system are mesembrine alkaloids. A standardized commercial extract of *S. tortuosum*, Zembrin, is a dual serotonin reuptake inhibitor (SRI) and phosphodiesterase-4 (PDE4) inhibitor (Harvey et al. 2011). PDE4 inhibitors may exert antidepressant effect via enhancement of cyclic adenosine monophosphate (cAMP) signaling (Zhang 2009). The combination of an SRI with a PDE4 inhibitor may have synergistic antidepressant potential (Cashman et al. 2009). PDE4 inhibitors also may play a role in regulating cognition via PDE4-cAMP cascade signaling involving phosphorylated cAMP response element binding protein.

Animal Studies

Veterinarian studies report that *Sceletium* reduced cage and travel stress in cats and decreased excessive nocturnal crying and barking of aged cats and dogs with dementia (Hirabayashi et al. 2002, 2004, 2005). In a model of restraint-induced psychological stress, low-dose *Sceletium* decreased stress-induced self-soothing behavior and stress-induced elevated corticosterone levels (Smith 2011). A recent pharmacoelectroencephalograph study (Dimpfel et al. 2016) reported that a *Sceletium* extract produced an electroencephalographic signature similar to that of rolipram, a synthetic research PDE4 inhibitor with antianxiety, antidepressant, and cognitive-enhancing activities. *Sceletium* did not show addictive potential in vivo (Loria et al. 2014), consistent with its mechanisms of action, anecdotal clinical experience, and the *African Herbal Pharmacopoeia* (Brendler et al. 2010).

Animal studies found *Sceletium* plant material to be safe at doses of 10–100 mg/kg body weight per day (Gericke and Viljoen 2008). *S. tortuosum* (Zembrin) has been shown to be safe in rats at 600 mg/kg body weight per day in a 90-day subchronic toxicity study and at 5,000 mg/kg body weight per day in a 14-day repeated-dose toxicity study (Murbach et al. 2014).

Human Studies

A randomized placebo-controlled study in healthy adults found that 25 mg/day of Zembrin for 3 months was safe and well tolerated (Nell et al. 2013). A single 25-mg dose of Zembrin in a pilot randomized placebo-controlled pharmaco–magnetic resonance imaging study in healthy young adults had acute effects: amygdalar reactivity to fearful faces under low perceptual load conditions was significantly attenuated, and connectivity analysis showed reduced amygdala-hypothalamic coupling, results consistent with anxiolytic potential (Terburg et al. 2013). In a double-blind, crossover, randomized placebo-controlled study in 21 healthy subjects (ages 45–61), 25 mg/day of Zembrin or placebo was taken for 3 weeks, followed by a 3-week washout, and then a switch to either placebo or extract for 3 weeks. The *Sceletium* extract significantly improved executive function and cognitive set flexibility compared with placebo and improved mood and sleep (Chiu et al. 2014).

Case Example: *S. tortuosum* for Depression and Anxiety

A 40-year-old married homemaker with two children, ages 6 and 9, was referred to a psychiatrist for medication review. Her history included recurrent major depressive disorder since age 17, postpartum depression, and social anxiety disorder. For the previous 8 years, she had been taking citalopram 20 mg/day, which adequately treated her depression and social anxiety. However, the side effects were difficult to tolerate: loss of libido, emotional blunting. and weight gain. Two attempts to discontinue citalopram resulted in recurrence of depression, necessitating medication resumption. The patient was determined to wean herself off citalopram. After the psychiatrist counseled her on pharmaceutical and botanical options, the patient chose a trial of 25 mg of *S. tortuosum*

(Zembrin). Citalopram was reduced to 10 mg/day for 1 week and then discontinued while she started 50 mg/day of *Sceletium*, which was increased to 75 mg/day.

At 1-month follow-up, the patient reported no anxiety or depressive symptoms, although she had occasional mild social anxiety, which was easily tolerated. Her libido returned to normal, she felt more in touch with her feelings, and she lost 2 kg of weight. During the next month, a slight lowering of mood responded well to increased *Sceletium* (100 mg/day). Eight months later, she remained in remission, taking 100 mg/day of Zembrin with no side effects.

Integrating *Sceletium* Into Clinical Practice

Clinical trials of *Sceletium* for patients with mood disorders have not yet been published. This section is based on anecdotal, cumulative clinical practice experience of one of us (O.G.) who has prescribed *Sceletium* for more than 15 years in more than 30 patients and one of the editors of this book, Richard P. Brown (R.P.B.), a psychopharmacologist who has prescribed it in more than 30 patients during the past 4 years. PDE4 inhibition may reinforce SRI antidepressant and anxiolytic activity. Thus, *Sceletium* may be useful in conditions known to respond to selective SRIs (SSRIs) and those with symptoms of anxiety and depression. Most practitioners use *Sceletium* primarily in patients with mild to moderate symptoms, as well as in those who prefer herbal agents rather than synthetic antidepressants. However, R.P.B. prescribes *Sceletium* in patients with mild to severe depression, with good effects in about 80% of cases. Candidates for a trial of *Sceletium* may include patients whose symptoms have previously responded to SSRIs but who discontinued treatment because of side effects, such as sexual dysfunction, emotional blunting, sleep disturbances, or weight gain. *Sceletium* does not appear to cause these SSRI-induced side effects. However, it can cause nausea, particularly at doses higher than 100 mg. Therefore, patients are advised to take *Sceletium* with food.

Anecdotally, *Sceletium* can augment non-SSRI antidepressants, including bupropion and mirtazapine, in patients whose symptoms are not responding adequately or who do not tolerate pharmaceuticals. In clinical practice, *Sceletium* has been combined with trazodone successfully without adverse effects. Some practitioners combine *Sceletium* with SSRIs, but this is not recommended, and caution is advised because of the potential for serotonin syndrome, although we have seen no such cases, and none has been reported to date.

The usual starting dose of standardized *Sceletium* extract is 25 mg in the morning (equivalent to 50 mg botanical raw material), which is titrated up to 50–100 mg in the morning within a few days. In more severe cases, R.P.B. has used dose increases in 25-mg increments every 3 days up to a maximum of 400 mg twice daily.

Sceletium has a rapid-onset activating effect, which tails off by late afternoon and then promotes good-quality sleep at night. The activating or stimulant effect becomes apparent at 50 mg standardized extract; lower doses may be mildly sedating in some patients. Nonstandardized *Sceletium* products (milled botanical material and uncharacterized extracts) with highly variable alkaloid content and composition (Shikanga et al. 2012) may increase anxiety on initiation of treatment and may contain adulterants. However, Zembrin does not show anxiogenic activity. The onset of anxiolytic and mood-elevating action of *Sceletium* is usually rapid, typically within a few days. Some patients report improved mood and anxiety from day 1. The rapid onset of action enables patients with intermittent symptoms to use *Sceletium* on an as-needed basis rather than daily.

Side effects of conventional SSRIs, such as emotional blunting and lethargy, can negatively affect the ability and motivation of patients to engage in psychotherapy. *Sceletium* can facilitate therapy by improving mood and anxiety without reducing emotional responsivity.

Guidelines for length of treatment with prescription antidepressants are applicable to *Sceletium*. In O.G.'s experience and per discussions with other practitioners, when *Sceletium* is prescribed at no more than 100 mg/day, no discontinuation symptoms are observed. However, R.P.B. reports that with doses greater than 100 mg/day, withdrawal symptoms similar to those of SSRI withdrawal can occur. He therefore recommends reducing the dose by 25-mg increments every 3 days.

Anecdotal reports from retail pharmacists in South Africa and Brazil indicate that *Sceletium* is being used by students and scholars to enhance concentration during examination time and by middle-aged people to enhance cognitive function. PDE4 inhibition is a pharmaceutical target for cognitive enhancement, and emerging evidence suggests that *Sceletium* may have cognitive-enhancing potential (Chiu et al. 2014; Dimpfel et al. 2016). To be more widely integrated into clinical practice, standardized *Sceletium* extracts must be evaluated in randomized clinical trials targeting mood disorders, anxiety disorders, attention-deficit disorder, attention-deficit/hyperactivity disorder, and mild cognitive impairment.

KEY POINTS

- *Sceletium* alkaloids, key active compounds, have serotonin reuptake inhibitor and phosphodiesterase-4 inhibitory activity, potentially useful in treating anxiety, depression, and cognitive impairment.

- Animal and human studies show an excellent safety profile. Preliminary human studies and clinical experience suggest efficacy in anxiety, depression, and cognitive impairment.

- Clinical experience suggests that commercial products of a standardized extract of *Sceletium* have a rapid onset of action and a low side-effect profile.

References

Brendler T, Eloff JN, Gurub-Fakim A, et al: African Herbal Pharmacopoeia. Association for African Medicinal Plant Standards. Port Louis, Mauritius, Graphic Press, 2010, pp 205–208
Cashman JR, Voelker T, Johnson R, et al: Stereoselective inhibition of serotonin re-uptake and phosphodiesterase by dual inhibitors as potential agents for depression. Bioorg Med Chem 17(1):337–343, 2009 19014888

Chiu S, Gericke N, Farina-Woodbury M, et al: Proof-of-concept randomized controlled study of cognition effects of the proprietary extract Sceletium tortuosum (Zembrin) targeting phosphodiesterase-4 in cognitively healthy subjects: implications for Alzheimer's dementia. Evid Based Complement Alternat Med 2014:682014, 2014 25389443

Dimpfel W, Schombert L, Gericke N: Electropharmacogram of Sceletium tortuosum extract based on spectral local field power in conscious freely moving rats. J Ethnopharmacol 177:140–147, 2016 26608705

Gericke N, Viljoen AM: Sceletium—a review update. J Ethnopharmacol 119(3):653–663, 2008 18761074

Harvey AL, Young LC, Viljoen AM, et al: Pharmacological actions of the South African medicinal and functional food plant Sceletium tortuosum and its principal alkaloids. J Ethnopharmacol 137(3):1124–1129, 2011 21798331

Hirabayashi M, Ichikawa K, Fukushima R, et al: Clinical application of South African tea on dementia dog [in Japanese]. Japanese Journal of Small Animal Practice 21:109–113, 2002

Hirabayashi M, Ichikawa K, Yoshi A, et al: Clinical effects of South African tea for cat [in Japanese]. Japanese Journal of Small Animal Practice 23:85–89, 2004

Hirabayashi M, Ichikawa K, Yoshi A, et al: Clinical effects of South African tea for dementia animal [in Japanese]. Japanese Journal of Small Animal Practice 24:27–31, 2005

Loria MJ, Ali Z, Abe N, et al: Effects of Sceletium tortuosum in rats. J Ethnopharmacol 155(1):731–735, 2014 24930358

Murbach TS, Hirka G, Szakonyiné IP, et al: A toxicological safety assessment of a standardized extract of Sceletium tortuosum (Zembrin®) in rats. Food Chem Toxicol 74:190–199, 2014 25301237

Nell H, Siebert M, Chellan P, et al: A randomized, double-blind, parallel-group, placebo-controlled trial of extract Sceletium tortuosum (Zembrin) in healthy adults. J Altern Complement Med 19(11):898–904, 2013 23441963

Shikanga EA, Viljoen AM, Combrinck S, et al: The chemotypic variation of Sceletium tortuosum alkaloids and commercial product formulations. Biochem Syst Ecol 44:364–373, 2012

Smith C: The effects of Sceletium tortuosum in an in vivo model of psychological stress. J Ethnopharmacol 133(1):31–36, 2011 20816940

Terburg D, Syal S, Rosenberger LA, et al: Acute effects of Sceletium tortuosum (Zembrin), a dual 5-HT reuptake and PDE4 inhibitor, in the human amygdala and its connection to the hypothalamus. Neuropsychopharmacology 38(13):2708–2716, 2013 23903032

Zhang HT: Cyclic AMP-specific phosphodiesterase-4 as a target for the development of antidepressant drugs. Curr Pharm Des 15(14):1688–1698, 2009 19442182

CHAPTER 18

Bacopa monnieri for Cognitive Support

Carlo Calabrese, N.D., M.P.H.

> Ayurvedic medicine regards Brahmi as having rejuvenating properties (Rasayana) specific to brain (Medhya) function.
>
> *R.H. Singh* (Singh et al. 2008)

The herb *Bacopa monnieri* (L.) Pennell (family Scrophulariaceae), a nootropic (brain enhancer), is available as a dietary supplement. A bitter herb, it appears in Vietnamese grocery stores as *rau dang*. In the West, it is called thyme-leaved gratiola, water hyssop, herb of grace, moneywort, or Indian pennywort. *Bacopa* is known as *Brahmi* in Ayurvedic medicine; it is cited in the *Charaka Samhita* (600 B.C. to 100 A.D.). *Brahmi* translates as "related to knowledge of god or reality." An alternative name is *saraswata*, after the goddess of learning. The single most important constituent in Ayurveda formulas for mental development and cognitive function, it is also used for concentration, mood, memory, anxiety, psychosis, sleep, epilepsy, and skin disorders.

Indications

Animal studies and clinical trials provide consistent signs of *Bacopa*'s nootropic effects. Evidence for *Bacopa* is most suggestive in cognitive decline of aging. No U.S. Food and Drug Administration–approved treatment is available for mild cognitive impairment or to slow the progression of dementia. Several uncontrolled clinical studies (e.g., Agarwal et al. 2006 in elders with memory loss; Goswami et al. 2011 in Alzheimer's disease), as well as more rigorous double-blind, randomized controlled trials (RCTs) reviewed later in this chapter showed positive effects of *Bacopa* on cognitive decline.

Studies of single-dose administration show mixed results in memory, but Benson et al. (2014) found nootropic effects in multitasking and sustained performance. In a study by Stough et al. (2001), effects were evident at 12 weeks but not at 5 weeks. Overall, these studies suggest that memory effects may take 3 months to appear.

Controlled Clinical Trials

Bacopa extracts have been tested in nine published double-blind, randomized placebo-controlled trials with cognitive measures (see Table 18–1). Treatment duration was usually about 3 months, with similarly standardized extracts (40%–55% bacosides) at doses between 250 and 600 mg/day. Signs of cognitive benefit appeared in eight of the nine trials. Seven trials, including participants older than 60, had positive results for aspects of memory enhancement. In two RCTs, patients had age-associated memory impairment (Barbhaiya et al. 2008; Raghav et al. 2006). One study in 72 healthy men and women ages 35–60 years found no difference in cognitive function (Sathyanarayanan et al. 2013). A systematic review of six of the trials concluded that *Bacopa* improved performance on 9 of 17 tests in the free recall domain (Pase et al. 2012). A 2014 meta-analysis of eight of the trials (total $N=437$) with low risk of bias noted differences in test procedures but concluded that there may be benefit in improving cognitive function (shortened Trail Making Test B; $P<0.001$) and speed of attention (decreased choice reaction time; $P<0.001$) (Kongkeaw et al. 2014).

Other RCTs have used herbal formulas that included *Bacopa*. A three-herb combination of 47% *Bacopa* with 450 mg of *Bacopa* extract (Sadhu et al. 2014) was given for 12 months to 60- to 75-year-old participants who either were healthy ($n=109$) or had senile dementia of the Alzheimer's type (SDAT; $n=123$). Healthy participants took *Bacopa* or placebo; SDAT patients received the herbal formula or donepezil 10 mg. The herbal group showed improvement over donepezil in SDAT patients in three of four cognitive tests ($P\leq0.02$), functional activities, and depression (both $P<0.0001$) but not in the Mini-Mental State Examination (MMSE) or delayed word recall. In the healthy group, there were significant improvements over placebo in MMSE, delayed word recall, functional activities, and depression.

Comparing cognitive effect sizes (Cohen's d) for *Bacopa*, modafinil, and *Ginkgo biloba*, *Bacopa* administration over time produced the most consistent and largest effects, with almost a standard deviation greater improvement for delayed word recall ($d=0.950$) and for protection from interference during delayed memory ($d=1.010$) (Neale et al. 2013).

Multiple Mechanisms of Action

Bacopa shows a range of possible molecular pathways to the benefits shown in clinical studies (Calabrese and Soumyanath 2012). *Bacopa* is a rare nonstimulant that shows cognitive enhancement. The mechanisms suggest enhancement of current cognitive function as well as slowing of cognitive degeneration, although long-term studies beyond 3 months have not been done.

TABLE 18–1. Double-blind, placebo-controlled randomized trials >6 weeks: *Bacopa* effects on memory and cognition

Reference	Length	Subjects	Extract and dose	Measures	Results vs. placebo
Stough et al. (2001)	12 weeks	$N=46$; 18–59 years; healthy	KeenMind 300 mg; 55% bacosides	RAVLT, learning and forgetting rate, TMT A and B, digit span, simple and choice reaction time	↑ Visual information processing speed ($P<0.02$), learning rate and memory consolidation on RAVLT ($P<0.05$), state anxiety ($P<0.001$)
Roodenrys et al. (2002)	3 months	$N=84$; 40–65 years; healthy	KeenMind 300 mg; 55% bacosides	Memory questionnaire, story recall, delayed recall of word pairs, DS, VS, coding	↑ Word pair delayed recall ($P<0.05$); no improvement in DS, VS, coding, general knowledge, memory questionnaire, or story recall
Raghav et al. (2006)	16 weeks	$N=40$; 55–70 years with memory loss	125 mg twice a day; 55% bacosides	>20% improvement in age-associated memory impairment score at 12 weeks	56% *Bacopa* subjects, 0% placebo improved >20% ($\chi^2=13.2$; $P<0.01$)
Barbhaiya et al. (2008)	12 weeks, 24-week follow-up	$N=62$; 50–75 years; memory complaints ≥1 year	BacoMind 450 mg; 40%–50% bacosides	Modified RAVLT, Wechsler Memory Scale	Improved ($P<0.05$) on 4 of 17 tests
Calabrese et al. (2008)	12 weeks	$N=54$; ≥65 years; healthy	Laila Impex 300 mg; 50% bacosides	RAVLT, Stroop, divided attention, WAIS	↑ RAVLT delayed word recall ($P=0.03$); Stroop ($P=0.003$), composite score ($P=0.01$)

TABLE 18–1. Double-blind, placebo-controlled randomized trials >6 weeks: *Bacopa* effects on memory and cognition *(continued)*

Reference	Length	Subjects	Extract and dose	Measures	Results vs. placebo
Stough et al. (2008)	90 days	$N=107$; 18–50 years; healthy	KeenMind 300 mg/ day	RAVLT, CDR assessment battery	↑ Visual information processing ($P=0.029$), working memory ($P=0.035$) on 11 subtests
Morgan and Stevens (2010)	12 weeks	$N=98$; >55 years; healthy	BacoMind 300 mg/ day	RAVLT, CFT, TMT, MAC-Q memory complaints	↑ RAVLT verbal learning, memory, delayed recall ($P<0.001$) on CFT, MAC-Q, TMT trend to improvement
Peth-Nui et al. (2012)	12 weeks	$N=60$; healthy elderly (62.6±6.5 years), 2 doses vs. placebo	300 and 600 mg proprietary standardized alcohol extract	Attention, continuity of attention, memory speed and quality, AChE and MAO, event-related potentials	↑ Continuity of attention and memory quality at both doses ($P<0.001$); ↓ AChE and MAO activity ($P<0.001$); ↓ latency of ERP ($P<0.05$)
Sathyanarayanan et al. (2013)	12 weeks	$N=72$; 35–60 years; healthy	450 mg extract standardized	Verbal learning and memory, inspection time, attention and interference, state and trait anxiety	Cognitive measures: no significant differences between groups; a trend for lower state anxiety

Note. AChE=acetylcholinesterase; CDR=Cognitive Drug Research; CFT=Complex Figure Test; DS=digit span; ERP=event-related potentials; MAC-Q=Memory Assessment Clinic-Q; MAO=monoamine oxidase; RAVLT=Rey Auditory-Verbal Learning Test; TMT=Trail Making Test; VS=visual span; WAIS=Wechsler Adult Intelligence Scale. ↑=improves or increases; ↓=reduces.

Bacopa affects neurotransmitter systems, including the cholinergic system, modulating acetylcholine release, acetylcholinesterase inhibition, and muscarinic cholinergic receptor binding. A trial by Peth-Nui et al. (2012) showed a decrease in acetylcholinesterase activity in humans. Neural protein metabolism appears to be enhanced by bacosides A and B with increased protein kinase activity and protein content in the hippocampus. Arborization and growth of dendrites also has been found. Increases in levels of the antioxidants superoxide dismutase, catalase, and glutathione peroxidase in the prefrontal cortex, striatum, and hippocampus followed chronic *Bacopa* administration in rats. Anticlastogenic activity in human lymphocytes was attributed to antioxidant properties. In rodents, suppression of inflammation (implicated in the pathogenesis of Alzheimer's disease and vascular dementia) by *Bacopa* extract was comparable to that by indomethacin. *Bacopa* selectively inhibited prostaglandin E2–induced inflammation in mice. *Bacopa* or its saponins showed neuroprotection against toxicities, including nicotine, sodium nitrite, diazepam, and scopolamine in mice; aluminum and hypoxia in rats; phenytoin-induced cognitive deficit in epileptic patients; and β-amyloid-induced cell death in primary cortical culture, as well as disruption of amyloid aggregation. It dose-dependently decreased levels of β-amyloid in cortex and hippocampus in the PSAPP Alzheimer's mouse model (Dhanasekaran et al. 2004).

Administration and Safety

Bacopa, usually available as encapsulated dried extract, should be standardized to a specific content of bacoside A or A and B, the active saponins. Several somewhat standardized commercial extracts of *Bacopa*, including Baccdrix, Bacognize (Verdure, Geni Herbs), BacoMind, Bacopa55 (Laila Impex), Bacopin (Sabinsa), and KeenMind (CDRI 08), are available. Most extracts have recommended doses of 300–450 mg/day, with some up to 600 mg/day. In addition, many combination products contain *Bacopa*.

Human and animal studies show *Bacopa* to be quite safe. However, long-term studies on safety and efficacy have yet to be done. The most frequent side effects are mild gastrointestinal symptoms (Calabrese et al. 2008; Morgan and Stevens 2010). Interactions with other drugs are theoretical, but *Bacopa* may interact additively with calcium channel blockers and thyroid hormones and increase effects of drugs metabolized by cytochrome P450. It may reduce the effects of phenytoin and anticholinergic medications used for allergies and depression. Because information is insufficient, *Bacopa* should not be used by women who are pregnant or nursing. No standard recommendations are available for children.

KEY POINTS

- *Bacopa* shows more consistent clinical trial evidence for cognitive enhancement in early cognitive decline than do other popular dietary supplements.

- Purported mechanisms of action by *Bacopa* include antioxidant, anti-inflammatory, and neuroprotective mechanisms, as well as effects on cholinergic systems and central protein metabolism.

References

Agarwal A, Sharma A, Rajamanickam GV, et al: Age consistent cognitive decline: an Ayurvedic pharmacological management. Indian Journal of Gerontology 20(4):317–336, 2006

Barbhaiya HC, Desai PD, Saxena VS, et al: Efficacy and tolerability of BacoMind on memory improvement in elderly participants—a double blind placebo controlled study. Journal of Pharmacology and Toxicology 3(6):425–434, 2008

Benson S, Downey LA, Stough C, et al: An acute, double-blind, placebo-controlled cross-over study of 320 mg and 640 mg doses of Bacopa monnieri (CDRI 08) on multitasking stress reactivity and mood. Phytother Res 28(4):551–559, 2014 23788517

Calabrese C, Soumyanath A: Brahmi: traditional botanical medicine for cognitive decline, in Phytochemicals: Health Promotion and Therapeutic Potential. Edited by Carkeet C, Grann K, Randolf RK, et al. Boca Raton, FL, CRC Press, 2012, pp 205–226

Calabrese C, Gregory WL, Leo M, et al: Effects of a standardized Bacopa monnieri extract on cognitive performance, anxiety, and depression in the elderly: a randomized, double-blind, placebo-controlled trial. J Altern Complement Med 14(6):707–713, 2008 18611150

Dhanasekaran M, Holcomb L, Young KA, et al: Bacopa monnieri extract reduces beta-amyloid deposition in the doubly transgenic PSAPP Alzheimer's disease mouse model. Neurology 63(8):1548, 2004

Goswami S, Sanji A, Kumar N, et al: Effect of Bacopa monnieri on cognitive functions in Alzheimer's disease patients. Int J Collab Res Intern Med Public Health 3(4):285–290, 2011

Kongkeaw C, Dilokthornsakul P, Thanarangsarit P, et al: Meta-analysis of randomized controlled trials on cognitive effects of Bacopa monnieri extract. J Ethnopharmacol 151(1):528–535, 2014 24252493

Morgan A, Stevens J: Does Bacopa monnieri improve memory performance in older persons? Results of a randomized, placebo-controlled, double-blind trial. J Altern Complement Med 16(7):753–759, 2010 20590480

Neale C, Camfield D, Reay J, et al: Cognitive effects of two nutraceuticals Ginseng and Bacopa benchmarked against modafinil: a review and comparison of effect sizes. Br J Clin Pharmacol 75(3):728–737, 2013 23043278

Pase MP, Kean J, Sarris J, et al: The cognitive-enhancing effects of Bacopa monnieri: a systematic review of randomized, controlled human clinical trials. J Altern Complement Med 18(7):647–652, 2012 22747190

Peth-Nui T, Wattanathorn J, Muchimapura S, et al: Effects of 12-week Bacopa monnieri consumption on attention, cognitive processing, working memory, and functions of both cholinergic and monoaminergic systems in healthy elderly volunteers. Evid Based Complement Alternat Med 2012(7):606424, 2012 23320031

Raghav S, Singh H, Dalal PK, et al: Randomized controlled trial of standardized Bacopa monniera extract in age-associated memory impairment. Indian J Psychiatry 48(4):238–242, 2006 20703343

Roodenrys S, Booth D, Bulzomi S, et al: Chronic effects of Brahmi (Bacopa monnieri) on human memory. Neuropsychopharmacology 27(2):279–281, 2002 12093601

Sadhu A, Upadhyay P, Agrawal A, et al: Management of cognitive determinants in senile dementia of Alzheimer's type: therapeutic potential of a novel polyherbal drug product. Clin Drug Investig 34(12):857–869, 2014 25316430

Sathyanarayanan V, Thomas T, Einöther SJ, et al: Brahmi for the better? New findings challenging cognition and anti-anxiety effects of Brahmi (Bacopa monniera) in healthy adults. Psychopharmacology (Berl) 227(2):299–306, 2013 23354535

Singh RH, Narsimhamurthy K, Singh G: Neuronutrient impact of Ayurvedic Rasayana therapy in brain aging. Biogerontology 9(6):369–374, 2008 18931935

Stough C, Lloyd J, Clarke J, et al: The chronic effects of an extract of Bacopa monniera (Brahmi) on cognitive function in healthy human subjects. Psychopharmacology (Berl) 156(4):481–484, 2001 11498727

Stough C, Downey LA, Lloyd J, et al: Examining the nootropic effects of a special extract of Bacopa monniera on human cognitive functioning: 90 day double-blind placebo-controlled randomized trial. Phytother Res 22(12):1629–1634, 2008 18683852

SECTION IV

Neurohormones

CHAPTER 19

Melatonin and Melatonin Analogues for Psychiatric Disorders

Amirhossein Modabbernia, M.D.

All men whilst they are awake are in one common world: but each of them, when he is asleep, is in a world of his own.

Plutarch

Melatonin (*N*-acetyl-5-methoxytryptamine) is a versatile hormone synthesized primarily by the pineal gland from tryptophan. Secretion of melatonin by the pineal follows a circadian rhythm regulated by the suprachiasmatic nuclei (SCN) in the hypothalamus (Dubocovich et al. 2003). As a result of inhibition of SCN by light, peak melatonin secretion occurs during the night. Melatonin is known for regulating sleep and circadian rhythm. Recent studies show that melatonin has strong radical scavenging and antioxidant properties (Ramis et al. 2015), regulates energy metabolism (Cipolla-Neto et al. 2014), and modulates immune function (Calvo et al. 2013). As such, the potential therapeutic uses of melatonin encompass a wide range of conditions, from diseases of the central nervous system to cancer and metabolic disorders. In this chapter, I offer an evidence-based review of melatonin and its analogues in psychiatric treatment.

Melatonin

Pharmacodynamics and Pharmacokinetics

Two G-protein-coupled receptors (MT_1 and MT_2) in SCN are responsible for mediating most of melatonin's actions in the brain. Melatonin suppresses the firing of SCN neurons during nighttime through its interaction with MT_1. MT_2 is responsible for melatonin's effect on SCN's circadian rhythm. After exposure to supranormal concentrations of melatonin, both MT_1 and MT_2 receptors are rapidly desensitized (Gerdin et al. 2004a, 2004b).

In clinical settings, melatonin is usually administered orally, although intravenous and sublingual routes have been used. About 9%–33% of orally administered melatonin is absorbed into the bloodstream (Harpsøe et al. 2015). The half-life of melatonin is 20–50 minutes. The peak plasma concentration is reached after 50 minutes (T_{max}=50 min). The most important enzyme in metabolizing melatonin is cytochrome P450 (CYP) 1A2 (Ma et al. 2005). The pharmacokinetics of melatonin are affected by factors such as age, smoking, and use of oral contraceptives, caffeine, and fluvoxamine. In elderly populations, a marked decrease in melatonin secretion occurs, whereas in critically ill patients, absorption is accelerated and elimination is compromised (Harpsøe et al. 2015).

Treatment with melatonin during pregnancy and breast-feeding is not recommended. Melatonin should not be used with other sedative-hypnotics and should be used with caution in patients with epilepsy because it might increase the frequency of seizures.

Sleep Disorders

A large proportion of clinical trials of melatonin have investigated its efficacy for insomnia. A meta-analysis of 19 randomized controlled trials (RCTs; N=1,683) showed that melatonin 0.3–5.0 mg/day modestly improved sleep-onset latency by 7 minutes, total sleep time (TST) by 8 minutes, and both subjective and objective sleep quality compared with placebo (Ferracioli-Oda et al. 2013). Longer duration and higher doses of melatonin were associated with a stronger therapeutic effect. Ferracioli-Oda et al. concluded that although melatonin effects are modest, they do not diminish with time.

Melatonin should be considered for insomnia if nonpharmacological interventions (e.g., sleep hygiene) are not successful. Doses of 0.1–3.0 mg and 0.3–5.0 mg produce physiological levels of melatonin sufficient for promoting sleep and phase- shifting circadian rhythms, respectively. Melatonin can be started at the lowest effective dose (0.3–0.5 mg), particularly in older adults (Vural et al. 2014); however, larger doses (up to 10 mg/day) might be needed and are well tolerated for treatment of insomnia, rapid eye movement (REM) sleep behavior disorder, tardive dyskinesia, and other conditions (Brown et al. 2009). Prolonged-release melatonin (Circadin) is licensed for treatment of insomnia in New Zealand and other countries for individuals older than 55 years. This formulation, which introduces melatonin into the bloodstream over a period of 8–10 hours, is generally well tolerated and is associated with minimal withdrawal or hangover. It does not interact with commonly used medications and does not affect cognition, memory, or postural stability (Lemoine and Zisapel 2012); however, it can have additive sedative effects if it is taken with other sedating medications or alcohol.

Melatonin is remarkably effective in jet lag, a condition that affects air travelers who cross multiple time zones. In a Cochrane review of 10 RCTs (N=975), 9 of 10 studies reported significant benefit from melatonin (0.5–5 mg taken between 10 P.M. and midnight destination time) versus placebo. Lower efficacy was observed for the slow-release preparation and during westward flights (Herxheimer and Petrie 2002).

There have been extensive efforts to study melatonin in neurodevelopmental and neurodegenerative disorders. Autism spectrum disorder is associated with altered circadian rhythm, frequent nighttime awakening, longer sleep-onset latency, reduced TST (Tordjman et al. 2015), and disturbances in melatonin secretion (Rossignol and Frye 2014). Several RCTs showed that melatonin (2–15 mg) significantly improved TST and sleep-onset latency in patients with autism spectrum disorder and sleep problems with minimal side effects (Tordjman et al. 2015). In a meta-analysis of five crossover RCTs (N=57), melatonin increased TST by 73 minutes and decreased sleep-onset latency by 66 minutes compared with placebo (Rossignol and Frye 2011). In a multicenter RCT of 146 children with neurodevelopmental disorders and concurrent severe sleep disorders that did not respond to usual sleep hygiene, melatonin (45 minutes before bedtime) increased TST by 22 minutes and decreased sleep-onset latency by 37 minutes (Gringras et al. 2012). In a meta-analysis of studies of patients with intellectual disability, melatonin decreased sleep-onset latency by 34 minutes, increased TST by 50 minutes, and significantly decreased the number of nighttime awakenings (Braam et al. 2009). For patients with autism spectrum disorder who have difficulty sleeping despite behavioral modification and sleep hygiene, melatonin can be started at 0.5–1 mg and titrated up in 1-mg increments to a maximum of 10 mg.

A meta-analysis of nine RCTs (Zhang et al. 2016) showed that melatonin improved subjective sleep quality in patients with Alzheimer's and Parkinson's disease, but it did not affect objective sleep outcomes. Melatonin effectively improved REM sleep behavior disorder associated with neurodegenerative diseases. In a meta-analysis of seven RCTs in dementia patients, melatonin improved TST by 24 minutes and sleep-onset latency marginally. The beneficial effect was stronger with longer treatment (Xu et al. 2015). Melatonin has been considered an alternative to clonazepam for treatment of REM sleep behavior disorder because of its beneficial effects and better tolerability profile (McGrane et al. 2015). Although the number of high-quality studies of melatonin in REM sleep behavior disorder is small, the evidence is expanding (McGrane et al. 2015). Current evidence suggests that melatonin might have a more direct effect on pathophysiology of this disorder than does clonazepam.

Melatonin also has been studied in sleep disturbances caused by shift work. In a meta-analysis of seven trials, melatonin (1–10 mg) after a night shift increased daytime sleep by 24 minutes compared with placebo. In a meta-analysis of three studies, melatonin increased nighttime sleep time by 17 minutes. The quality of evidence was generally low (Liira et al. 2014). No dose-response effect was present, and sleep-onset latency was unchanged.

Anxiety and Agitation

A meta-analysis of 12 RCTs (N=774) found that premedication with melatonin significantly reduced preoperative anxiety in adults. Melatonin efficacy was comparable to that of midazolam in preoperative anxiety, although effects on postoperative anxiety were mixed (Hansen et al. 2015). A meta-analysis of four RCTs (N=358) yielded low-grade evidence for melatonin premedication for postoperative anxiety in children (Mihara et al. 2015).

Prevention of Delirium and Sundowning

A meta-analysis of four RCTs (N=609 elderly patients) showed that melatonin (0.5–5 mg) or ramelteon (8 mg) given at 9 P.M. for several days might prevent some cases of delirium (Chen et al. 2016). Melatonin decreased the incidence of delirium in general by 56% (95% confidence interval [CI]=−13%–85%) and on medical wards by 75% (95% CI=12%–93%) but not in surgical patients. Findings from this small number of studies were interpreted cautiously. Patients with dementia can experience sundowning, worsening confusion, and agitation at the end of the day and into the night. A meta-analysis found that melatonin (2.5–10 mg/day) reduced sundowning in two of four RCTs and five case series (de Jonghe et al. 2010).

Counteracting the Metabolic Effects of Atypical Antipsychotics

In patients taking atypical antipsychotics such as olanzapine, common side effects are weight gain, hypertriglyceridemia, and glucose intolerance, possibly caused by disturbing circadian rhythm (Cohrs 2008). Melatonin may reduce metabolic side effects of antipsychotics by restoring normal circadian rhythm. Melatonin enhances oxidative phosphorylation (Martín et al. 2002) and interacts with the appetite-regulating hormone leptin (Szewczyk-Golec et al. 2015). Studies suggest that melatonin improves insulin resistance (Gonciarz et al. 2013; McMullan et al. 2013; Tresguerres et al. 2013). Small RCTs show that melatonin (3–5 mg every night) can counteract metabolic side effects of atypical antipsychotics (especially weight gain) (Modabbernia et al. 2014; Mostafavi et al. 2014; Romo-Nava et al. 2014) while causing minimal side effects compared with other options (e.g., metformin).

Other Uses

Clinicians find melatonin modestly helpful for tardive dyskinesia in some patients (Castro et al. 2011). A double-blind RCT in 22 patients with schizophrenia and tardive dyskinesia reported that melatonin 10 mg/day for 6 weeks reduced Abnormal Involuntary Movement Scale scores significantly more than did placebo (Shamir et al. 2001). However, the American Academy of Neurology guidelines found insufficient evidence to support or refute the efficacy of melatonin for tardive dyskinesia (Bhidayasiri et al. 2013). Small studies suggest that coadministration of melatonin and fluoxetine might improve sleep in patients with major depression (Hansen et al. 2014; Serfaty et al. 2010). Systematic reviews found insufficient evidence for melatonin treatment of cognitive impairment, depression, or epilepsy (Brigo and Del Felice 2012; Hansen et al. 2014; Jansen et al. 2006).

Safety and Tolerability

Melatonin, considered a safe supplement, is not regulated by the U.S. Food and Drug Administration (FDA). In a 28-day placebo-controlled RCT, melatonin 10 mg was not associated with significant side effects or changes in biochemical or hormonal parameters (Seabra et al. 2000). Several studies reported slight daytime sleepiness and drowsiness as melatonin side effects in small proportions of patients (Rossignol and Frye 2011).

Overview of the Synthetic Analogues of Melatonin

Ramelteon, an MT_1 and MT_2 receptor agonist (Kato et al. 2005) approved for insomnia by the FDA, was found by the European Medicines Agency to have insufficient evidence of efficacy in insomnia. A meta-analysis of 13 RCTs concluded that ramelteon slightly improved subjective sleep-onset latency and objective TST without affecting REM sleep architecture or awakenings (Kuriyama et al. 2014). In a multicenter double-blind, randomized placebo-controlled trial in elderly patients with serious medical conditions, those given ramelteon had significantly lower incidence of delirium compared with placebo (3% vs. 32%) (Hatta et al. 2014).

Tasimelteon, a melatonin receptor agonist (greater affinity for MT_2 than for MT_1), was FDA approved for non-24-hour sleep-wake disorder, a rare circadian rhythm disorder in blind people. In a 27-center RCT, tasimelteon 20 mg 1 hour before sleep entrained 20% of non-24-hour sleep-wake disorder participants compared with 3% given placebo (Lockley et al. 2015).

Agomelatine, an atypical antidepressant approved by the European Medicines Agency for treatment of depression, is not available in the United States. Evidence suggests that it improves depressive symptoms through a synergistic effect on MT_1/ MT_2 (agonist) and serotonin type 2C receptors (antagonist) (Racagni et al. 2011). In a meta-analysis of 20 RCTs ($N=7,460$ participants), agomelatine was more effective than placebo, with a small effect size (standardized mean difference=0.24; 95% CI=0.12–0.35) (Taylor et al. 2014). Three large RCTs suggested that agomelatine (25–50 mg/day for 12–24 weeks) was superior to placebo for generalized anxiety disorder. Although agomelatine is generally safe, hepatotoxicity occurs occasionally (Gahr et al. 2015).

KEY POINTS

- Melatonin can be beneficial for insomnia (including in children with neurodevelopmental disorders), rapid eye movement sleep behavior disorder, sundowning, jet lag, perioperative anxiety and delirium, and metabolic side effects of antipsychotics.

- Melatonin and its analogues have minimal, transient side effects, except for agomelatine, which rarely causes hepatotoxicity.

References

Bhidayasiri R, Fahn S, Weiner WJ, et al: Evidence-based guideline: treatment of tardive syndromes: report of the Guideline Development Subcommittee of the American Academy of Neurology. Neurology 81(5):463–469, 2013 23897874

Braam W, Smits MG, Didden R, et al: Exogenous melatonin for sleep problems in individuals with intellectual disability: a meta-analysis. Dev Med Child Neurol 51(5):340–349, 2009 19379289

Brigo F, Del Felice A: Melatonin as add-on treatment for epilepsy. Cochrane Database Syst Rev 6(6):CD006967, 2012 22696363

Brown RP, Gerbarg PL, Muskin PR: How to Use Herbs, Nutrients and Yoga in Mental Health Care. New York, WW Norton, 2009

Calvo JR, González-Yanes C, Maldonado MD: The role of melatonin in the cells of the innate immunity: a review. J Pineal Res 55(2):103–120, 2013 23889107

Castro F, Carrizo E, Prieto de Rincón D, et al: Effectiveness of melatonin in tardive dyskinesia. Invest Clin 52(3):252–260, 2011 21950196

Chen S, Shi L, Liang F, et al: Exogenous melatonin for delirium prevention: a meta-analysis of randomized controlled trials. Mol Neurobiol 53(6):4046–4053, 2016 26189834

Cipolla-Neto J, Amaral FG, Afeche SC, et al: Melatonin, energy metabolism, and obesity: a review. J Pineal Res 56(4):371–381, 2014 24654916

Cohrs S: Sleep disturbances in patients with schizophrenia: impact and effect of antipsychotics. CNS Drugs 22(11):939–962, 2008 18840034

de Jonghe A, Korevaar JC, van Munster BC, et al: Effectiveness of melatonin treatment on circadian rhythm disturbances in dementia: are there implications for delirium? A systematic review. Int J Geriatr Psychiatry 25(12):1201–1208, 2010 21086534

Dubocovich ML, Rivera-Bermudez MA, Gerdin MJ, et al: Molecular pharmacology, regulation and function of mammalian melatonin receptors. Front Biosci 8:d1093–d1108, 2003 12957828

Ferracioli-Oda E, Qawasmi A, Bloch MH: Meta-analysis: melatonin for the treatment of primary sleep disorders. PLoS One 8(5):e63773, 2013 23691095

Gahr M, Zeiss R, Lang D, et al: Hepatotoxicity associated with agomelatine and other antidepressants: disproportionality analysis using pooled pharmacovigilance data from the Uppsala Monitoring Centre. J Clin Pharmacol 55(7):768–773, 2015 25650773

Gerdin MJ, Masana MI, Dubocovich ML: Melatonin-mediated regulation of human MT(1) melatonin receptors expressed in mammalian cells. Biochem Pharmacol 67(11):2023–2030, 2004a 15135299

Gerdin MJ, Masana MI, Rivera-Bermúdez MA, et al: Melatonin desensitizes endogenous MT2 melatonin receptors in the rat suprachiasmatic nucleus: relevance for defining the periods of sensitivity of the mammalian circadian clock to melatonin. FASEB J 18(14):1646–1656, 2004b 15522910

Gonciarz M, Bielański W, Partyka R, et al: Plasma insulin, leptin, adiponectin, resistin, ghrelin, and melatonin in nonalcoholic steatohepatitis patients treated with melatonin. J Pineal Res 54(2):154–161, 2013 22804755

Gringras P, Gamble C, Jones AP, et al: Melatonin for sleep problems in children with neurodevelopmental disorders: randomised double masked placebo controlled trial. BMJ 345:e6664, 2012 23129488

Hansen MV, Danielsen AK, Hageman I, et al: The therapeutic or prophylactic effect of exogenous melatonin against depression and depressive symptoms: a systematic review and meta-analysis. Eur Neuropsychopharmacol 24(11):1719–1728, 2014 25224106

Hansen MV, Halladin NL, Rosenberg J, et al: Melatonin for pre- and postoperative anxiety in adults. Cochrane Database Syst Rev 4(4):CD009861, 2015 25856551

Harpsøe NG, Andersen LP, Gögenur I, et al: Clinical pharmacokinetics of melatonin: a systematic review. Eur J Clin Pharmacol 71(8):901–909, 2015 26008214

Hatta K, Kishi Y, Wada K, et al: Preventive effects of ramelteon on delirium: a randomized placebo-controlled trial. JAMA Psychiatry 71(4):397–403, 2014 24554232

Herxheimer A, Petrie KJ: Melatonin for the prevention and treatment of jet lag. Cochrane Database Syst Rev (2):CD001520, 2002 12076414

Jansen SL, Forbes DA, Duncan V, et al: Melatonin for cognitive impairment. Cochrane Database Syst Rev (1):CD003802, 2006 16437462

Kato K, Hirai K, Nishiyama K, et al: Neurochemical properties of ramelteon (TAK-375), a selective MT1/MT2 receptor agonist. Neuropharmacology 48(2):301–310, 2005 15695169

Kuriyama A, Honda M, Hayashino Y: Ramelteon for the treatment of insomnia in adults: a systematic review and meta-analysis. Sleep Med 15(4):385–392, 2014 24656909

Lemoine P, Zisapel N: Prolonged-release formulation of melatonin (Circadin) for the treatment of insomnia. Expert Opin Pharmacother 13(6):895–905, 2012 22429105

Liira J, Verbeek JH, Costa G, et al: Pharmacological interventions for sleepiness and sleep disturbances caused by shift work. Cochrane Database Syst Rev 8(8):CD009776, 2014 25113164

Lockley SW, Dressman MA, Licamele L, et al: Tasimelteon for non-24-hour sleep-wake disorder in totally blind people (SET and RESET): two multicentre, randomised, double-masked, placebo-controlled phase 3 trials. Lancet 386(10005):1754–1764, 2015 26466871

Ma X, Idle JR, Krausz KW, et al: Metabolism of melatonin by human cytochromes p450. Drug Metab Dispos 33(4):489–494, 2005 15616152

Martín M, Macías M, León J, et al: Melatonin increases the activity of the oxidative phosphorylation enzymes and the production of ATP in rat brain and liver mitochondria. Int J Biochem Cell Biol 34(4):348–357, 2002 11854034

McGrane IR, Leung JG, St Louis EK, et al: Melatonin therapy for REM sleep behavior disorder: a critical review of evidence. Sleep Med 16(1):19–26, 2015 25454845

McMullan CJ, Curhan GC, Schernhammer ES, et al: Association of nocturnal melatonin secretion with insulin resistance in nondiabetic young women. Am J Epidemiol 178(2):231–238, 2013 23813704

Mihara T, Nakamura N, Ka K, et al: Effects of melatonin premedication to prevent emergence agitation after general anaesthesia in children: a systematic review and meta-analysis with trial sequential analysis. Eur J Anaesthesiol 32(12):862–871, 2015 26225499

Modabbernia A, Heidari P, Soleimani R, et al: Melatonin for prevention of metabolic side-effects of olanzapine in patients with first-episode schizophrenia: randomized double-blind placebo-controlled study. J Psychiatr Res 53:133–140, 2014 24607293

Mostafavi A, Solhi M, Mohammadi MR, et al: Melatonin decreases olanzapine induced metabolic side-effects in adolescents with bipolar disorder: a randomized double-blind placebo-controlled trial. Acta Med Iran 52(10):734–739, 2014 25369006

Racagni G, Riva MA, Molteni R, et al: Mode of action of agomelatine: synergy between melatonergic and 5-HT2C receptors. World J Biol Psychiatry 12(8):574–587, 2011 21999473

Ramis MR, Esteban S, Miralles A, et al: Protective effects of melatonin and mitochondria-targeted antioxidants against oxidative stress: a review. Curr Med Chem 22(22):2690–2711, 2015 26087763

Romo-Nava F, Alvarez-Icaza González D, Fresán-Orellana A, et al: Melatonin attenuates antipsychotic metabolic effects: an eight-week randomized, double-blind, parallel-group, placebo-controlled clinical trial. Bipolar Disord 16(4):410–421, 2014 24636483

Rossignol DA, Frye RE: Melatonin in autism spectrum disorders: a systematic review and meta-analysis. Dev Med Child Neurol 53(9):783–792, 2011 21518346

Rossignol DA, Frye RE: Melatonin in autism spectrum disorders. Curr Clin Pharmacol 9(4):326–334, 2014 24050742

Seabra ML, Bignotto M, Pinto LR Jr, et al: Randomized, double-blind clinical trial, controlled with placebo, of the toxicology of chronic melatonin treatment. J Pineal Res 29(4):193–200, 2000 11068941

Serfaty MA, Osborne D, Buszewicz MJ, et al: A randomized double-blind placebo-controlled trial of treatment as usual plus exogenous slow-release melatonin (6 mg) or placebo for sleep disturbance and depressed mood. Int Clin Psychopharmacol 25(3):132–142, 2010 20195158

Shamir E, Barak Y, Shalman I, et al: Melatonin treatment for tardive dyskinesia: a double-blind, placebo-controlled, crossover study. Arch Gen Psychiatry 58(11):1049–1052, 2001 11695951

Szewczyk-Golec K, Woźniak A, Reiter RJ: Inter-relationships of the chronobiotic, melatonin, with leptin and adiponectin: implications for obesity. J Pineal Res 59(3):277–291, 2015 26103557

Taylor D, Sparshatt A, Varma S, et al: Antidepressant efficacy of agomelatine: meta-analysis of published and unpublished studies. BMJ 348:g1888, 2014

Tordjman S, Davlantis KS, Georgieff N, et al: Autism as a disorder of biological and behavioral rhythms: toward new therapeutic perspectives. Front Pediatr 3:1, 2015 25756039

Tresguerres JA, Cuesta S, Kireev RA, et al: Beneficial effect of melatonin treatment on age-related insulin resistance and on the development of type 2 diabetes. Horm Mol Biol Clin Investig 16(2):47–54, 2013 25436746

Vural EM, van Munster BC, de Rooij SE: Optimal dosages for melatonin supplementation therapy in older adults: a systematic review of current literature. Drugs Aging 31(6):441–451, 2014 24802882

Xu J, Wang LL, Dammer EB, et al: Melatonin for sleep disorders and cognition in dementia: a meta-analysis of randomized controlled trials. Am J Alzheimers Dis Other Demen 30(5):439–447, 2015 25614508

Zhang W, Chen XY, Su SW, et al: Exogenous melatonin for sleep disorders in neurodegenerative diseases: a meta-analysis of randomized clinical trials. Neurol Sci 37(1):57–65, 2016 26255301

SECTION V

Mind-Body Practices

CHAPTER 20

Polyvagal Theory and the Social Engagement System

Neurophysiological Bridge Between Connectedness and Health

Stephen W. Porges, Ph.D.
C. Sue Carter, Ph.D.

The Polyvagal Theory helps us understand how cues of risk and safety, continuously monitored by our nervous system, influence physiological and behavioral states. The theory emphasizes the human quest to calm neural defense systems by detecting features of safety.

S.W. Porges, "Making the World Safe for Our Children"
(Porges 2015)

We wish to thank Dr. Patricia L. Gerbarg for assisting in the preparation of this chapter.

Polyvagal Theory: Neural Mechanisms That Mediate Effects of Mind-Body Treatments

Polyvagal theory is a reconceptualization of how autonomic state and behavior are intertwined (Porges 1995, 2007, 2011). Body practices within complementary, alternative, and integrative medicine (CAIM) involve active behaviors, which exercise neural regulation of the autonomic nervous system and are facilitated by procedures that conform to our quest to feel safe. This quest may be conceptualized as a core biological imperative that underlies the actions of mental, physical, and neurophysiological processes.

Polyvagal theory explains how cues of risk and safety promote states of safety and calmness or states of defense. The theory shows how features of mind-body therapies trigger physiological states that calm neural defense systems, improve mental and physical health, and support feelings of safety and connectedness with others. Polyvagal theory proposes that physiological state is a fundamental part, not a correlate, of emotion and mood. The theory emphasizes a bidirectional link between brain and viscera, which would explain how thoughts and emotions can change our physiological state and how our physiological state influences our thoughts and emotions.

The human nervous system provides two paths to trigger neural mechanisms capable of downregulating defense and enabling states of calmness that support health, spontaneous social behavior, and connectedness. One path is *passive* and does not require conscious awareness (see the subsection "Neuroception" later in the chapter), and the other is *active* and requires *conscious voluntary behaviors* to trigger specific neural mechanisms that change physiological state. Positive patient-therapist interactions recruit the passive pathway (Geller and Porges 2014). This involves the therapist's ability to use positive facial expressions and to speak in a prosodic voice that conveys benevolent feelings of concern toward the patient. The calming of the patient through social engagement is supplemented by the features of the clinical context in which the treatment is delivered, such as a quiet space secure from intrusion, a comfortable chair, or soothing music. Both the animate features of the therapist's engagement and the inanimate features of the clinical context trigger the passive pathway to promote the physiological state associated with feeling safe. Mind-body practices recruit the active pathway by performing voluntary behaviors such as voluntarily regulated breathing practices, movements and postures (e.g., yoga, qigong, tai chi), and vocalizations (e.g., sounds, chants, songs) that exercise the neural circuits that promote neurophysiological states supporting health. These volitional behaviors, which are part of mind-body practices, are directly wired into vagal circuits that efficiently alter the physiological state (see the subsection "Polyvagal Theory: Overview" later in this chapter).

The Role of the Vagus Nerves in Bidirectional Brain-Body Communication

During the phylogenetic transition from ancient reptiles to mammals, the autonomic nervous system changed. In primitive reptiles, the autonomic nervous system regulated bodily organs via two subsystems: the sympathetic nervous system and the parasympathetic nervous system. The sympathetic nervous system provided the neural pathways for visceral changes that support fight-or-flight behaviors. This physiological adjustment to support mobilization was associated with increases in heart rate and inhibition of digestive processes, which required suppression of parasympathetic (i.e., vagal) influences to the heart and the gut. Complementing the sympathetic nervous system, the reptilian parasympathetic nervous system serves two functions. First, when not recruited as a defense system, it supports processes of health, growth, and restoration. Second, when recruited as a defense system, the parasympathetic nervous system reduces metabolic activity by dampening heart rate and respiration, enabling immobilized reptiles to appear inanimate to potential predators. When reptiles are not under threat, the two components of the autonomic nervous system function antagonistically to innervate several of the body organs to coordinate bodily functions. This synergism between the sympathetic and the parasympathetic nervous systems is maintained in mammals but only when mammals are safe. In this safe state, the potential of the autonomic nervous system being recruited in support of defense is greatly reduced. Polyvagal theory considers being safe as a biobehavioral state determined by the nervous system, often independent of awareness and actual threat. Thus, removal of threat may not change physiological state or enable an individual to feel safe.

Most of the neural pathways of the parasympathetic nervous system travel through the vagus nerves, the large tenth cranial nerves that originate in the brain stem and provide a bidirectional connection between visceral organs and the brain. The vagus contains motor fibers that regulate the function of visceral organs and sensory fibers that provide the brain with continuous information about the status of these organs. The flow of information between body and brain informs specific brain circuits that regulate target organs. Bidirectional communication provides a plausible neural basis for a mind-body science and a brain-body medicine by providing bodily portals of intervention to correct brain dysfunction through peripheral vagal stimulation (e.g., electronic vagal nerve stimulation for treatment of epilepsy or depression) and plausible explanations for exacerbation of physical symptoms by psychological stressors, such as stress-related episodes of irritable bowel syndrome. In addition, bidirectional communication between the brain and specific visceral organs provides an anatomical basis for historical concepts within physiology and medicine, such as Walter Cannon's homeostasis (Cannon 1932) and Claude Bernard's internal milieu (Bernard 1872).

Polyvagal Theory: Overview

Polyvagal theory emphasizes a hierarchical relation among components of the autonomic nervous system that evolved to support adaptive behaviors in response to environmental conditions of safety, danger, and life threat (Porges 2011). The theory is named *polyvagal* to highlight the existence of two vagal circuits: an ancient vagal circuit associated with "immobilization" defense and a phylogenetically newer circuit related to feeling safe and engaging in spontaneous social behavior. The theory articulates two defense systems: 1) the commonly known fight-or-flight system associated with activation of the sympathetic nervous system and 2) a lesser-known system of immobilization and dissociation associated with activation of a phylogenetically more ancient vagal pathway.

Polyvagal theory describes the neural mechanisms through which physiological states communicate feelings of safety and threat to oneself and to others. Bodily feelings contribute to an individual's capacity either to feel safe and spontaneously engage with others or to feel threatened and recruit defensive strategies. The theory explains how each of three phylogenetic stages, during the development of the vertebrate autonomic nervous system, is associated with a distinct and measurable autonomic subsystem. Each of these three subsystems remains active and is expressed in humans under certain conditions (Porges 2009). The three autonomic subsystems are phylogenetically ordered and behaviorally linked to three global adaptive domains of behavior: 1) social communication (facial expression, vocalization, listening), 2) defensive strategies associated with mobilization (fight-or-flight behaviors), and 3) defensive immobilization (feigning death, vasovagal syncope, behavioral shutdown, dissociation). On the basis of their phylogenetic emergence during the evolution of the vertebrate autonomic nervous system, these neuroanatomically based subsystems form a response hierarchy.

Most of the neural fibers in the vagus are sensory (approximately 80% of the total fibers); however, most scientific interest has been directed to the motor fibers that regulate the visceral organs, including the heart and the gut. Of these motor fibers, only about 15% are myelinated (approximately 3% of the total vagal fibers). Myelin, a fatty coating over the neural fiber, is associated with faster and more tightly regulated neural control circuits. The myelinated vagal pathway to the heart is a rapidly responding component of a neural feedback system, involving brain and heart, which rapidly adjusts heart rate to challenges.

Humans and other mammals have two functionally distinct vagal circuits. One vagal circuit is phylogenetically older and unmyelinated. It originates in a brain stem area called the dorsal motor nucleus of the vagus. The other vagal circuit is uniquely mammalian and myelinated. It originates in the brain stem area nucleus ambiguus. The phylogenetically older unmyelinated vagal motor pathways are shared with most vertebrates and, when not recruited as a defense system, function to support health, growth, and restoration via neural regulation of subdiaphragmatic organs (internal organs below the diaphragm). The "newer" myelinated vagal motor pathways, found only in mammals, regulate the supradiaphragmatic organs (heart and lungs). This newer vagal circuit, which slows heart rate and supports states of calmness, mediates the physiological state necessary for mind-body treatments to have positive effects.

The Vagal Brake

Through evolution, the primary vagal regulation of the heart shifted in mammals from unmyelinated pathways to include myelinated pathways. Because the nucleus ambiguus is ventral to the dorsal motor nucleus, the regulation of myelinated vagal pathways to the heart is frequently included as part of a ventral vagal complex. The myelinated vagus functions as a brake on the heart's pacemaker, resulting in a substantially slower heart rate than the intrinsic rate of the pacemaker. Thus, the myelinated vagus via rapid inhibition and disinhibition of the pacemaker can quickly calm or mobilize an individual. Consistent with the calming function, the myelinated vagus actively inhibits the influence of the sympathetic nervous system on the heart and dampens hypothalamic-pituitary-adrenal (HPA) axis activity (see Porges 2001). Thus, the vagal brake, by modulating visceral state, enables the individual to rapidly engage and disengage with objects and other individuals and to promote self-soothing behaviors and calm states.

Breathing is the only autonomic function that can be easily controlled voluntarily. Thus, it is an efficient, easily accessible voluntary behavior that regulates the vagal brake by reducing and increasing the influence of the vagus on the heart. Hering (1910) reported that cardioinhibitory vagal pathways had a respiratory rhythm that reflected dynamic adjustments of vagal control of the heart. More recently, this phenomenon was described as a "respiratory gate" by Eckberg (2003), who emphasized enhancement of vagal influences on the heart during exhalation and dampening of vagal cardiac influences during inhalation. Numerous mind-body practices involve shifts in voluntarily regulated breathing patterns (see Chapter 21, "Breathing Techniques in Psychiatric Treatment"). These include changes in the rate and depth of respiration; vocalizations such as sounds (e.g., "om"), chants, and songs; breath holds; and changes in the relative duration of inhalation and expiration, which manipulate the respiratory gate. Other practices, such as meditation, also affect breath patterns. Posture shifts, which trigger baroreceptors (blood pressure receptors) to adjust blood flow to the brain, also recruit systematic changes in vagal regulation of the heart to avoid dizziness and fainting (vasovagal syncope). These manipulations of the vagal brake exercise the inhibitory influence of the vagus on the heart as an efficient calming mechanism.

The Face-Heart Connection: Emergence of the Social Engagement System

The face-heart connection enabled mammals to detect whether an animal of the same species was in a calm physiological state and "safe" to approach or in a highly mobilized and reactive physiological state during which engagement would be dangerous. The face-heart connection concurrently enabled an individual to signal "safety" through patterns of facial expression and vocal intonation, potentially calming an agitated conspecific to enable formation of a social relationship. When the newer mammalian vagus is optimally functioning in social interactions (inhibiting the sympathetic excitation that promotes fight-or-flight behaviors), emotions are well regulated, vocal prosody is rich, and the autonomic state supports calm, spontaneous social engagement behaviors. Thus, it is highly advantageous to become adept at managing social interactions by using the "newer" mammalian vagus rather than the more limited options of recruiting the sympathetic nervous system to support fight-or-flight behaviors or the "older" vagus to support immobilization and death feigning.

The face-heart system is bidirectional such that the newer myelinated vagal circuit influences social interactions, and positive social interactions influence vagal function to optimize health, dampen stress-related physiological states, and support positive reciprocal social interactions. As individuals change facial expressions, the intonation of their voices, the pattern of breathing, and their posture, they are also changing their physiology through "neural exercises" affecting the influence of the myelinated vagus on the heart and state of mind.

When an individual feels safe, two important features are expressed. First, bodily state is regulated more efficiently to promote growth and restoration (visceral homeostasis). Functionally, this is accomplished through an increase in the influence of myelinated vagal motor pathways on the cardiac pacemaker to slow heart rate, inhibit the fight-or-flight mechanisms of the sympathetic nervous system, dampen the stress response system of the HPA axis (e.g., cortisol), and reduce inflammation by modulating immune reactions (e.g., cytokines). Second, through evolution, the brain stem nuclei that regulate the myelinated vagus became integrated with the nuclei that regulate the muscles of the face and head via special visceral efferent pathways. These neuroanatomical developments provide a face-heart connection involving mutual interactions between the vagal influences on the heart and the neural regulation of the striated muscles of the face and head. The phylogenetically novel face-heart connection provided mammals with an ability to convey physiological state via facial expression and prosody (intonation of voice), enabling facial expression and voice to calm physiological state (Porges 2011; Porges and Lewis 2010; Stewart et al. 2013). Social communication, employing the face-heart system for social engagement, provides a mechanism through which individuals can coregulate one another's behavior and physiology.

The Social Engagement System

The phylogenetic origin of behaviors associated with the social engagement system is intertwined with the phylogeny of the autonomic nervous system. As the muscles of the face and head emerged as social engagement structures, the myelinated vagus evolved and was regulated by the nucleus ambiguus. This convergence of neural mechanisms produced an integrated social engagement system with synergistic behavioral (somatomotor) and visceral components, as well as interactions between ingestion, state regulation, and social engagement. The neural pathways originating in several cranial nerves that regulate the striated muscles of the face and head (special visceral efferent pathways) and the myelinated vagal fibers form the neural substrate of the social engagement system (see Porges 1998, 2001, 2003). As illustrated in Figure 20–1, the somatomotor component includes the neural structures involved in social and emotional behaviors. Special visceral efferent nerves innervating striated muscles regulate structures derived from ancient gill arches (Truex and Carpenter 1969). The social engagement system has a motor control component in the cortex (upper motor neurons) that regulates brain stem nuclei (lower motor neurons) to control eyelid opening (looking), facial muscles (emotional expression), middle ear muscles (extracting human voice from background noise), muscles of mastication (ingestion), laryngeal and pharyngeal muscles (e.g., prosody, intonation), and head-turning muscles (social gesture and orientation). Collectively, these muscles function both as determinants of engagement with the social environment and as filters that limit social stimuli. The neural pathway involved in raising the eyelids (the facial nerve) also tenses the stapedius muscle in the middle ear, which facilitates hearing human voice. Thus, the neural mechanisms for making eye contact are shared with those needed to listen to human voice. As a cluster, poor eye gaze, difficulties extracting human voice from background sounds, blunted facial expression, minimal head gesture, limited vocal prosody, and poor state regulation are common features of individuals with autism and other psychiatric disorders.

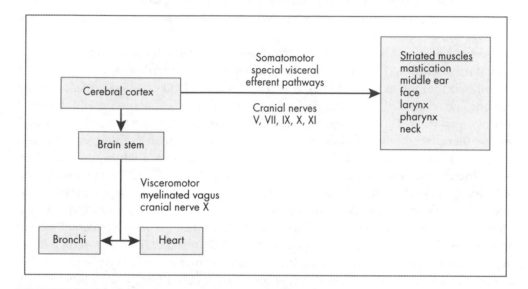

FIGURE 20–1.   Motor pathways of the social engagement system.

The social engagement system includes a somatomotor component (special visceral efferent pathways that regulate the striated muscles of the face and head) and a visceromotor component (myelinated vagus that regulates the heart and bronchi).

Afferents from the target organs of the social engagement system, including the muscles of the face and head, provide potent input to the brain stem source nuclei regulating both visceral and somatic components of the social engagement system. Thus, activation of the somatomotor component (e.g., listening, ingestion, lifting eyelids) can influence the visceral state via myelinated vagal efferents to the sinoatrial node (increasing or decreasing the influence of the vagal brake). These changes in visceral state will either promote or impede social engagement behaviors. For example, reducing the influence of the vagal brake promotes mobilization (fight-or-flight behaviors), which impedes expression of social engagement behaviors. Conversely, increasing the influence of the vagal brake promotes spontaneous social engagement behaviors and feelings of safety and trust.

Recruiting Active and Passive Pathways

The pathways defining the social engagement system enable the effects of mind-body practices (e.g., vocalizing, breathing practices, shifting postures, movements) to influence the physiological state via myelinated pathways within the vagus. Features of the social engagement system are recruited by passive and active pathways. The passive pathway recruits the social engagement system through cues of safety such as a quiet environment, positive and compassionate therapist-patient interactions, prosodic quality (e.g., melodic intonation) of the therapist's vocalizations, and music modulated across frequency bands that overlap with vocal signals of safety used by a mother to calm her infant. Successful therapists, regardless of their orientation, often intuitively manipulate the passive pathway in treatment. In contrast, the active pathway recruits the social engagement system when the patient engages in mind-body practices, such as vocalizations, voluntarily controlled breathing practices, movements, or postures.

Perhaps the most potent method for influencing the myelinated vagus is through voluntarily controlled breathing practices. Research documents that breathing gates the influence of the myelinated vagus on the heart (see Eckberg 2003). Vagal efferent inhibition of the heart's pacemaker is potentiated during exhalation and dampened during inhalation. Thus, although several therapeutic techniques (e.g., dialectical behavior therapy, cognitive-behavioral therapy) involve slow breathing, calming is a function of breath rate and inhalation-to-exhalation ratio. Techniques that slow breathing and expand the duration of exhalation relative to inhalation enhance the inhibitory effect of the vagus on the heart. This strategy of prolonging exhalation relative to inhalation is embedded in certain breathing practices, chants, and singing. Moreover, as the phrases of vocalizations become longer, breathing becomes slower and deeper. Breathing movements expand from the chest toward the abdomen in order to inhale a sufficient volume of air. With abdominal or belly breathing, the diaphragm must be pushed downward, stimulating vagal afferents and functionally influencing the vagal outflow to the heart. Similarly, modulation of breathing during chants and meditation provides a potent mechanism to regulate and exercise vagal efferent influence on the heart.

Vocalizations, including chanting and singing, and playing a wind instrument may be conceptualized as CAIM treatments that require not only active manipulation of breathing but also recruitment of additional components of the social engagement system. For example, chants require production and monitoring of sounds while regulating breath. Modulation of vocalizations requires the active involvement of laryngeal and pharyngeal nerves (see Figure 20–1) to change pitch and to regulate resonance. Breath is critical because the sounds are produced by controlled expiration passing air at a sufficient velocity across structures in the larynx. Moreover, control of vocalizations requires monitoring of acoustic properties via middle ear structures. Without sufficient neural tone to the middle ear muscles, the sounds of human vocalizations will be lost in the background of low-frequency sounds. Playing a wind instrument could be conceptualized as a CAIM treatment because it involves listening and voluntary control of breathing and of muscles of the face and mouth. Thus, virtually all the neural pathways involved in the social engagement system (see Figure 20–1) are recruited and coordinated with breathing practices, chanting, vocalizing, or playing a wind instrument. This includes regulation of muscles of the mouth, face, neck, middle ear (acoustic monitoring), larynx, and pharynx. Thus, vocalization may provide an "active pathway" to recruit and exercise several aspects of the social engagement system while promoting a calm state through the ventral vagal pathway.

Mind-body practices may involve voluntary posture shifts, which influence blood pressure receptors known as baroreceptors. Baroreceptors send signals to the brain stem that either increase heart rate by downregulating vagal efferent output (and often stimulating sympathetic output) or decrease heart rate by increasing vagal efferent output. Postures can efficiently shift physiological states, often enabling a visceral feeling of activation (due to transitory withdrawal of the ventral vagus) that is rapidly followed by calming (after reengagement of the ventral vagus). Functionally, voluntary behaviors of breathing, vocalizing, and postures provide a way to regulate and exercise all the neural circuits of the social engagement system. As an individual becomes more proficient in using the active pathway as a neural exercise of autonomic regulation, the autonomic nervous system becomes more resilient. This resilience is manifested in a greater capacity to downregulate defense and to support more flexible, adaptive emotional states, social behaviors, and health.

Consistent with the polyvagal theory, treatments, including CAIM, are optimized during biobehavioral states associated with feeling safe. In this neurophysiological safe state, it is easier to inhibit the neurobiological defense strategies, which may be interfering with the patient's ability to trust and feel safe enough to explore thoughts and feelings in therapy. Thus, treatment is facilitated when the patient is in a physiological state that supports feelings of safety. This can be mediated through the passive pathway, which simultaneously downregulates the involuntary defense subsystems and potentiates the physiological state associated with the evolutionarily newer social engagement system.

Although the provision of a safe, quiet environment is important, it is not always possible. In noisy clinics or emergency departments, or during and after disasters, a quiet environment cannot be achieved. Even when in a quiet office, patients often feel unsafe, anxious, defensive, and inhibited. Nevertheless, certain mind-body practices, particularly slow breathing practices, can be effectively used to shift the patient into a state of mental and physical calmness even under adverse conditions (see Chapter 21). Furthermore, when the instructions for the practices are given in a soft prosodic voice, the passive pathway is activated. In mind-body interventions, breath, posture, and vocalization engage the active pathway as neural exercises of circuits within the social engagement system. By enhancing the efficiency and reliability of pathways inhibiting defense systems, the individual acquires greater feelings of safety such that the body shifts to a neurophysiological state that supports health, growth, and restoration.

To understand how the passive pathway is recruited, it is necessary to understand two additional features of polyvagal theory: dissolution and neuroception. First, through the process of dissolution (see the following subsection, "Dissolution"), the theory describes autonomic reactivity as a phylogenetically organized response hierarchy in which evolutionarily newer circuits inhibit older circuits. *Dissolution* explains how specific autonomic states have the capacity to support either defensive or calm behaviors. The autonomic state that supports calm behavior also has the capacity to actively downregulate reactivity and defense. Thus, it is not sufficient for an individual to solely refrain from defensive behaviors. He or she also must be in an autonomic state that is incompatible with defensive behaviors. Second, through the process of neuroception (see subsection "Neuroception" below), context can influence autonomic state. *Neuroception* is a complex neural process that evaluates risk in the environment independent of cognitive awareness. Neuroception detects risk from sensory patterns in the environment and reflexively shifts autonomic state to support either defense or safe interactions. Neuroception provides clues to how the passive pathway is elicited. Dissolution provides an understanding of emergent properties, related to both resilience and vulnerability, associated with the various autonomic states elicited via neuroception.

DISSOLUTION

The three circuits defined by polyvagal theory are organized and respond to challenges in a phylogenetically determined hierarchy consistent with the Jacksonian principle of dissolution. Jackson proposed that higher (phylogenetically newer) neural circuits inhibit lower (phylogenetically older) circuits, and "when the higher are suddenly rendered functionless, the lower rise in activity" (Jackson 1882, p. 412). Although Jackson proposed dissolution to explain changes in brain function due to damage and illness, polyvagal theory proposes a similar phylogenetic hierarchical model to describe the sequence of autonomic responses to challenges.

In addition to the myelinated vagal pathway, in order to survive in dangerous and life-threatening situations, the mammalian nervous system retained two more primitive neural circuits to regulate defensive strategies: *fight-flight* and *death-feigning*. It is important to note that social behavior, social communication, and visceral homeostasis are incompatible with neurophysiological states that support defense. In the hierarchy of adaptive responses, the newest circuit is used first; if that circuit fails to provide safety, older circuits are recruited sequentially. Thus, from a polyvagal perspective, the objective of CAIM treatments is to recruit the phylogenetically newest circuit that downregulates defense and uses the social engagement system and the myelinated vagus. Mind-body procedures, via the active pathway, can exercise the social engagement system, including the myelinated vagus. Mind-body practices provide more efficient neural exercises when the individual is in a calm and safe physiological state, wherein the active pathway is not in conflict with adaptive defense reactions elicited through the passive pathway. Thus, understanding how to regulate the passive pathway to maintain a calm physiological state is important for optimizing the effectiveness of CAIM. Neuroception provides insight into mechanisms that enable or disable the passive pathway.

NEUROCEPTION

The nervous system processes sensory information from the environment and from the viscera to evaluate risk continuously. Polyvagal theory proposes that this neural evaluation of risk does not require conscious awareness and functions through neural circuits that are shared with our phylogenetic ancestors. The term *neuroception* (Porges 2004) was introduced to emphasize a neural process, distinct from conscious perceptions or sensations, capable of distinguishing environmental (and visceral) features that indicate safety, danger, or life threat. In safe environments, the autonomic state adaptively dampens sympathetic activation and protects the oxygen-dependent central nervous system, especially the cortex, from the metabolically conservative reactions of the dorsal vagal complex (e.g., vasovagal syncope).

Neuroception mediates both the expression and the disruption of positive social behavior, emotion regulation, and visceral homeostasis (Porges 2004, 2007). Triggered by feature detectors in the brain, neuroception may involve areas of temporal cortex that communicate with the central nucleus of the amygdala and the periaqueductal gray. Accordingly, neuroception is proposed as a mechanism through which limbic reactivity is modulated by temporal cortex responses to biological movements, including voices, faces, and hand gestures. Embedded in the construct of neuroception is the capacity of the nervous system to detect and react to the "intention" of movements and sounds by decoding and interpreting the intuited goal of the movements and sounds of animate and inanimate objects. This process occurs without awareness. Although we are often unaware of the stimuli that trigger neuroceptive responses, we are usually profoundly aware of our body's reactions (e.g., rapid heart rate, shaking, sweating). Thus, the neuroception of familiar individuals and those with appropriately prosodic voices and warm, expressive faces promotes a calm physiological state and a sense of safety that translate into a positive social interaction.

Navigating in a potentially precarious environment, neuroception is involved in regulating the nervous system to perform two important adaptive tasks: 1) assessment of risk and 2) if the environment is safe, inhibition of the more primitive limbic structures involved in defensive fight, flight, or immobilization (e.g., death feigning). Any stimulus that can signal cues of safety through neuroception has the potential to recruit the evolutionarily advanced social engagement system that promotes calm behavioral states and supports prosocial behaviors.

Removing cues of danger is not sufficient for ensuring that everyone feels safe. Many experience quiet spaces as safe and restful, but others become anxious and hypervigilant in anticipation of an undefined intrusion. One method to enable safe feelings is slow, regulated breathing practices, preferably with eyes closed, while sitting or lying in a physically comfortable supported position. Vagal afferent messages from the respiratory system can override anxiety and hypervigilance (see Chapter 21). Another method for attaining a neuroception of safety is to process additional sensory features in the environment, such as acoustic stimulation modulated in the frequency band of a mother's lullaby. Humans are hardwired to be calmed by modulated voices (Porges and Lewis 2010). The acoustic features that calm infants are universal and have been repurposed by composers of classical music (Porges 2010). Composers implicitly understood that they could lull the audience into a state of safety (via neuroception) by constructing melodic themes that duplicate the vocal range of a mother soothing her infant, while limiting the contribution of low-frequency sounds. Similarly, the acoustic structure of liturgical vocal music minimizes low-frequency sounds and emphasizes voices in the range of the nurturing mother calming her infant. In contrast, organs with large pipes generating low-frequency tones do not create a feeling of safety but trigger a feeling of awe. These low tones have acoustic features that overlap with our immobilization reactions to a predator.

In most situations, the passive pathway is activated during social interactions by prosodic vocalizations, gestures, and facial expressions. Violations of a "neural expectancy" for reciprocal interactions can shift the physiological state from calmness to defensiveness that would, by disrupting homeostasis, interfere with healing processes (see Geller and Porges 2014). The reciprocal behaviors and intersubjective experiences that define therapeutic interactions may greatly influence a patient's physiological state and thereby contribute to treatment outcomes. In addition to physiological state shifts in response to the interactions between social engagement systems of the patient and the therapist, neuroception monitors features of the *context* in which treatment is delivered. Polyvagal theory helps identify optimal contexts for delivering CAIM. Contexts that enable the individual to reduce hypervigilance and maintain a state of calmness provide 1) protection from others when one is in a physically vulnerable state (e.g., supine or eyes closed) and 2) reduction of sensory cues of danger by attenuating low- and high-frequency sounds associated with danger and by limiting distracting visual cues. Such contexts are characteristic of traditional forms of psychotherapy and psychoanalysis in which the therapist uses a warm prosodic voice to regulate the state of the patient even when the patient is unable to make direct eye contact.

Visceral cues as triggers of defense.   Potent visceral feedback from organs below the diaphragm often occurs during illness and injury. Unlike specifically localized sensory feedback through spinal nerves, for example, when our gut is distended, our brain interprets *interoceptive* signals through vagal afferent pathways from subdiaphragmatic organs as generalized. It is often difficult to identify the precise origin of visceral signals (Craig 2002; Porges 1993). During illness, injury, inflammation, or any serious challenge to the normal "homeostatic" function of a visceral organ, signals travel from the organ through vagal sensory fibers to a brain stem area, the nucleus of the solitary tract. This nucleus contributes to central regulation of autonomic state and the function of visceral organs. As the primary sensory nucleus of the vagus, the nucleus of the solitary tract sends information to higher brain centers and vagal "motor" nuclei (nucleus ambiguus and dorsal nucleus of the vagus) to selectively modulate specific target organs.

When using *mobilization* as a defense (fight-or-flight behaviors), vagal afferent pathways, via the nucleus of the solitary tract, impact the nucleus ambiguus, enabling sympathetic activation by turning off the inhibitory action of the myelinated ventral vagal pathway on the heart (i.e., withdrawing the vagal brake) (Porges et al. 1996). However, when using *immobilization* as a defense, vagal sensory pathways, via the nucleus of the solitary tract, activate the dorsal nucleus of the vagus. Thus, trauma inflicted directly on the subdiaphragmatic area (via surgery, birthing, rape, illness, or injury) may trigger dorsal vagal responses (e.g., immobilization with fear) that are manifested psychologically as depression or dissociation, behaviorally as fatigue, and medically as problems in blood pressure regulation, fainting (vasovagal syncope), fibromyalgia, or digestive disorders, including irritable bowel syndrome. With higher-level defensive strategies, the social engagement system and the ventral vagus (e.g., vagal brake) are downregulated, and physiological states do not support health, growth, and restoration. Mind-body practices can be used to enhance physiological resilience and to optimize homeostasis by strengthening higher-level neural systems and reducing dependence on lower-level defense systems.

Potential discrepancies between feelings and cognitions. *Neuroception* refers to those neural processes involved in risk evaluation that are not conscious. Functionally, this can lead to discrepancies between conscious perceptions and feelings. We may be aware of how we feel, but we may not be aware of the antecedent features in the environment that trigger the neuroceptive processes that change our physiological state and form the neural substrate of our feelings. For example, lowering pitch and reducing prosody may trigger a neuroceptive response similar to a fear response to a predator. The words may be benign, but the tonal qualities of voice may trigger a physiological state that supports aggressive behaviors (Pell et al. 2015). During such states, higher brain processes attempt to make sense of discrepancies between feelings and cognitions. In most situations, feelings take priority because the feelings are wired into our brain's adaptive survival strategies. In contrast, hostile words delivered via melodic vocalizations may have less negative effect.

Once feelings are driving defenses, higher brain structures build a cohesive personal narrative that justifies being defensive. When we are in these physiologically vulnerable states, our attempts to engage socially may be aggressive, and we may misinterpret the social cues of others as aggressive. In vulnerable people, even subtle behavioral changes, such as mild exercise or walking, may reduce the calming influence of the vagal brake and put the individual into a state in which the social engagement behaviors of others may be misinterpreted as aggressive. Pausing to breathe slowly (at 4.5–6 breaths per minute) can rapidly calm such defensive reactions, providing time for higher cognitive processes and social engagement to take effect. This technique is embedded in therapeutic strategies such as cognitive-behavioral therapy and dialectical behavior therapy.

Regardless of an individual's age, the social engagement system is vulnerable to environmental cues of danger and life threat. Even with the removal of danger cues, the social engagement system may remain dormant unless it is appropriately stimulated with safety cues during critical developmental stages. Research with infants of depressed mothers (Tronick and Reck 2009) illustrates that a lack of opportunity for reciprocal interactions changes the emotional and social profile and trajectory of the infant. For the social engagement system to function, the cues of interaction that are processed by both the visual (facial expressions, gestures) and the auditory (prosodic vocalizations) systems are critical. This redundancy of sensory domains (visual and auditory) enables cues of safety to regulate the child, even if one of these sensory systems is damaged. Although gentle tactile cues may communicate safety, they are often preceded by prosodic voice or warm facial expressions. Without the antecedent vocal and facial signaling of safety, even gentle touch may trigger a neuroceptive state of danger, and the child may recoil from the touch.

The emergence of the social engagement system provides humans with the opportunity to use social behavior to coregulate physiological state and to reciprocally experience a state of safety. During this mutually shared state of feeling safe, the expansive capacities of the human experience can be optimized. The social engagement system functions as a bidirectional conduit between sensory cues from others and the motor systems that express our thoughts and feelings. Although this conduit of connectedness can efficiently downregulate defensive states through potent features of voice and face, it is vulnerable to diffuse and potent sensory stimuli coming from our bodily organs. Thus, engagement behaviors may be relatively inefficient in calming when directed at an individual who is in a physiological state of defense. Under these conditions, facial expressions and syntax may be misinterpreted and, instead of calming, may elicit aggression. Nevertheless, the auditory channel may be more accessible in regulating state. The prepotent influence of a mother's voice in calming a fussy infant shows this effect. A mother's smile alone is unlikely to soothe the child.

Social behavior, including patient-therapist interactions, is supported by biological components that were repurposed or co-opted through mammalian evolution, thereby enabling mutually adaptive coregulation in which individuals optimized one another's physiological states. The phylogenetic shifts in the autonomic nervous system may explain how neuroception triggers states that support either coregulation or defense. Clinically, we observe that past trauma often leads to biased neuroception that detects risk when there is no risk. In the short term, biased neuroception is protective by minimizing exposure to potential predators. In the long term, this hyper-defensiveness makes it difficult for individuals to fulfill their biological imperative to connect, which would enable them to coregulate and to develop enduring social relationships.

Oxytocin and Vasopressin: The Neurochemistry Underlying Polyvagal States

Coregulation is not entirely neural because it includes behavioral features and biochemical changes. Throughout the life span of mammals, the neuropeptide oxytocin plays a prominent role in the biochemistry of social relationships. In mammals, oxytocin is involved in reproduction by helping expel the large-headed newborn from the uterus, expressing milk, and establishing a selective and lasting bond between mother and offspring (Carter 2014). Mammals depend on their mothers' milk for some time after birth. Human mothers form a strong and lasting bond with their newborns immediately after birth during the time that is essential for nourishment and survival of the infant; however, women who give birth by cesarean delivery without going through labor, or who opt not to breast-feed, still form strong emotional bonds with their children. Furthermore, fathers, grandparents, and adoptive parents also form lifelong attachments to children. Preliminary evidence suggests that the mere presence of an infant increases the release of oxytocin in adults (Feldman 2012; Kenkel et al. 2012). The infant's gaze triggers neurophysiological events (social engagement system and oxytocin) that support the strong social bonds that we interpret as love and trust. Research supporting the role of oxytocin in the establishment and maintenance of strong social bonds has, until recently, been based on parental behavior (Feldman 2012) or social behaviors in animals (Carter 1998; Kenkel et al. 2012). However, recent human studies documented that administration of intranasal oxytocin facilitated social behaviors, including eye contact and social cognition (Meyer-Lindenberg et al. 2011). This convergence between physiological state (release of oxytocin and an optimized neural regulation of the autonomic nervous system) and social behavior provides a plausible mechanism whereby social behaviors optimize physiological state and promote feelings of trust and love. Moreover, this convergence emphasizes the bidirectionality between social behavior and physiological state. For example, calm physiological states promote spontaneous social engagement behaviors, and social engagement behaviors can lead to calm physiological states. From a CAIM perspective, the clinical environment provides a "social" portal through which the therapist can calm and optimize the patient's physiological state by improving regulation of the autonomic nervous system and prosocial hormones (e.g., oxytocin).

Just as the activation of the social engagement system is not the equivalent of trust and love, neither is oxytocin the molecular equivalent of trust and love. Both are components of a complex, interactive neural system that allows the body to adapt and co-regulate even during highly emotive and challenging situations. The mechanisms for reciprocal social interactions involve extensive neural networks throughout the brain and autonomic nervous system that are dynamic and constantly changing during the life span. The properties of oxytocin are neither predetermined nor fixed. Other hormones and epigenetic factors regulate oxytocin's cellular receptors. These receptors change and adapt in response to life experiences. Both the oxytocin system and the experience of safe social interactions change over time (Carter et al. 2009).

Oxytocin often interacts with a related peptide, vasopressin. The neural circuits regulated by oxytocin and vasopressin are sometimes redundant. Both neuropeptides are implicated in behaviors that require social engagement by either males or females, such as huddling over an infant (Kenkel et al. 2012). Regulation of the social engagement system, oxytocin, and vasopressin occurs in the brain stem. Interactions among these systems are documented by the presence of receptors for oxytocin and vasopressin in the brain stem source nuclei of the afferent vagal circuit and both efferent vagal circuits (Porges 2001). Research in several mammalian species documented the critical role of oxytocin and vasopressin in the establishment of selective social bonds, parenting, and mate protection. These studies linked oxytocin and vasopressin to the biological imperative of connectedness. Oxytocin and vasopressin potentiate the dynamic behaviors expressed via the social engagement system. These neuropeptides regulate crucial visceral feelings expressed through the autonomic nervous system, which we associate with trusting, loving relationships.

Central vasopressin is associated with the polyvagal state of mobilization. The effects of vasopressin are associated with an increase in sympathetic excitation and, in most cases, with a decrease in the influence of the myelinated vagus via pathways originating in the nucleus ambiguus. Central vasopressin raises the set point of the baroreceptor reflex (a circuit regulating blood pressure), enabling heart rate and blood pressure to rise to higher levels in support of movement, without a reflexive downregulation (Porges 2001). This biobehavioral state supports vigilance and defensive behaviors needed to guard self (Ferris 2008), partner, or territory (Carter 1998).

Peripheral vasopressin acts on a different system. Peripheral vasopressin may support immobilization and death feigning through the dorsal vagus shutdown response described in the polyvagal theory. Peripheral vasopressin also increases the magnitude of the baroreceptor reflex, which immediately decreases heart rate and may cause fainting such that the individual appears to be dead or inanimate. This involuntary response is a primitive biological reflex that we inherited from our reptilian ancestors. Perhaps most relevant to mind-body practices, oxytocin is associated with immobility without fear. This includes relaxed physiological states and postures that enable birth, breast-feeding, and consensual sexual behavior.

Although oxytocin is not essential for parenting, the increase of oxytocin associated with birth and lactation may enable a woman to be less anxious around her newborn and express loving feelings (Carter and Altemus 1997). When oxytocin is absent (e.g., because of a mutation in the oxytocin gene), vasopressin may stimulate the oxytocin receptor, with consequences similar to those of oxytocin. The dynamic interaction between oxytocin and vasopressin is essential for complex social behaviors (e.g., parenting). In humans and other socially monogamous mammals such as the prairie vole, the intricate molecular dance between oxytocin and vasopressin fine-tunes the coexistence of calm caregiving with protective aggression.

Summary

Polyvagal theory provides an innovative model that links the mechanisms mediating feelings of safety to social behavior and health. It helps us understand how cues of risk and safety, continuously monitored by our nervous system (neuroception), influence physiological and behavioral states. As illustrated in Table 20–1, neuroception of environmental cues triggers different physiological states to adapt to features of safety, danger, and life threat. Each biobehavioral state has a neurophysiological profile involving a specific autonomic pathway and neuropeptide that in combination support different clusters of adaptive behaviors. Neurophysiological circuits, disrupted during stress and trauma, impair our abilities to feel connected and to coregulate. The human quest to calm neural defense systems by detecting features of safety is initiated at birth when the infant is dependent on the mother for soothing and nurture and continues throughout the life span with needs for trusting relationships. This innate quest for a safe relationship can be facilitated by mind-body practices that regulate physiological state and by aspects of patient-therapist interaction. Polyvagal theory provides a plausible explanation for how mind-body treatments use both passive (via neuroception) and active (via neural exercises) pathways to enhance homeostatic function, emotion regulation, and social engagement.

TABLE 20–1. Neuroception of environmental conditions

Safety	Danger	Life threat
Parasympathetic system: myelinated vagus	Sympathetic system	Parasympathetic system: unmyelinated vagus
↑ Heart rate variability	↓ Heart rate variability	↓ Heart rate variability
↑ Body awareness	↓ Body awareness	↓ Body awareness
↑ Social engagement	↓ Social engagement	↓ Social engagement
Immobilization without fear	Mobilization	Immobilization with fear
Flexible and adaptive	Approach or withdrawal	Death-feign, collapse
Bond, connect, love, intimacy, soothing, healing, cooperative	Emotion dysregulation, hypervigilance, overactivity	Disconnect, dissociate
↑ Oxytocin	↑ Central vasopressin	↑Peripheral vasopressin?

Note. The polyvagal theory postulates three levels of autonomic response to perceived environmental conditions.

KEY POINTS

- Polyvagal theory emphasizes bidirectional communication between brain and viscera, which would explain how thoughts and emotions affect physiological states, how physiological states influence thoughts and emotions, and how mind-body practices affect physiological state, thoughts, and emotions.

- The therapist's use of positive facial expressions and prosodic voice conveys benevolent feelings of concern toward the patient and recruits the passive neuroceptive pathway.

- Mind-body practices recruit the active pathway through voluntary behaviors that are directly wired into vagal circuits, promoting neurophysiological states that support health.

- The peripheral vagal system provides portals of intervention for correcting dysfunctions of the central and autonomic nervous systems.

- Specific mind-body treatments may recruit the phylogenetically newest circuits to downregulate defense and favor use of the social engagement system and myelinated vagus.

References

Bernard C: De la Physiologie Générale. Paris, Hachette, 1872

Cannon WB: The Wisdom of the Body. New York, WW Norton, 1932

Carter CS: Neuroendocrine perspectives on social attachment and love. Psychoneuroendocrinology 23(8):779–818, 1998 9924738

Carter CS: Oxytocin pathways and the evolution of human behavior. Annu Rev Psychol 65:17–39, 2014 24050183

Carter CS, Altemus M: Integrative functions of lactational hormones in social behavior and stress management. Ann N Y Acad Sci 807(1):164–174, 1997 9071349

Carter CS, Boone EM, Pournajafi-Nazarloo H, et al: Consequences of early experiences and exposure to oxytocin and vasopressin are sexually dimorphic. Dev Neurosci 31(4):332–341, 2009 19546570

Craig AD: How do you feel? Interoception: the sense of the physiological condition of the body. Nat Rev Neurosci 3(8):655–666, 2002 12154366

Eckberg DL: The human respiratory gate. J Physiol 548 (Pt 2):339–352, 2003 12626671

Feldman R: Oxytocin and social affiliation in humans. Horm Behav 61(3):380–391, 2012 22285934

Ferris CF: Functional magnetic resonance imaging and the neurobiology of vasopressin and oxytocin. Prog Brain Res 170:305–320, 2008 18655891

Geller SM, Porges SW: Therapeutic presence: neurophysiological mechanisms mediating feeling safe in therapeutic relationships. Journal of Psychotherapy Integration 24(3):178–192, 2014

Hering HE: A functional test of heart vagi in man [in German]. Menschen Munchen Medizinische Wochenschrift 57:1931–1933, 1910

Jackson JH: On some implications of dissolution of the nervous system. Medical Press and Circular 2:411–414, 1882

Kenkel WM, Paredes J, Yee JR, et al: Neuroendocrine and behavioural responses to exposure to an infant in male prairie voles. J Neuroendocrinol 24(6):874–886, 2012 22356098

Meyer-Lindenberg A, Domes G, Kirsch P, et al: Oxytocin and vasopressin in the human brain: social neuropeptides for translational medicine. Nat Rev Neurosci 12(9):524–538, 2011 21852800

Pell MD, Rothermich K, Liu P, et al: Preferential decoding of emotion from human non-linguistic vocalizations versus speech prosody. Biol Psychol 111:14–25, 2015 26307467

Porges SW: The infant's sixth sense: awareness and regulation of bodily processes. Zero to Three 14(2):12–16, 1993

Porges SW: Orienting in a defensive world: mammalian modifications of our evolutionary heritage. A Polyvagal Theory. Psychophysiology 32(4):301–318, 1995 7652107

Porges SW: Love: an emergent property of the mammalian autonomic nervous system. Psychoneuroendocrinology 23(8):837–861, 1998 9924740

Porges SW: The polyvagal theory: phylogenetic substrates of a social nervous system. Int J Psychophysiol 42(2):123–146, 2001 11587772

Porges SW: The Polyvagal Theory: phylogenetic contributions to social behavior. Physiol Behav 79(3):503–513, 2003 12954445

Porges SW: Neuroception: a subconscious system for detecting threats and safety. Zero to Three 24(5):19–24, 2004

Porges SW: The polyvagal perspective. Biol Psychol 74(2):116–143, 2007 17049418

Porges SW: Music therapy and trauma: insights from the polyvagal theory, in Symposium on Music Therapy and Trauma: Bridging Theory and Clinical Practice. New York, Satchnote Press, 2010, pp 3–15

Porges SW: The polyvagal theory: new insights into adaptive reactions of the autonomic nervous system. Cleve Clin J Med 76 (suppl 2):S86–S90, 2009 19376991

Porges SW: The Polyvagal Theory: Neurophysiological Foundations of Emotions, Attachment, Communication, and Self-Regulation (Norton Series on Interpersonal Neurobiology). New York, WW Norton, 2011

Porges SW: Making the world safe for our children: down-regulating defence and up-regulating social engagement to 'optimise' the human experience. Children Australia 40(2):114–123, 2015

Porges SW, Lewis GF: The polyvagal hypothesis: common mechanisms mediating autonomic regulation, vocalizations and listening. Handbook of Behavioral Neuroscience 19:255–264, 2010

Porges SW, Doussard-Roosevelt JA, Portales AL, et al: Infant regulation of the vagal "brake" predicts child behavior problems: a psychobiological model of social behavior. Dev Psychobiol 29(8):697–712, 1996 8958482

Stewart AM, Lewis GF, Heilman KJ, et al: The covariation of acoustic features of infant cries and autonomic state. Physiol Behav 120:203–210, 2013 23911689

Tronick E, Reck C: Infants of depressed mothers. Harv Rev Psychiatry 17(2):147–156, 2009 19373622

Truex RC, Carpenter MB: Human Neuroanatomy. Baltimore, MD, Williams & Wilkins, 1969

CHAPTER 21

Breathing Techniques in Psychiatric Treatment

Stress, Anxiety, Depression, Attention, Relationships, Trauma, and Mass Disasters

Richard P. Brown, M.D.

Patricia L. Gerbarg, M.D.

> Breath is the bridge which connects life to consciousness, which unites your body to your thoughts.
>
> *Thích Nhất Hạnh*

Imbalances of the autonomic nervous system underlie and exacerbate stress-related conditions, including anxiety disorders, posttraumatic stress disorder (PTSD), depression, substance abuse, attention-deficit/hyperactivity disorder (ADHD), and behavioral disorders of childhood. The vagaries of the autonomic nervous system drive oxidative damage, inflammation, aging, and the progression of stress-related medical conditions. Restoring sympathovagal balance and resiliency is fundamental to treatment of most disorders seen in psychiatric, pediatric, and general medical practices. The most efficient way to balance the sympathetic and parasympathetic branches of the autonomic nervous system is through voluntarily regulated breathing practices (VRBPs).

Chanting is one of the most ancient breath-regulating practices, used by religious and tribal leaders to calm the mind and strengthen the sense of communal bonding. Shamans and medicine men knew how to use the breath to promote healing and to induce altered states of mind. Warriors developed intense breath practices to focus their minds; to enhance situational awareness, endurance, and strength; to endure painful wounds; and to heal themselves. Awareness or mindfulness of breath is fundamental to Buddhist meditation, yoga, qigong, and other mind-body traditions. Mind-body practices are being developed with specific VRBPs that can be integrated into all mental health treatment modalities and settings. Properly done VRBPs cause very few adverse effects, even in elderly or ill patients, and cost very little. They can be easily taught, are nonstigmatizing, and are accepted across diverse cultures.

In this chapter, we review simple, safe, effective VRBPs that can relieve anxiety and improve emotion regulation, cognitive function, performance, behavior, and relationships. For more extensive discussion and references, see Brown and Gerbarg 2012a; Brown et al. 2013; Gerbarg and Brown 2016a; Gerbarg et al. 2011; and Streeter et al. 2012.

Neurophysiology of Voluntarily Regulated Breathing Practices and Polyvagal Theory

Breath and emotion are bidirectional. Each emotional state is associated with a particular breathing pattern. By consciously changing the pattern of breath, one can shift emotional states (Philippot et al. 2002). In Chapter 20, "Polyvagal Theory and the Social Engagement System," Porges and Carter explained the role of the vagus nerves in bidirectional mind-body communication. *Polyvagal theory* describes afferent parasympathetic nervous system pathways that transmit interoceptive information from visceral organs to the brain. Afferent information from the respiratory system provides an enormous amount of data from millions of receptors (e.g., each alveolus contains three types of stretch receptors); bronchial, laryngeal, pharyngeal, and nasal passages; baroreceptors; chemoreceptors (registering changes in pO_2 and pCO_2); and receptors in the diaphragm, thoracic cavity, and chest wall. Every millisecond, respiratory information streams up vagal pathways to brain stem nuclei and from there to central nervous system networks regulating emotion, perception, cognitive processing, and behavior (see Figure 21–1) (Brown and Gerbarg 2005; 2016a; Brown et al. 2009).

Evidence indicates that slow breathing practices (through vagal afferents) could reduce overactivity in the amygdala, increase underactivity in prefrontal emotion regulatory centers, modulate hypothalamic-pituitary-adrenal function, increase levels of the inhibitory neurotransmitter γ-aminobutyric acid, stimulate oxytocin release, and improve cognitive function (Brown and Gerbarg 2012a; Brown et al. 2013; Gerbarg and Brown 2016a, 2016b; Streeter et al. 2012).

Voluntarily Regulated Breathing Practices

Respiratory sinus arrhythmia and heart rate variability are derived mathematically from the normal changes in the heart's beat-to-beat interval between inspiration and expiration (Lehrer and Gevirtz 2014). These changes reflect the flexibility of the cardiovascular system. High respiratory sinus arrhythmia and heart rate variability are associated with better health and longevity. Low respiratory sinus arrhythmia and

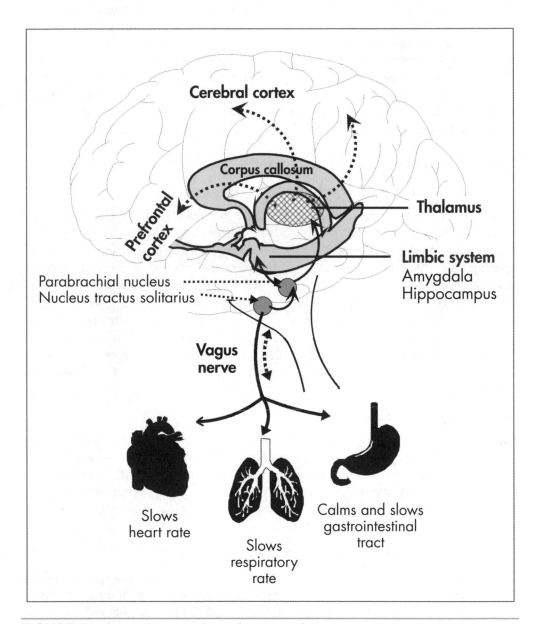

FIGURE 21–1. Bidirectional vagal nerve pathways.

Vagal afferent pathways transmit information from the lungs (and other organs) to brain stem nuclei (nucleus tractus solitarius and parabrachial nucleus). From these nuclei, pathways ascend to the limbic system (amygdala and hippocampus), hypothalamus, insular cortex, thalamus, and thalamocortical projections to prefrontal cortex and other areas of the cerebral cortex (Brown et al. 2009).

heart rate variability are associated with chronic stress, anxiety, panic disorder, PTSD, depression, and aging. The effects of paced breathing on respiratory sinus arrhythmia and heart rate variability have been well documented. For an average adult man, a respiratory rate of 15 cycles per minute (cpm) produces a small difference in heart rate of about 4 beats per minute; at a rate of 5 cpm, the difference in heart rate increases to as much as 35–40 beats per minute in a very healthy man. For most adults, gentle breathing at 4.5–6 cpm increases heart rate variability, as indicated by heart rate variability high-frequency spectrum activity (Lehrer and Gevirtz 2014), leading to a calm state. Slow VRBPs are the most useful clinically because they can rapidly reduce the sympathetic overdrive associated with states of stress and anxiety while increasing parasympathetic activity. Studies show that slow VRBPs are associated with reduction in perceived stress, anxiety, and insomnia (Brown et al. 2013; Gerbarg and Brown 2016b).

Slow Voluntarily Regulated Breathing Practices

UNILATERAL AND ALTERNATE NOSTRIL BREATHING

Two forms of slow breathing are *unilateral nostril breathing* (UNB) and *alternate nostril breathing* (ANB). During UNB, one hand is held over the nose while the fingers close one nostril (either the right or the left). For ANB, the fingers alternate closing and opening the right and left nostrils. The duration of each phase of the breath cycle can be regulated. For a review of studies on unilateral nostril breathing and alternate nostril breathing, see Brown et al. (2013). In clinical practice, alternate nostril breathing can effectively calm someone who is very anxious; however, alternate nostril breathing may be impractical in some situations because it requires holding one hand over the nose, a conspicuous activity in public settings. In certain situations, such as combat, using one hand for alternate nostril breathing is not feasible, thus limiting the usefulness of these techniques.

QIGONG BREATH 4-4-6-2

Respiratory rates can be slowed by adjusting one or more of the four phases of the breath cycle: inhale, pause, exhale, pause. One well-known pattern is called *4-4-6-2* because each phase is counted: four on the inhale, four during a pause, six on the exhale, and two during a pause. Extending the expiratory phase increases parasympathetic activation. We have found it effective clinically in rapidly reducing anxiety, rage, and suicidal thoughts.

COHERENT BREATHING OR RESONANT BREATHING

Coherent breathing, also called *resonant breathing*, is gentle, natural breathing in and out through the nose with equal length of inspiration and expiration at a rate that optimizes sympathovagal balance (heart rate variability), between 4.5 and 6 cpm for adults. Performed without straining, coherent breathing creates a mental state of emotional calmness with mental alertness and enhanced cognitive processing (Brown and Gerbarg 2012a). Coherent breathing is easily taught to individuals or groups in about 20–30 minutes. Ideally, the eyes are closed to focus inward, and breath is paced with a recorded chime tone or other sound (e.g., ocean wave). Coherent breathing can be done with coordinated arm movements while standing, sitting, or supine.

BREATH MOVING

An advanced practice found in qigong and other traditions entails moving the breath and attention to different parts of the body in circuits, for example, closing the eyes and imagining that as one breathes in, breath moves to the top of the head, and as one breathes out, breath moves to the base of the spine (see www.robertpeng.com). Breath moving combined with coherent breathing can be used in treating psychological conditions, physical injuries, and pain. In patients with severe asthma and other respiratory problems, breath moving is used to prevent transient bronchiolar constriction during slow breathing practices.

RESISTANCE BREATHING

Resistance breathing techniques create resistance to the flow of breath. For example, in ocean breath (*ujjayi*), slightly contracting pharyngeal muscles create a sound similar to the ocean while stimulating the vagus nerve and thus enhancing parasympathetic nervous system tone (Brown et al. 2013; Gerbarg and Brown 2016a). Chanting and singing are also resistance breathing in which vocal cord contractions create turbulence to air flow, resulting in sound. Bernardi et al. (2001) showed that chanting the Hail Mary prayer in Latin, breathing at 6 cpm, resulted in increased baroreflex sensitivity and vagal respiratory response.

Rapid, Forceful Breathing Practices or High-Frequency Breathing

Rapid, forceful breathing increases alertness, energy, and attention and includes "Ha" breath, bellows breath (*bhastrika*), and breath of fire (*kapalabhati*) (see review by Telles and Singh 2013). High-frequency breathing should be done only for a few minutes, interspersed with normal breathing and rest, to avoid hyperventilation effects, such as altered mental states. Contraindications include uncontrolled hypertension, seizure disorder, recent surgery, panic, PTSD, flashbacks, dissociative disorders, and respiratory conditions. Rapid, forceful breathing is contraindicated in bipolar disorder because activating practices can trigger hypomanic or manic symptoms, which may occur immediately or be delayed.

Ha breath uses sharp, moderately forceful inhalation and exhalation, and the sound "Ha" is made on the exhale. This activates and focuses the mind. It can be done at moderate rates between 15 and 20 cpm. For most people, Ha breath should be limited to 20 breaths per round with 60 seconds of rest between rounds for no more than 3 rounds.

Voluntarily Regulated Breathing Practices in Clinical Practice

Treatment of Anxiety Disorders, Stress, Insomnia, Posttraumatic Stress Disorder, and Depression

Stress-related and anxiety disorders respond well to slow VRBPs. A clinician can teach coherent breathing within 20 minutes by using a paced chime track on a compact disc or smartphone and instruct the patient to practice daily starting with 5–10 minutes and increasing to 20 minutes, the minimal therapeutic dose. Very anxious patients may need 20 minutes twice a day until symptoms improve. Literature is available on therapeutic breathing practices and how to use them for a wide range of conditions (Brown and Gerbarg 2012a, 2012b). In the short term, coherent breathing can quiet the mind, reduce anxiety, and facilitate sleep. In the long term, daily practice improves autonomic system resiliency, emotion regulation, and social relationships. After 1 or 2 months of practice, patients can do coherent breathing with eyes open while engaged in everyday activities, because it can be done anywhere without anyone knowing that the patient is engaged in a calming, self-regulatory practice.

Slow VRBPs are particularly effective for alleviating symptoms of trauma- and stressor-related disorders such as PTSD: intrusive memories, avoidance, negative emotional states, hypervigilance, poor concentration, and sleep disturbance. Quiet but painful symptoms of trauma and military service are emotional numbing and disconnectedness, which distort family relationships and the sense of self. Slow VRBPs reduce defensive states and support social engagement and bonding (see Chapter 20). The following case illustrates how breathing practices may permanently restore the sense of meaningful connection to self and others.

> After serving for 2 years as a mental health specialist in Iraq, Nancy returned home to her husband with symptoms of posttraumatic stress. Unable to get help through the Department of Veterans Affairs system, she tried numerous forms of therapy, including eye movement desensitization and reprocessing and mindfulness-based cognitive-behavioral therapy. This enabled her to rationally observe and control her overreactions such that she could function, but she felt numb and emotionally disconnected.
>
> Nancy felt well enough to start a family, and she became pregnant. But when her daughter was born, Nancy felt painfully detached, unable to experience a maternal bond. For 4 more years, she continued to search for relief, until she attended a 2-day Breath-Body-Mind (BBM) workshop with Dr. Richard P. Brown, during which she felt a fleeting sensation of wholeness. She began daily breath and movement practices and described the following effects: "I was able to calm my body and mind. I began to thrive. I began to feel life inside me after feeling disconnected and detached for so long. The love known only to my intellect began to fill my heart. For the first time, I was able to embrace my child and truly experience shared love and motherhood. For the first time, I felt profound, deep closeness with my husband, who had waited so long for us to bond. Tapping into my inner resources, I found new meaning and purpose. I have arrived and feel welcome home."

As with Nancy, many survivors of trauma, military service, and mass disasters experience permanent resolution of trauma-related symptoms through specific breath and movement practices (Carter et al. 2013; Descilo et al. 2010; Gerbarg 2008; Gerbarg and Brown 2011, 2012a; Gerbarg et al. 2014).

Studies of yoga programs with prominent regulated breathing components showing significant improvements in depression include five RCTs, one RCT dose-finding study, and two open pilot studies (Brown et al. 2013; Chu et al. 2017; Janakiramaiah et al. 2000; Sharma et al., in press; Streeter et al. 2017). For example, in an RCT of 26 women (BDI>14), those who participated in a 12-week yoga program (breathing exercises, yoga poses, and supine meditation/relaxation) showed increased parasympathetic tone and reduced depressive symptoms and perceived stress compared with a control group (Chu et al. 2017). In another 12-week dose-finding RCT (Iyengar yoga and coherent breathing) of 30 depressed subjects randomly assigned to a high-dose group and a low-dose group, BDI-II scores declined significantly from screening (24.6 ± 1.7) through week 12 for the high-dose group (-18.6 ± 6.6, $p < 0.001$) and from screening (27.7 ± 2.1) to week 12 for the low-dose group (-17.7 ± 9.3, $p < 0.001$) (Streeter et al. 2017).

Children and Youth

Children respond well to breathing practices that can be used in classrooms and after-school programs. A few minutes of Ha breath can be used to focus attention quickly, or coherent breath at age-appropriate rates can be used to reduce anxiety and overre-activity (Brown and Gerberg 2012a, 2012b; for information on children's programs, see www.breath-body-mind.com).

Mass Disasters

Short programs of breathing practices are being used for immediate and long-term re-lief of trauma from mass disasters worldwide. A small number of trainers can pro-vide rapid emotional relief to vast numbers of survivors and can train local residents to continue teaching others. These interventions require no equipment or electricity and are low in cost (Brown and Gerberg 2012a; Gerberg et al. 2011; www.breath-body-mind.com; www.stws.org).

Stress-Related Medical Conditions

Mind-body treatments and VRBPs have the potential to ameliorate physical and psychological pathogenic processes contributing to stress-related conditions, such as inflammatory bowel disease (IBD), a disorder of immune response exacerbated by stress that can be life-threatening. In a double-blind, randomized controlled trial, 29 patients with IBD at the Cornell-Weill Medical Center IBD Center were randomly assigned to either a BBM workshop (breathing, movement, and open focus attention training; see Chapter 25, "Open Focus Training for Stress, Pain, and Psychosomatic Illness") or an educational seminar of equal duration (Gerberg et al. 2015). Both groups continued their usual IBD treatments. The interventions required 9 hours during 2 days plus a 1-hour follow-up per week for 6 weeks, then once a month. At 6 months, the BBM group had significantly greater improvements on the Brief Symptom Inventory ($P=0.04$), Beck Anxiety Inventory ($P=0.03$), Beck Depression Inventory (BDI; $P=0.01$), IBD Questionnaire ($P=0.01$), Perceived Disability Scale ($P=0.001$), and Perceived Stress Questionnaire ($P=0.01$) compared with no significant change on any measure in the control group. The BBM group had significant reduction in measures of IBD symptoms and the inflammatory marker C-reactive protein ($P=0.01$) compared with no change in the control group. Slow VRBPs (coherent breathing), through vagal activation of the cholinergic anti-inflammatory pathway, may trigger anti-inflammatory cascades within the gastrointestinal tract and promote healing. This study validates the potential to heal numerous conditions by counteracting disease-promoting processes at both psychological and physical levels.

KEY POINTS

- Voluntarily regulated breathing practices (VRBPs), by restoring autonomic balance, can relieve symptoms of stress, anxiety, depression, and trauma.

- Intensive practice of specific VRBPs with movement and attention training can potentially resolve long-standing symptoms of trauma.

- VRBPs can improve attention and cognitive function.

- Coherent breathing is a low-risk, low-cost, effective intervention that can be easily integrated into mental health care, medical treatments, school programs, and disaster response.

References

Bernardi L, Porta C, Gabutti A, et al: Modulatory effects of respiration. Auton Neurosci 90(1–2):47–56, 2001 11485292

Brown RP, Gerbarg PL: Sudarshan Kriya yogic breathing in the treatment of stress, anxiety, and depression: part I-neurophysiologic model. J Altern Complement Med 11(1):189–201, 2005 15750381

Brown RP, Gerbarg PL: Yoga breathing, meditation, and longevity. Ann N Y Acad Sci 1172:54–62, 2009 19735239

Brown RP, Gerbarg PL: The Healing Power of the Breath. Boston, MA, Shambhala Press, 2012a

Brown RP, Gerbarg PL: Non-Drug Treatments for ADHD: Options for Kids, Adults, and Clinicians. New York, WW Norton, 2012b

Brown RP, Gerbarg PL, Muskin PR: How to Use Herbs, Nutrients, and Yoga in Mental Health Care. New York, WW Norton, 2009

Brown RP, Gerbarg PL, Muench F: Breathing practices for treatment of psychiatric and stress-related medical conditions. Psychiatr Clin North Am 36(1):121–140, 2013 23538082

Carter J, Gerbarg PL, Brown RP, et al: Multi-component yoga breath program for Vietnam veteran post traumatic stress disorder: randomized controlled trial. J Trauma Stress Disord Treat 2(3):1–10, 2013

Chu IH, Wu WL, Lin IM, et al: Effects of yoga on heart rate variability and depressive symptoms in women: a randomized controlled trial. J Altern Complement Med Jan 4, 2017 [Epub ahrad of print] 28051319

Descilo T, Vedamurtachar A, Gerbarg PL, et al: Effects of a yoga breath intervention alone and in combination with an exposure therapy for post-traumatic stress disorder and depression in survivors of the 2004 South-East Asia tsunami. Acta Psychiatr Scand 121(4):289–300, 2010 19694633

Gerbarg PL: Yoga and neuro-psychoanalysis, in Bodies in Treatment: The Unspoken Dimension. Edited by Anderson FS. Hillsdale, NJ, Analytic Press, 2008, pp 127–150

Gerbarg PL, Brown RP: Mind-body practices for recovery from sexual trauma, in A Guide to Recovery and Empowerment. Edited by Bryant-Davis T. Lanham, MD, Rowman & Littlefield, 2011, pp 199–216

Gerbarg PL, Brown RP: Neurobiology and neurophysiology of breath practices in psychiatric care. Psychiatric Times 33(11):22–25, 2016a

Gerbarg PL, Brown RP: Breathing practices for mental health and aging, in Complementary and Integrative Therapies for Mental Health and Aging. Edited by Lavretsky H, Sajatovic M, Reynolds C. New York, Oxford University Press, 2016b, pp 239–256

Gerbarg PL, Wallace G, Brown RP: Mass disasters and mind-body solutions: evidence and field insights. Int J Yoga Therap 2(21):97–107, 2011 22398351

Gerbarg P, Gootjes L, Brown RP: Mind-body practices and the neuro-psychology of well-being, in Religion and Spirituality Across Cultures (Cross-Cultural Advancements in Positive Psychology; Delle Fave A, series ed). Edited by Kim-Prieto C. New York, Springer, 2014, pp 227–246

Gerbarg PL, Jacob VE, Stevens L, et al: The effect of breathing, movement, and meditation on psychological and physical symptoms and inflammatory biomarkers in inflammatory bowel disease: a randomized controlled trial. Inflamm Bowel Dis 21(12):2886–2896, 2015 26426148

Janakiramaiah N, Gangadhar BN, Naga Venkatesha Murthy PJ: Antidepressant efficacy of Sudarshan Kriya Yoga (SKY) in melancholia: a randomized controlled comparison with electroconvulsive therapy (ECT) and imipramine. Affect Disord 57(1–3):255–259, 2000 10708840

Lehrer PM, Gevirtz R: Heart rate variability biofeedback: how and why does it work? Front Psychol 5(5):756, 2014 25101026

Philippot P, Chapelle G, Blairy S: Respiratory feedback in the generation of emotion. Cogn Emot 16(5):605–627, 2002

Sharma A, Barrett MS, Cucchiara AJ, et al: A breathing-based meditation intervention for patients with major depressive disorder following inadequate response to antidepressants: a ramdomized pilot study. J Clin Psychiatry (in press)

Streeter CC, Gerbarg PL, Saper RB, et al: Effects of yoga on the autonomic nervous system, gamma-aminobutyric-acid, and allostasis in epilepsy, depression, and post-traumatic stress disorder. Med Hypotheses 78(5):571–579, 2012 22365651

Streeter CC, Gerbarg PL, Whitfield TH, et al: Treatment of major depressive disorder with Iyengar yoga and coherent breathing: a randomized controlled dosing study. J Altern Complement Med 23(3):201–207, 2017 28296480

Telles S, Singh N: Science of the mind: ancient yoga texts and modern studies. Psychiatr Clin North Am 36(1):93–108, 2013 23538080

CHAPTER 22

Use of Yoga in Managing Posttraumatic Stress Disorder

Nilkamal Singh, M.Sc.

Shirley Telles, Ph.D.

Acharya Balkrishna

The goal of yoga is to cut the seed of sorrow before it sprouts.

Svāmi Svātmārāma, Hatha Yoga Pradīpikā *(fifteenth century)*

Individuals who have posttraumatic stress disorder (PTSD) can experience irrational responses, such as intense fear, panic, helplessness, rage, or feeling paralyzed, to seemingly innocuous events. Exposure to traumatic reminders can stimulate stress hormone secretion and influence the activation of brain regions involved in the trauma response. Imaging studies indicate an associated increase in cerebral blood flow in the right medial orbitofrontal cortex, insula, amygdala, and anterior temporal pole and a relative deactivation in the left anterior prefrontal cortex and Broca's area, the expressive speech center (Hull 2002). Hence, when an individual with PTSD is exposed to reminders of the trauma, this exposure may activate brain regions that engender intense emotions (e.g., the amygdala) and simultaneously deactivate brain regions involved in the inhibition of emotions (e.g., prefrontal cortex), sustained attention, working memory, rational thinking, and translation of experience into communicable language. Consequently, traumatized individuals are prone to overreact to reminders of the past by automatically engaging in defensive reactions (fight, flight, freeze, or dissociate) that occurred at the time of the trauma but that are inappropriate reactions to their current reality.

Severe psychological trauma can cause dysfunction in neuroendocrine and autonomic stress response systems, with excessive sympathetic activation, parasympathetic suppression, and increased levels of cortisol. Severe childhood trauma can affect all aspects of development, including cognitive, social, emotional, physical, psychological, and moral development (Harris et al. 2004). Serious consequences of trauma can emerge during adolescence and persist into adult life.

Nonpharmacological therapeutic techniques that enable the person to regulate internal states and responses to stressors can augment psychotherapeutic or pharmacological management of trauma-related disorders (Brown et al. 2009; Saeed et al. 2010). The Indian science of yoga includes physical postures (*asanas*), voluntary regulated breathing (*pranayama*), meditation, conscious sensory withdrawal (*pratyahara*), and philosophical principles (Taimini 1986). Studies have shown that practicing yoga can bring functional and structural changes in brain areas associated with PTSD (Cohen et al. 2009; Hölzel et al. 2010). Even though these studies were completed in healthy individuals, the findings suggest that yoga practice may reduce activity within the amygdala in people with PTSD. Concomitantly, practicing yoga has been shown to activate areas of the brain involved in the inhibition of emotions, as well as to improve sustained attention and working memory (Rajesh et al. 2014; Sheela et al. 2013). Many studies have shown that practicing yoga can be beneficial for depression (Schuver and Lewis 2016), stress (Fares and Fares 2016), and anxiety (de Manincor et al. 2016). Studies suggest that these effects of yoga may result from restoration of the balance between the functioning of the sympathetic and parasympathetic divisions of the autonomic nervous system. In this chapter, we review randomized controlled studies of the effects of yoga on persons with PTSD diagnoses and discuss possible mechanisms through which yoga can be beneficial in managing PTSD.

Yoga and Posttraumatic Stress Disorder

A search in two bibliographic databases, PubMed and Google Scholar, for "yoga and PTSD" yielded 42 articles, of which we selected 11 for review on the basis of the following criteria: randomized controlled trials (RCTs), use of yoga as the primary intervention, and English language. Review articles and feasibility studies were excluded. Among the 11 RCTs, 4 reported reduction in specific PTSD symptom clusters, including reexperiencing, hyperarousal, and emotional arousal. The remaining 7 found improvement in PTSD-related symptoms (Table 22–1).

In an RCT, 100 adults who had armed combat–related PTSD were randomly assigned to either a Satyananda yoga group or a control group that received the mandatory ordinary assistance protocol designed by the Colombian Agency for Reintegration (Quiñones et al. 2015). After 16 weeks of yoga practice, scores on the Posttraumatic Stress Disorder Checklist–Civilian (PCLC) improved significantly more than scores for the control group ($P < 0.05$); the highest percentage improvement occurred in the reexperiencing symptom cluster in the yoga group ($P < 0.05$) (Quiñones et al. 2015). In an 8-week study, 80 individuals with PTSD symptoms caused by various types of trauma were randomly assigned to a yoga group and a wait-list con-

TABLE 22–1. Summary of randomized controlled studies of yoga for posttraumatic stress disorder (PTSD)

Study	N	Screening tool(s)	Intervention	Duration	Outcomes	Significance
Quiñones et al. (2015)	100	Clinical observation by psychologists	Satyananda yoga	16 weeks	Yoga group: ↓ PCLC; highest percent improvement in reexperiencing	$P < 0.05$ for both groups
Jindani et al. (2015)	80	PCL-17	Kundalini yoga	8 weeks	Yoga group: ↑ improvement in sleep, positive affect, perceived stress, anxiety, stress resilience	$P < 0.05$ for all measures
Culver et al. (2015)	76	PTSD	Yoga	8 weeks	Yoga group: ↓ symptoms of PTSD	$F_{2,28} = 3.30$; $P = 0.05$
Martin et al. (2015)	38	PSS-I and DSM	Yoga	1/week×12 weeks or 2/week×6 weeks	Yoga group: ↓ external motivation	$P < 0.05$
Reddy et al. (2014)	38	PSS-I	Kripalu-based Hatha yoga, trauma sensitive	12 sessions	Yoga group: ↓ AUDIT and DUDIT scores	$P < 0.001$ for both measures
Carter et al. (2013)	31	DSM-IV	Sudarshan Kriya, modified	6 months	Yoga group: CAPS, CES-D, and PCLM-17 improved	CAPS: $P < 0.05$; CES-D: $P < 0.01$; PCLM-17: $P < 0.001$

TABLE 22–1. Summary of randomized controlled studies of yoga for posttraumatic stress disorder (PTSD) *(continued)*

Study	N	Screening tool(s)	Intervention	Duration	Outcomes	Significance
Seppälä et al. (2014)	21	Screening tool not mentioned	Sudarshan Kriya yoga	7 days	Yoga group:↓ PTSD scores, anxiety, respiration rate; ↓ startle correlated with ↓ hyperarousal symptoms	PTSD: $P < 0.001$; anxiety: $P < 0.001$; respiration: $P < 0.05$; startle, hyperarousal: $P < 0.001$
Mitchell et al. (2014)	38	PC-PTSD	Kripalu yoga	1/week×12 weeks or 2/week×6 weeks	Yoga group: ↓ reexperiencing and hyperarousal symptoms	$P < 0.01$ for both measures
Telles et al. (2010)	22	SQD	Patañjali yoga	1 week	Yoga group: ↓ sadness; control group: ↑ anxiety	$P < 0.05$ for both changes
Catani et al. (2009)	31	DSM-IV	Meditation-relaxation	6 sessions	PTSD ↓ symptoms, ↓ impaired functioning in both groups	$P < 0.001$ for both groups
Gordon et al. (2008)	82	HTQ Trauma symptom list	Mind-body group	6 weeks	Yoga group: ↓ PTSD scores	$P < 0.001$

Note. AUDIT=Alcohol Use Disorder Identification Test; CAPS=Clinician Administered PTSD Scale; CES-D=Center for Epidemiologic Studies Depression Scale; DSM=*Diagnostic and Statistical Manual of Mental Disorders*; DUDIT=Drug Use Disorder Identification Test; HTQ=Harvard Trauma Questionnaire; PCL-17=Posttraumatic Stress Disorder Checklist; PCLC=Posttraumatic Stress Disorder Checklist–Civilian; PCLM-17=Posttraumatic Stress Disorder Checklist–Military version; PC-PTSD=Primary Care PTSD screen; PSS-I=PTSD Symptom Scale–Interview; SQD=Screening Questionnaire for Disaster Mental Health; ↓=decreased; ↑=increased.

trol group (Jindani et al. 2015). Changes in PTSD symptoms were observed in both groups; however, participants in the yoga group showed greater changes in measures of sleep ($P<0.05$), positive affect ($P<0.05$), perceived stress ($P<0.05$), anxiety ($P<0.05$), stress ($P<0.05$), and resilience ($P<0.05$). Approximately 57% of the wait-list control group was involved in other treatments (e.g., cognitive-behavioral therapy or exposure therapy), excluding contemplative components.

Seventy-six orphaned children in Haiti were randomly assigned to a yoga group and an aerobic dance group. An additional nonrandomized wait-list control group was included (Culver et al. 2015). After 8 weeks of intervention, significant improvement in PTSD symptoms was observed in the yoga group ($F_{2,28}=3.30$; $P=0.05$); non-significant reduction in PTSD symptoms was seen in the aerobic dance group ($P>0.05$). An RCT of 38 women with PTSD found no change in physical activity or self-efficacy in either a yoga group or an assessment-only control group (Martin et al. 2015). The yoga group had significant reduction in external motivation ($P<0.05$).

Individuals with PTSD are at high risk for drug and alcohol abuse. In an RCT (Reddy et al. 2014), 38 veteran and civilian women with alcohol and drug use disorders diagnosed with PTSD randomly assigned to a yoga group and a control group. After 12 yoga sessions, scores on the Alcohol Use Disorder Identification Test (AUDIT) and Drug Use Disorder Identification Test (DUDIT) declined significantly in the yoga group ($P<0.001$). In the control group, AUDIT scores increased, and DUDIT scores remained stable. Hence, for individuals with PTSD, yoga can help increase positive coping strategies and may reduce alcohol and drug abuse.

In an RCT, 31 Australian Vietnam War veterans who were 100% disabled as a result of military service–related PTSD and who failed numerous trials of psychotropic medication combinations and individual and group therapies were randomly assigned to a group that received a 22-hour, 5-day Sudarshan Kriya yoga intervention modified for veterans (followed by home practice and 90-minute follow-up sessions weekly for 6 weeks and then monthly) or to a control group (Carter et al. 2013). After 6 weeks, the intervention group showed significantly greater reductions on the Clinician Administered Posttraumatic Stress Disorder Scale (CAPS) compared with the wait-list control group ($P<0.05$), with a large effect size of 0.91. At 6-month follow-up, repeat CAPS showed further improvements. Six-week scores on the Center for Epidemiologic Studies Depression Scale (CES-D) and Posttraumatic Stress Disorder Checklist–Military version (PCLM-17) showed significant improvement ($P<0.01$ and $P<0.001$, respectively) compared with control participants. In a similar subsequent study, 21 Afghanistan war veterans were randomly assigned to yoga and wait-list control groups (Seppälä et al. 2014). Sudarshan Kriya yoga was given for 7 days, and follow-up was done at 1 month and 1 year. The yoga group showed reductions in PTSD scores ($P<0.001$), anxiety symptoms ($P<0.001$), and respiration rate ($P<0.05$). A reduction in eyeblink startle reflex was correlated with reductions in symptoms of hyperarousal ($P<0.001$).

Another study randomly assigned 38 women with PTSD diagnoses to a yoga group and an assessment control (Mitchell et al. 2014). After 12 weeks of Kripalu-based yoga, participants had a reduction in re-experiencing ($P<0.01$) and hyperarousal ($P<0.01$). A sample of 22 adult survivors of the 2008 flood in Bihar, India, were randomly assigned to two groups: a 7-day yoga intervention and a control group who continued their regular activities (Telles et al. 2010). The yoga group showed a significant decrease in sadness ($P<0.05$). Anxiety significantly increased ($P<0.05$) in the control group but not in the yoga group, suggesting that yoga might help prevent development of anxiety disorders following mass disasters.

Children (ages 8–14 years) in a refugee camp in Sri Lanka following the 2004 Southeast Asian tsunami were randomly assigned to two groups. One group received six sessions of narrative exposure therapy for children (KIDNET); the other received six sessions of meditation-relaxation (MED-RELAX; Catani et al. 2009). PTSD symptoms and impairment in functioning were significantly reduced at 1 month in both groups and remained stable over time. Follow-up at 6 months showed recovery rates of 81% for the children given KIDNET and 71% for those receiving MED-RELAX. In another RCT, 82 adolescents affected by war in Kosovo who met criteria for PTSD (Harvard Trauma Questionnaire) were randomly assigned to a wait-list control group or a 12-session mind-body group program (meditation, guided imagery, and breathing techniques; self-expression through words, drawings, and movement; autogenic training and biofeedback; and genograms) (Gordon et al. 2008). After 12 sessions, the intervention group had significantly lower PTSD symptoms ($P<0.001$) compared with the control group. After adolescents in the control group received the same intervention, their symptoms of PTSD diminished.

These randomized controlled studies suggest that yoga can help reduce symptoms of PTSD regardless of the type of the trauma or population. The main limitations of most of the studies were small sample sizes, lack of an active control group, and insufficient details about the specific yoga practices. Unlike pharmaceutical studies, it is virtually impossible to blind subjects to yoga interventions effectively. Because most outcome measures in these studies were psychological tools and because most of the controls were inactive wait-list groups, the psychological effects of participating in a group intervention and interaction with the instructor(s) on the variables measured should be considered. Two of the studies used active control groups (Catani et al. 2009; Culver et al. 2015) and found reductions in PTSD symptoms in both yoga and active control groups. Therefore, although this evidence is promising, it is not conclusive. RCTs with active control groups, physiological measures, and imaging techniques would contribute to understanding the effects of yoga on the brain regions involved in PTSD and its symptomatology.

Possible Mechanisms for Yoga Reduction of Posttraumatic Stress Disorder Symptoms

Given the possibility of using yoga to positively modify mental state following trauma, it is interesting to speculate about the mechanisms underlying the observed benefits. The proposed mechanisms have been presented elsewhere (Telles et al. 2012) and are summarized here.

During a stressful situation, changes in regulation of the serotonin (5-HT) transporter in the amygdala may alter the stress response (Murrough et al. 2011). The amygdala of individuals with PTSD shows increased activity. These patients also have abnormally reduced amygdala 5-HT binding, which correlates with higher symptoms of anxiety and depression. Hence, abnormal 5-HT signaling within neural systems possibly underlies threat detection and fear learning. In a case series in which four patients were given 12 weeks of yoga plus slow breathing, single-photon emission computed tomography (baseline and postintervention) found significant decreases in activity in the right amygdala, dorsal medial cortex, and sensorimotor areas (Cohen et al. 2009). Another study found that healthy individuals who participated for 8 weeks in a mindfulness-based stress reduction program showed a decline in amygdala gray matter (Hölzel et al. 2010). These studies support a plausible mechanism whereby yoga could reduce symptoms of PTSD by reducing the overactivation of the amygdala while increasing activity of prefrontal and insular areas.

Studies in which yoga practices increase activity in the "higher" centers, such as prefrontal cortex, insula, and anterior cingulate, suggest that yoga could modulate amygdalar activity. Thus, through direct input to the limbic structures as well as higher emotion regulatory systems, yoga could significantly reduce PTSD symptoms. For example, whole blood serotonin levels and mood state changes were assessed before and after focused attention on tanden breathing in 15 healthy right-handed participants (Yu et al. 2011). Tanden breathing, part of Zen meditation, focuses attention on breathing movements in the lower abdomen, with a breath rate of three to four breaths per minute. During focused attention on tanden breathing, participants had a significant increase in oxyhemoglobin level in the anterior prefrontal cortex, an increase in alpha activity with decreased theta activity, and an increase in whole blood serotonin levels that correlated with increased alpha activity and reduced negative feelings.

Imbalance within the ascending dopaminergic tracts may cause rapid fluctuations in the level of arousal and in associated mood, drive, and motivation. Stress reduction, positive affect, and plasma catecholamines were assessed in 67 regular meditators and 57 nonmeditators with a meditation practice called brain wave vibration mind-body training, which is thought to change negative thoughts into positive ones (Jung et al. 2010). Members of the meditation group had higher scores on positive affect and lower scores on negative affect compared with nonmeditators. Their plasma dopamine levels also were higher. The control group showed a negative correlation between stress and positive affect. A positive correlation was also found between somatization of stress and norepinephrine-to-epinephrine and dopamine-to-epinephrine ratios in the control group. Hence, meditation can lower stress levels and increase positive affect and plasma dopamine levels.

The anxiety-lowering effect of yoga practices also may involve the inhibitory neurotransmitter γ-aminobutyric acid (GABA). Two studies reported that thalamic GABAergic activity increased after yoga practice. In the earlier study, 8 experienced yoga practitioners were compared with 11 nonpractitioners (Streeter et al. 2007). All subjects were evaluated with the Structural Clinical Interview for DSM-IV Axis I Disorders, Research Version, Patient Edition (First et al. 1997), and the Addiction Severity Index. The yoga group completed a 60-minute session that included yoga postures and associated breathing practices, whereas the comparison subjects read periodicals and popular fiction during a 60-minute session. The GABA levels in the thalamus increased by 27% in the yoga practitioners after the yoga session, but the comparison group showed no change. The second study addressed the issue of whether changes in thalamic GABA levels are specific to yoga or related to physical activity (Streeter et al. 2010). Participants were randomly assigned to a yoga group ($n=19$) or a metabolically matched physical exercise group ($n=15$) for 60 minutes 3 times a week for 12 weeks. Magnetic resonance spectroscopy scans found that thalamic GABA levels increased in the yoga group and were positively correlated with improved mood. Acute changes in GABA levels in the yoga group approached significance ($P=0.09$; t test). Increases in thalamic GABA levels were associated with improved mood and decreased anxiety—changes that usually occur with pharmacological agents for mood and anxiety. These studies suggest that certain changes in neurotransmitters following yoga practice contributed to the improved psychological state in trauma victims who practiced yoga. This is probably one of several ways that yoga can influence psychological state in trauma victims. Studies of changes in neurotransmitter levels in response to yoga in patients with PTSD are needed.

Streeter et al. (2010) hypothesized that stress can induce 1) decreased parasympathetic nervous system (PNS) and increased sympathetic nervous system (SNS) activity, 2) underactivity of the inhibitory neurotransmitter GABA, and 3) increased allostatic load. They further hypothesized that the positive effect of yoga may be the result of 1) increased activity of the PNS and GABA system, partly through stimulation of the vagus nerves, and 2) reduced allostatic load resulting in symptom relief. Conditions such as PTSD are exacerbated by stress, have low PNS and low GABA system activity, respond to pharmacological agents that increase GABAergic activity, and improve in response to yoga-based interventions. In a 12-week Phase I randomized controlled dosing study of 30 patients with moderate major depressive disorder, Beck Depression Inventory–2 scores declined significantly, correlating with increased number of minutes that patients practiced Iyengar yoga and coherent breathing at five breaths per minute (see Chapter 21, "Breathing Techniques in Psychiatric Treatment") ($P=0.02$). In addition, respiratory sinus arrhythmia, a measure of sympathetic and parasympathetic activity, increased significantly ($P=0.03$), indicating increased parasympathetic activity. Moreover, subnormal thalamic GABA levels increased to normal range (Streeter et al. 2016).

KEY POINTS

The improvement in posttraumatic stress disorder (PTSD) symptoms after yoga practice may be attributed to the following:

- Increased levels of neurotransmitters such as serotonin, dopamine, and γ-aminobutyric acid

- Improved regulation of the autonomic nervous system by increasing parasympathetic effects on numerous brain structures involved in stress response and emotion processing

- Reduction in the hyperactivity of the amygdala, as reflected in reduced PTSD symptoms

References

Brown RP, Gerbarg PL, Muskin PR: How to Use Herbs, Nutrients, and Yoga in Mental Health Care. New York, WW Norton, 2009

Carter JJ, Gerbarg P, Brown RP, et al: Multi-component yoga breath program for Vietnam veteran post traumatic stress disorder: randomized controlled trial. J Trauma Stress Disord Treat 2(3):1–10, 2013

Catani C, Kohiladevy M, Ruf M, et al: Treating children traumatized by war and tsunami: a comparison between exposure therapy and meditation-relaxation in north-east Sri Lanka. BMC Psychiatry 9:22, 2009 19439099

Cohen DL, Wintering N, Tolles V, et al: Cerebral blood flow effects of yoga training: preliminary evaluation of 4 cases. J Altern Complement Med 15(1):9–14, 2009 19769471

Culver KA, Whetten K, Boyd DL, et al: Yoga to reduce trauma-related distress and emotional and behavioral difficulties among children living in orphanages in Haiti: a pilot study. J Altern Complement Med 21(9):539–545, 2015 26090580

de Manincor M, Bensoussan A, Smith CA, et al: Individualized yoga for reducing depression and anxiety, and improving well-being: a randomized controlled trial. Depress Anxiety 33(9):816–828, 2016 27030303

Fares J, Fares Y: The role of yoga in relieving medical student anxiety and stress. N Am J Med Sci 8(4):202–204, 2016 27213148

First MB, Spitzer RL, Gibbon M, et al: Structured Clinical Interview for DSM-IV Axis I Disorders, Research Version, Patient Edition (SCID-I/P). New York, Biometrics Research, New York State Psychiatric Institute, 1997

Gordon JS, Staples JK, Blyta A, et al: Treatment of posttraumatic stress disorder in postwar Kosovar adolescents using mind-body skills groups: a randomized controlled trial. J Clin Psychiatry 69(9):1469–1476, 2008 18945398

Harris WW, Putnam FW, Fairbank JA: Mobilizing trauma resources for children. Presented at the meeting of the Johnson & Johnson Pediatric Institute: Shaping the Future of Children's Health, San Juan, Puerto Rico, February 12–16, 2004

Hölzel BK, Carmody J, Evans KC, et al: Stress reduction correlates with structural changes in the amygdala. Soc Cogn Affect Neurosci 5(1):11–17, 2010 19776221

Hull AM: Neuroimaging findings in posttraumatic stress disorder: systematic review. Br J Psychiatry 181:102–110, 2002 12151279

Jindani F, Turner N, Khalsa SB: A yoga intervention for posttraumatic stress: a preliminary randomized control trial. Evid Based Complement Alternat Med 2015:351746, 2015 26366179

Jung YH, Kang DH, Jang JH, et al: The effects of mind-body training on stress reduction, positive affect, and plasma catecholamines. Neurosci Lett 479(2):138–142, 2010 20546836

Martin EC, Dick AM, Scioli-Salter ER, et al: Impact of a yoga intervention on physical activity, self-efficacy, and motivation in women with PTSD symptoms. J Altern Complement Med 21(6):327–332, 2015 25973554

Mitchell KS, Dick AM, DiMartino DM, et al: A pilot study of a randomized controlled trial of yoga as an intervention for PTSD symptoms in women. J Trauma Stress 27(2):121–128, 2014 24668767

Murrough JW, Huang Y, Hu J, et al: Reduced amygdala serotonin transporter binding in posttraumatic stress disorder. Biol Psychiatry 70(11):1033–1038, 2011 21855859

Quiñones N, Maquet YG, Vélez DM, et al: Efficacy of a Satyananda yoga intervention for reintegrating adults diagnosed with posttraumatic stress disorder. Int J Yoga Therap 25(1):89–99, 2015 26667292

Rajesh SK, Ilavarasu JV, Srinivasan TM: Effect of Bhramari pranayama on response inhibition: evidence from the stop signal task. Int J Yoga 7:138–141, 2014

Reddy S, Dick AM, Gerber MR, et al: The effect of a yoga intervention on alcohol and drug abuse risk in veteran and civilian women with posttraumatic stress disorder. J Altern Complement Med 20:750–756, 2014

Saeed SA, Antonacci DJ, Bloch RM: Exercise, yoga, and meditation for depressive and anxiety disorders. Am Fam Physician 81(8):981–986, 2010 20387774

Schuver KJ, Lewis BA: Mindfulness-based yoga intervention for women with depression. Complement Ther Med 26:85–91, 2016 27261987

Seppälä EM, Nitschke JB, Tudorascu DL, et al: Breathing-based meditation decreases posttraumatic stress disorder symptoms in U.S. military veterans: a randomized controlled longitudinal study. J Trauma Stress 27(4):397–405, 2014 25158633

Sheela, Nagendra HR, Ganpat TS: Efficacy of yoga for sustained attention in university students. Ayu 34(3):270–272, 2013

Streeter CC, Jensen JE, Perlmutter RM, et al: Yoga Asana sessions increase brain GABA levels: a pilot study. J Altern Complement Med 13(4):419–426, 2007 17532734

Streeter CC, Whitfield TH, Owen L, et al: Effects of yoga versus walking on mood, anxiety, and brain GABA levels: a randomized controlled MRS study. J Altern Complement Med 16(11):1145–1152, 2010 20722471

Streeter CC, Whitfield TH, Owen L, et al: Effects of Iyengar yoga and coherent breathing on mood and brain GABA levels in patients with MDD: Phase 1 randomized controlled dosing study. Paper presented at the 169th annual meeting of the American Psychiatric Association, Atlanta, GA, May 14–18, 2016

Taimini K: The Science of Yoga. Madras, India, Theosophical Publishing House, 1986

Telles S, Singh N, Joshi M, et al: Post traumatic stress symptoms and heart rate variability in Bihar flood survivors following yoga: a randomized controlled study. BMC Psychiatry 10:18, 2010 20193089

Telles S, Singh N, Balkrishna A: Managing mental health disorders resulting from trauma through yoga: a review. Depress Res Treat 2012:401513, 2012 22778930

Yu X, Fumoto M, Nakatani Y, et al: Activation of the anterior prefrontal cortex and serotonergic system is associated with improvements in mood and EEG changes induced by Zen meditation practice in novices. Int J Psychophysiol 80(2):103–111, 2011 21333699

CHAPTER 23

Mind-Body Practices Tai Chi and Qigong in the Treatment and Prevention of Psychiatric Disorders

Ryan Abbott, M.D., J.D., MTOM

Donald D. Chang, Ph.D.

Harris Eyre, Ph.D., M.B.B.S.

Helen Lavretsky, M.D., M.S.

It furthers one
To undertake something.
It furthers one to cross the great water.

I Ching

In this chapter, we focus on tai chi and qigong for treating and preventing psychiatric disorders. A growing body of evidence supports the incorporation of mind-body practices, such as tai chi and qigong, into mental health treatment (Abbott and Lavretsky 2013). These practices have been shown to reduce symptoms associated with psychiatric disorders, to improve quality of life, and to positively affect several medical conditions (Abbott et al. 2007; Jahnke et al. 2010; Wang 2008; Woo et al. 2007). Emerging research suggests that tai chi and qigong may even reduce symptoms of psychiatric disorders to a greater extent than does conventional exercise. This may be attributable to meditative or other aspects of mind-body techniques.

Tai Chi and Qigong: An Overview

Qigong originated in China thousands of years ago. In traditional Chinese medical theory, qigong cultivates and circulates the natural energy known as *qi* (also *chi* or *ki*), which is considered essential for physiological and psychological function. Qigong consists of orchestrated body postures, movement sequences, breathing methods, vocalizations, and visualization techniques. According to traditional theory, qigong involves increasing awareness of subtle shifts in the flow and distribution of energy in the body and progresses to subtler and more complex exercises to direct the flow of this energy so that it can be used to strengthen internal organs, overcome blockages where injury or trauma has occurred, relieve pain and tension, cultivate a calm and peaceful state of mind, and fortify the body against future illness. A multitude of styles or schools of qigong practices are available.

Tai chi, a type of qigong, originated hundreds of years ago. First developed as a martial art, it is now practiced largely for health benefits (Liu et al. 2015). Compared with the simpler, more repetitive movements in qigong, tai chi tends to consist of lengthier, more complex choreographed movements. Although many types of tai chi exist, most people practice the forms identified with one of three schools: Sun, Yang, and Wu (Jahnke et al. 2010). Clinical trials have not consistently used a standardized version of tai chi, although many have used a simplified version, tai chi chih, or tai chi "easy." Because tai chi and qigong are similar in many respects, they may share similar mechanisms of action. In the absence of rigorous research comparing the efficacy of different types of practices, our discussion encompasses both unless otherwise specified. For details on clinical studies discussed later in this chapter, see Table 23–1.

Putative Physiological Mechanism of Action

Although the definitive mechanisms by which tai chi and qigong impart their therapeutic effects on neuronal function require further study, several physiological correlations have been observed that suggest potential biological pathways: 1) sympathetic output reduction and relaxation promotion (Cahn and Polich 2006; Irwin et al. 2008; Jevning et al. 1992; Motivala et al. 2006); 2) activation of anti-inflammatory pathways; 3) decreased expression of inflammation-related genes; 4) modulation of pro-inflammatory transcription factor NF-κB; 5) reduction in levels of inflammatory markers such as C-reactive protein; and 6) reduction in levels of adrenocorticotropic hormone and cortisol (Bower and Irwin 2016; Lavretsky et al. 2011; Lee et al. 2003; Ryu et al. 1996). Furthermore, tai chi and qigong have been observed to improve immune responses, vaccine responses, and baroreflex sensitivity (Irwin et al. 2007; Ryu et al. 1996; Sato et al. 2010).

Evidence also points to positive effects on neuronal activity. In electroencephalogram (EEG) studies, participation in tai chi and qigong was associated with increased frontal EEG theta wave activity (Field et al. 2010), indicating increased relaxation and mental focus. Similar changes were not observed in conventional exercise control

TABLE 23–1. Selected randomized controlled trials (RCTs) and reviews: effects of tai chi and qigong on psychiatric disorders

Study design: *n*, mean age (years), duration, interventions	Outcomes (CI, *P*)	Reference
Psychosocial well-being		
Evaluated 15 RCTs for tai chi effects on psychosocial well-being	Tai chi: significant effect in 13 of 15 studies. Improvements: management of depression and anxiety	W. C. Wang et al. (2009)
Evaluated 40 RCTs for tai chi effects on psychological well-being	Tai chi: significantly ↑ psychological well-being; ↓ stress, anxiety, depression, and mood disturbance; and ↑ self-esteem in 21 of 33 RCTs and non-RCTs	C. Wang et al. (2010b)
Stress		
RCT, *n*=252 patients with HIV, age=42.2: 10-week trial of tai chi vs. relaxation training vs. spiritual growth vs. wait-list control; stress assessed via Coping subscale of DIS	Tai chi and relaxation training: ↑ emotion-focused coping compared with wait-list control (*P*=0.030) Tai chi: ↓ emotion-focused subscale (−1.25±1.60; 95% CI=0.61–6.93; *P*<0.02)	McCain et al. (2008)
RCT, *n*=98, age=73.2: 24-week trial of tai chi 1 hour twice a week vs. wait-list control; psychological distress assessed via Subjective Exercise Experiences scale	Latent growth curve modeling analysis: significantly ↓ slope for tai chi (*P*<0.5) indicated greater decreases in stress vs. control	Li et al. (2001)
RCT, *n*=96, age=36.2: tai chi vs. brisk walking vs. meditation vs. reading group; assessment via mental arithmetic stress test and emotional stress detected while viewing stressful film	Tai chi: superior stress reduction (based on heart rate, blood pressure, state anxiety from POMS) compared with reading control (*P*<0.001)	Jin (1992)
RCT, *n*=152, age=59–85: 12-week trial of hydrotherapy vs. tai chi vs. wait-list control; stress assessed by WOMAC and DASS21 scores	Tai chi: significant improvements in WOMAC pain and function (30.7±18.9, change of 9.6; 95% CI=5.4–13.7) vs. control (40.0±16.2, change of 4.4; 95% CI=0.2–8.6) DASS21 scores: significantly ↓ stress in tai chi group (9.3±8.4) vs. control (13.7±9.7)	Fransen et al. (2007)

TABLE 23–1. Selected randomized controlled trials (RCTs) and reviews: effects of tai chi and qigong on psychiatric disorders *(continued)*

Study design: *n*, mean age (years), duration, interventions	Outcomes (CI, *P*)	Reference
Mood		
RCT, *n*=100 patients with systolic heart failure, age=67±11: 12-week trial of tai chi vs. health education control program	Tai chi: ↓ POMS score (median=−6) vs. control (median=−1): improved mood (*P*<0.05)	Yeh et al. (2011)
RCT, *n*=21 obese women, age=44.4: 10-week trial of tai chi vs. structured exercise control	Tai chi: ↓ BDI score	Dechamps et al. (2009)
RCT, *n*=38 male patients with HIV, age=20–60: 12-week trial of exercise vs. tai chi vs. control without intervention	Exercise and tai chi group: mood improvements vs. control (*P*<0.05)	Galantino et al. (2005)
Anxiety		
RCT, *n*=20 patients with rheumatoid arthritis, age=51±17: 12-week trial of tai chi vs. attention control; primary outcome: ACR 20 response	Tai chi: 50% achieved ACR 20 response (*P*=0.03) and ↓ EQ-5D score (*P*=0.09) Control: none achieved ACR 20 response	Wang (2008)
RCT, *n*=52 patients with chronic heart failure, mean age=68.9: 16-week trial of tai chi vs. standard care without exercise rehabilitation	Tai chi: ↑ mean walk distance (+14 m) vs. control (+5 m); SCL-90-R anxiety: no statistical difference	Barrow et al. (2007)
RCT, *n*=34 patients with CVD, age=77: 12-week trial of tai chi vs. rehabilitation once a week; quality of life assessed by GHQ-60 score	Tai chi: significant time-by-group interaction in GHQ-60 score for anxiety (*P*=0.034) compared with control group	W. Wang et al. (2010)
RCT, *n*=72, age=69.2±9.3: 12-week trial of tai chi vs. low-impact exercise vs. nonexercise control	Tai chi and low-impact exercise: anxiety ↓ significantly from control on STAI (*P*<0.01)	Frye et al. (2007)
RCT, *n*=76 patients with borderline hypertension or diastolic blood pressure, age=50: 12-week trial of tai chi vs. sedentary life control	Tai chi: STAI: ↓ trait anxiety (32.8±6.2), state anxiety (30.6±6.2) significant vs. control (*P*<0.01) Control: trait (39.8±6.6) and state (36.8±6.0) anxiety scores	Tsai et al. (2003)

TABLE 23–1. Selected randomized controlled trials (RCTs) and reviews: effects of tai chi and qigong on psychiatric disorders *(continued)*

Study design: *n,* mean age (years), duration, interventions	Outcomes (CI, *P*)	Reference
Depression		
RCT, *n*=66 patients with fibromyalgia, age=62.9±15.5: 12-week trial of tai chi vs. wellness education plus stretching control	Tai chi: significantly ↓ CES-D index (*P*=0.04)	C. Wang et al. (2010a)
RCT, *n*=40 patients with knee osteoarthritis, age=65: 12-week trial of tai chi vs. wellness education and stretching control twice a week	Tai chi: significantly improved CES-D score (−6.70, 95% CI=−11.63–−1.77; *P*=0.009)	C. Wang et al. (2009)
RCT, *n*=112 community-dwelling adults, age=70: 25-week trial of tai chi (*n*=59) vs. health education control (*n*=53)	Tai chi: improved (*P*<0.5) BDI score (−1.68; 95% CI=2.42 to −0.94) Control: −1.33 (95% CI=−2.28 to −0.38)	Irwin et al. (2007)
RCT, *n*=14 patients with clinical depression, age=72.6: 3-month trial of tai chi vs. inactive control	Tai chi: significantly ↓ CES-D index (15.3±9.8) vs. control (39.1±9.7; *P*<0.05)	Chou et al. (2004)
RCT, *n*=112 patients with major depressive disorder taking 10 mg escitalopram, age≥60: 4-week trial of tai chi vs. health education control	Tai chi: Patients with major depressive disorder treated with escitalopram had greater ↓ depression (94%; Ham-D score<10) vs. control (77%; Ham-D score<10; *P*<0.06)	Lavretsky et al. (2011)
Sleep disturbance		
RCT, *n*=118, age=75: 24-week trial of tai chi vs. low-impact exercise control	Tai chi: significant improvements in sleep quality on PSQI vs. control (*P* < 0.1)	Li et al. (2004)
RCT, *n*=112 volunteers, age=69: 16-week trial of tai chi vs. health education session; sleep quality assessed by PSQI	Tai chi: 63% achieved a PSQI score<5 (*P*<0.05 compared with control) Control: 32% achieved <5 PSQI score	Irwin et al. (2008)
RCT, *n*=34 patients with CVD, age≥50: 12-week trial of tai chi vs. rehabilitation sessions control	Tai chi: Sleep quality significantly improved compared with control (*P*<0.05)	W. Wang et al. (2010)

TABLE 23–1. Selected randomized controlled trials (RCTs) and reviews: effects of tai chi and qigong on psychiatric disorders *(continued)*

Study design: *n*, mean age (years), duration, interventions	Outcomes (CI, *P*)	Reference
Substance abuse		
RCT, *n*=86 heroin-addicted men, age=18–52: 10-day trial of qigong vs. medication vs. no treatment; outcomes: withdrawal symptoms, Ham-A score, urine morphine level	Qigong: ↓ mean symptom scores (*P*<0.01), ↓ anxiety scores (*P*<0.01) vs medication and no treatment	Li et al. (2002)
RCT, *n*=248 residents at an adult rehabilitation unit, age=34±10: 2-week trial of qigong vs. SMART; outcome: rehabilitation treatment completion rates	Qigong: significantly ↑ addiction treatment completion rate compared with the SMART group (92% vs. 78%; *P*<0.01)	Chen et al. (2010)
Cognitive functioning		
RCT, *n*=389 Chinese participants with a CDR Scale score of 0.5 or amnestic mild cognitive impairment, age=77±6: 1-year trial of tai chi vs. stretching exercise control; 2 months posttreatment, cognitive function assessed with visual scans and CDR Scale	Tai chi: significant correlation with stable CDR Scale score (OR=0.14; 95% CI=0.03–0.71; *P*=0.02)	Lam et al. (2011)
RCT, *n*=132, age=69: 6-month trial of tai chi vs. Western exercise vs. attention control cognitive function assessed via semantic fluency and digit span tests	Tai chi: ↑ cognitive function measure (F=7.75; *P*<0.001) vs. Western exercise and control groups	Taylor-Piliae et al. (2010)
RCT, *n*=96 participants from Vinh City, Vietnam, age=60–79: 6-month trial of tai chi daily practice vs. control	Tai chi: ↑ cognitive performance as assessed by the TMT (*P*<0.001)	Nguyen and Kruse (2012)

TABLE 23–1. Selected randomized controlled trials (RCTs) and reviews: effects of tai chi and qigong on psychiatric disorders *(continued)*

Study design: *n*, mean age (years), duration, interventions	Outcomes (CI, *P*)	Reference
Parkinson's disease		
RCT, *n*=195 patients with idiopathic Parkinson's disease, age=40–85: 24-week trial of tai chi vs. resistance training vs. stretching; outcome: change from baseline in limits-of-stability test	Tai chi: ↑ maximum excursion (5.55% change from baseline; 95% CI=1.12–9.97) and directional control (10.45% change from baseline; 95% CI=3.89–17.00)	Li et al. (2012)
RCT, *n*=33 Parkinson's patients, age≥40: 10- to 13-week trial of tai chi or control with no intervention; outcome assessed by Berg Balance Scale scores and UPDRS	Tai chi: significant change in UPDRS (*P*<0.025) and Berg Balance Scale (*P*<0.001) assessments	Hackney and Earhart (2008)
RCT, *n*=24 Parkinson's patients, age=62.25: 12-week trial of tai chi vs. nonexercise control; Parkinson's disease symptoms evaluated with UPDRS	Tai chi: significant changes in the Mentation, Behavior, and Mood subscale (*P*<0.025) and the Motor subscale (*P*<0.010) of the UPDRS	Choi et al. (2013)
TBI		
RCT, *n*=20 patients with TBI: 8-week trial of qigong vs. control group with no intervention; outcome was evaluated with General Health Questionnaire and Social Support for Exercise Habits Scale	Qigong: significant improvement in mood (*P*=0.02) vs. control and self-esteem improvement compared with baseline (*P*=0.01)	Blake and Batson (2009)
RCT, *n*=18 participants with TBI, mean age=45.7: 3-week trial of tai chi vs. wait-list control group; mood states evaluated with VAMS	Tai chi: improvements on all VAMS scores vs. control (all scales at least *P*<0.05, except fatigue)	Gemmell and Leathem (2006)

Note. ACR=American College of Rheumatology; BDI=Beck Depression Inventory; CDR=Clinical Dementia Rating; CES-D=Center for Epidemiologic Studies Depression Scale; CI=confidence interval; CVD=cerebrovascular disorder; DASS21=Depression, Anxiety and Stress Scale; DIS=Dealing With Illness Scale; EQ-5D=EuroQol 5-dimensions questionnaire; GHQ-60=General Health Questionnaire-60; Ham-A=Hamilton Anxiety Scale; Ham-D=Hamilton Depression Rating Scale; OR=odds ratio; POMS=Profile of Mood States; PSQI=Pittsburgh Sleep Quality Index; SCL-90-R=Symptom Checklist–90—Revised; SMART=Stress Management and Relaxation Training; STAI=State-Trait Anxiety Inventory; TBI=traumatic brain injury; TMT=Trail Making Test; UPDRS=Unified Parkinson's Disease Rating Scale; VAMS=Visual Analogue Mood Scales; WOMAC=Western Ontario and McMaster Universities Osteoarthritis Index; ↑=increased; ↓=decreased.

subjects (Chou et al. 2004; Liu et al. 2003), although conventional exercise has been linked with preserving neuronal structure and promoting synaptogenesis (Bugg and Head 2011; Kleim et al. 2002). In addition, two studies documented the influence of tai chi on brain remodeling. In a study of 22 individuals (mean age=52 years) who practiced tai chi, high-resolution magnetic resonance imaging showed increased thickness of brain regions related to motor and executive functions compared with a control group with no physical exercise (Wei et al. 2013). A year later, the same research group again studied 22 tai chi practitioners (mean age=52 years) and found significantly greater and more experience-dependent functional homogeneity in the right postcentral gyrus compared with control subjects (Wei et al. 2014).

Clinical Use of Tai Chi and Qigong for Mental Well-Being and Mental Health Disorders

Psychological and Social Well-Being

A comprehensive review of the effects of tai chi on psychological well-being included 40 studies (17 randomized controlled trials [RCTs], 16 nonrandomized comparison studies, and 7 observational studies) with a total of 3,817 individuals reporting at least 1 psychological health issue from a search of 11 English and Chinese databases (C. Wang et al. 2010b; W.C. Wang et al. 2009). Of these studies, 21 found that participants practicing tai chi for 1 year had significantly increased psychological well-being and reduced stress, anxiety, and depression. An RCT of 52 individuals with HIV found that those randomly assigned to tai chi showed improved psychosocial functioning compared with a cognitive-behavioral relaxation group, a spiritual growth group, and a wait-list control group (McCain et al. 2008). Similar improvements in psychological well-being were found in an extensive review of qigong (Chow and Tsang 2007).

Stress Management

Tai chi practice has been significantly correlated with reduced stress in RCTs. In one study, 96 adults (mean age=36.2 years) who underwent a single 1-hour session of tai chi experienced significant reductions in stress levels compared with adults practicing meditation, brisk walking, or neutral reading (Jin 1992). A second RCT involving 20 adults (mean age=67 years) who practiced tai chi for 2 hours once weekly for 10 weeks showed reduced stress compared with adults in a routine physical activity group (Sun et al. 1996). A similar study found that 72 adults (mean age=73 years) who practiced tai chi for 1 hour twice a week had reduced stress compared with those who did not (Li et al. 2001). However, an RCT of 152 adults with hip or knee osteoarthritis (mean age=70 years) who practiced tai chi for 1 hour twice weekly for 12 weeks found no significant difference in stress reduction compared with patients in a hydrotherapy or wait-list control group (Fransen et al. 2007). Nonetheless, the preponderance of evidence suggests that tai chi reduces stress and related physical and psychological symptoms, as the following case illustrates.

J.C., a 67-year-old African American woman, was depressed as a result of years of caring for her mother with Alzheimer's disease. J.C. had signs of moderate dementia, chronic stress, insomnia, and chronic pain from fibromyalgia and rheumatoid arthritis. She participated in a study comparing 30 minutes of daily tai chi with health education in depressed geriatric patients (Lavretsky et al. 2011). After J.C. was randomly assigned to the intervention group, she started daily tai chi practice. Her depression improved within the first month, with her Hamilton Rating Scale for Depression (Ham-D) score decreasing more than 50% below her initial score of 12, which was consistent with moderate depression. She reported increased ability to cope and assess stressful situations more objectively, with less anger and resentment than before. She also learned to allocate time to pleasurable activities and reported no longer feeling "trapped" or like a "victim of circumstances." J.C. became more aware of her needs for rest and relaxation, thus increasing her ability to cope with stress and chronic pain. Moreover, she felt empowered by concepts of resilience and self-reliance. Her strength was in being open to changing her attitude.

This case illustrates our experiences in recommending tai chi to patients. J.C. was an ideal candidate on the basis of her age, depressive symptoms, and medical comorbidities. As in many cases, tai chi improved mental health and quality of life without side effects. Therefore, we recommend it as a first-line treatment to any patient like J.C. who is motivated to practice a behavioral intervention and does not need immediate pharmacological treatment. We also recommend it as a complementary treatment for patients for whom we prescribe medications.

Anxiety, Mood, and Depression

Tai chi and qigong have significant positive effects on anxiety. Clinical trials evaluating anxiety have included diverse groups of patients, including healthy individuals (Tsai et al. 2003) as well as those with rheumatoid arthritis (Wang 2008), chronic heart failure (Barrow et al. 2007), cerebrovascular disorders (C. Wang et al. 2010a), and sedentary lifestyle coupled with advanced age (Frye et al. 2007). Several of these studies also reported improvements in sleep quality and insomnia. In most of the studies, tai chi was practiced for about 1 hour per week for at least 12 weeks. One study of 25 patients (mean age=69.9 years) who practiced tai chi and qigong during medical rehabilitation reported significant improvements in heart failure symptoms and psychological well-being with no adverse events (Barrow et al. 2007). However, one RCT found no significant difference between tai chi and wait-list control in stress management or anxiety, possibly because of high baseline scores in the control group (Fransen et al. 2007).

Comparative studies suggest that tai chi may be more effective than conventional care or exercise for reducing anxiety (Bond et al. 2002; Jin 1992). Seven RCTs of individuals with anxiety or depression (although not formally diagnosed with a psychiatric disorder) found that tai chi significantly improved mood:

1. One hundred outpatients (mean age=67 years) with systolic heart failure showed greater improvement in quality of life (Minnesota Living With Heart Failure Questionnaire) with 12 weeks of tai chi compared with a time-matched education program (Yeh et al. 2011).

2. Of 21 obese women (mean age=44 years) randomly assigned to either 2-hour weekly tai chi sessions or a conventional exercise program, only the tai chi group experienced improvements in mood (Dechamps et al. 2009).
3. A study of 38 adults (ages 20–60 years) with advanced HIV/AIDS who participated in 8 weeks of twice-weekly 1-hour tai chi showed improved psychological coping and social interactions compared with others who engaged in aerobic exercise or usual activity (Galantino et al. 2005).
4. One hundred thirty-five healthy sedentary adults (mean age=53 years) who practiced tai chi for 45 minutes three times a week for 16 weeks reported improved mood compared with the exercise and relaxation control groups (Brown et al. 1995).
5. A study of 96 adults (mean age=36 years) found that those who practiced 1 hour of tai chi had reduced stress levels compared with adults who practiced meditation, brisk walking, or neutral reading (Jin 1992).
6. Ninety-eight low-activity elderly adults (mean age=73 years) reported reduced psychological distress via the Subjective Exercise Experiences scale with twice a week tai chi sessions over 24 weeks compared with a control group who maintained normal routine activities (Li et al. 2001).
7. Of 252 adults with HIV infection (mean age=42 years), those who practiced tai chi over a 10-week period reported an increase in overall quality of life compared with a wait-list control group as measured by the Functional Assessment of HIV Infection scale (McCain et al. 2008).

To date, the only study finding no effect of tai chi on mood involved 22 individuals (mean age=68 years) with osteoarthritis (Hartman et al. 2000). However, pain and arthritis symptoms improved.

Among the trials of tai chi and qigong for anxiety, 13 of 14 RCTs found that tai chi groups showed greater improvements in depression than did control groups. For example, a single-blind 12-week study of 22 fibromyalgia patients (mean age=50 years) found greater improvements in scores on the Center for Epidemiologic Studies Depression Scale (CES-D) with tai chi compared with a stretching and wellness education group (C. Wang et al. 2010a). Another single-blind, 12-week trial randomly assigned 40 patients (mean age=65 years) with knee osteoarthritis to tai chi or wellness education and stretching and showed that patients in the tai chi group experienced greater improvements in depressive symptoms than did those given wellness education and stretching exercises (C. Wang et al. 2009). These observations are consistent with a review of 36 RCTs (total=3,799 older adults), which concluded that tai chi and qigong significantly improve depression and anxiety (Rogers et al. 2009). However, most of these studies were conducted in patient populations without a diagnosis of a mental disorder. Only two of these studies, involving participants with clinically diagnosed depression, found significant reduction in depressive symptoms associated with the practice of tai chi and qigong (Chou et al. 2004; Lavretsky et al. 2011). Thus, although existing data suggest that tai chi and qigong have a therapeutic effect, additional research is needed.

Sleep Disturbance

Several studies showed that tai chi and qigong improved sleep quality, with corresponding effects on mental health (Irwin et al. 2008; Li et al. 2004; Nguyen and Kruse 2012; W. Wang et al. 2010). One RCT of 112 participants (mean age=69 years) discovered that those who practiced tai chi were more likely to show improvements in sleep quality than were those given health education or conventional rehabilitation (Irwin et al. 2008). A second RCT studying 118 geriatric participants (mean age=75 years) saw improvements in not only sleep quality but also daytime sleepiness (Li et al. 2004). An RCT in Vietnam observed that 48 individuals (mean age=69 years) who practiced tai chi training for 6 months experienced significant improvements in sleep quality, balance, and cognitive performance compared with control participants who simply maintained their routine daily activities ($P<0.001$) (Nguyen and Kruse 2012).

Substance Abuse

One RCT found that qigong during rehabilitation helped alleviate withdrawal symptoms from substance abuse. In the trial, 86 patients (age=18–52 years) diagnosed with heroin abuse were randomly assigned to qigong, medication, or no-treatment control; qigong participants experienced comparatively fewer withdrawal symptoms (Li et al. 2002). Qigong was also credited with a lower relapse rate and improved anxiety scores. In another study of 248 adults (mean age=33.6 years), those who participated in a qigong meditation program had higher treatment completion rates in substance abuse programs and greater reductions in cravings compared with those who had a standard stress management plus relaxation program (Chen et al. 2010). Of interest, the women experienced greater reductions in anxiety and withdrawal symptoms than did the men.

Cognitive Functioning

Tai chi was found to improve cognitive function. A 1-year study in China randomly assigned 389 geriatric participants with dementia or amnestic cognitive impairment to receive either tai chi or strengthening and toning exercises (Lam et al. 2011). After 5 months, both groups showed improvements in global cognitive function, delayed recall, and subjective complaints, but only the tai chi group maintained a stable clinical dementia rating and experienced improvements in visual spans. Another RCT of 132 community-dwelling older adults found that tai chi imparted significant improvements in cognitive function over Western exercise or attention control, and the improvements persisted throughout a 12-month follow-up (Wayne et al. 2014). Similarly, an RCT of 96 elderly individuals (mean age=69) reported that tai chi training improved cognitive speed and auditory and visual attention (Nguyen and Kruse 2012). Another review of 12 studies in community-dwelling older adults concluded that tai chi offered positive cognitive benefits (Miller and Taylor-Piliae 2014). A recent systematic review of four RCTs and five nonrandomized trials found that tai chi showed a significant potential for cognitive protection in adults (Zheng et al. 2015). Altogether, these studies suggest that tai chi may have a beneficial effect on cognitive function, especially in elderly individuals.

Parkinson's Disease

Most of the research evaluating tai chi in the treatment of neurological diseases has focused on Parkinson's disease. An RCT of 195 patients (age=40–85 years) with Parkinson's disease compared whether a tailored tai chi program could improve postural control (Li et al. 2012). Patients were randomly assigned to tai chi, resistance training, or stretching groups. At the end of 24 weeks, patients assigned to practice tai chi consistently performed better on the primary outcome measure of maximum excursion and directional control compared with the resistance training and stretching groups. The tai chi group also performed better than the stretching group in all secondary balance measures, including strength, functional reach, timed up-and-go tests, motor scores, and number of falls. The beneficial effects of tai chi were maintained up to 3 months after intervention, and no adverse events were reported. Another study of 33 Parkinson's patients at least 40 years old observed that 1-hour sessions of tai chi improved several balance measures compared with no intervention, and a trial of 24 individuals with Parkinson's disease (mean age=62.25 years) found that a 12-week tai chi program improved behavior, mood, and motor symptoms (Choi et al. 2013; Hackney and Earhart 2008). The therapeutic effects of tai chi in patients with Parkinson's disease have been comprehensively reviewed (Gladfelter 2011).

Traumatic Brain Injury

Traumatic brain injury (TBI) often can result in impaired cognitive function. Tai chi and qigong have been shown to mitigate some of the symptoms associated with this condition. A study of 20 patients (mean age=45 years) with TBI showed that those who participated in qigong for 8 weeks had improved mood and self-esteem compared with a control group that engaged in nonexercise activities (Blake and Batson 2009). However, no difference in physical functioning was observed between the groups. Another RCT assigned 18 adults (mean age=45.7 years) with TBI to either tai chi or wait-list control and evaluated their moods with Visual Analogue Mood Scales (VAMS; Gemmell and Leathem 2006). The tai chi group had significantly improved VAMS scores after 3 weeks, with decreases in sadness, confusion, anger, tension, and fear and increasing trends in energy and happiness. However, these studies evaluated patients over only a short time frame; the long-term benefits of tai chi and qigong for TBI remain to be seen.

Special Populations

Tai chi and qigong are important in geriatric care for several reasons. First, low-intensity, low-impact practices take less physical toll on the body compared with many other exercises. The movements of tai chi and qigong are gentle enough for elderly individuals, who are often in poor physical condition, to practice without significant risk of adverse events. For example, patients are not required to lie down or contort into difficult postures. Second, tai chi and qigong offer not only psychological relief but also physical benefits for many symptoms that affect the elderly, such as pain from osteoarthritis or fibromyalgia (Field 2011). Third, tai chi and qigong improve balance and reduce the risk of falls (Deandrea et al. 2010). Depression and falls have a complex bi-directional relationship (Iaboni and Flint 2013). Antidepressants, especially selective serotonin reuptake inhibitors, increase the risk of falling and are associated with fragility fractures to a higher degree than other classes of psychotropic medications (Bolton et al. 2008; Vestergaard et al. 2008; Woolcott et al. 2009). In contrast, tai chi and qigong are safe, nonpharmacological alternative or adjunctive treatments.

Of note, the evidence for tai chi reducing the risk of falls is not entirely consistent. A Cochrane meta-analysis (Gillespie et al. 2009) found that tai chi and qigong had only a moderate effect on reducing falls in geriatric populations; another meta-analysis (Logghe et al. 2010) found insufficient evidence. A study of 684 community-residing older adults (mean age=74.5 years) in New Zealand found that tai chi did not significantly prevent falls compared with adults in general exercise control groups over a 17-month follow-up period (Taylor et al. 2012).

Tai chi and qigong also may be particularly useful in treating military personnel, such as veterans with mild TBI (Yost and Taylor 2013). Certain at-risk military populations have a high incidence of mental health, substance abuse, and pain issues.

Complementary Approach to Pharmacological Strategies

Tai chi and qigong are behavioral interventions that can be used in conjunction with pharmacological and other conventional treatments. Nonpharmacological approaches to mental disorders, such as tai chi and qigong, address the unmet need of patients who do not attain remission and functional recovery with pharmacotherapy alone (Charney et al. 2002; Thase 2003; Zajecka 2003). Furthermore, elderly patients are at higher risk for drug-drug interactions. Tai chi and qigong do not interact with drugs and rarely cause adverse events.

Limitations of Tai Chi and Qigong Research

Research on tai chi and qigong has not been well standardized. One systematic review found that more than half of the 42 RCTs on tai chi published from 1992 to 2007 used suboptimal quality of reporting (Li et al. 2011). Many studies used small sample sizes, different styles of tai chi and qigong, and variable practice times and intensities. Furthermore, there is no licensing or meaningful regulation of tai chi or qigong and no well-accepted organization that certifies qualified instructors. As such, it is difficult to rely on the results of a single study. Moreover, attempts at rigorous meta-analysis are hampered by the heterogeneity of practices and study designs. Such complexities in the literature may contribute to contradictory conclusions among meta-analyses.

Differences in efficacy among various forms of tai chi and qigong have not been studied. One review and meta-analysis of tai chi and qigong for depressive symptoms concluded that qigong was effective but tai chi was not (Liu et al. 2015). In contrast, two prior reviews concluded that tai chi had beneficial effects on depressive symptoms (Chi et al. 2013; C. Wang et al. 2010b).

Clinical Recommendations

Given that tai chi and qigong are low-intensity exercises that carry a minimal risk of adverse events and that they have been observed to positively affect qualify of life and a broad range of physical and psychiatric disorders, clinicians may consider recommending tai chi or qigong to any patient who is motivated to practice a mind-body intervention. On the basis of the average effective practice duration (dose) in the literature, clinicians should encourage patients to practice for a minimum of 30 minutes per session three times a week. Research suggests that patients may begin to experience benefits in a matter of weeks and that after a few weeks or months, they may attain sustained benefits, even without continued practice. Nevertheless, we advise patients that tai chi and qigong can be practiced indefinitely and that continued practice is likely to result in enhanced and sustained benefits. For patients with limited mobility, a qualified instructor should be able to teach modified versions of these exercises.

It is important to note the absence of strong evidence for the use of tai chi and qigong as primary treatments for mental disorders. Only select diseases and neurological disorders have been evaluated in clinical trials. Tai chi and qigong should not be substituted for examination by a qualified mental health professional and, when indicated, conventional medical treatment.

The lack of clear quality standards or clinical guidelines for tai chi and qigong is challenging for health care practitioners who wish to make appropriate referrals. Tai chi and qigong are often taught in group classes (sometimes in parks), adding a socialization benefit for patients. Usually, patients rely on word-of-mouth and community referrals (now aided by the Internet) to find instructors. Clinicians may contact local instructors to develop a referral network for patients, or they may observe (or participate in) classes to better assess the quality of the instructor and the setting for patients. Psychiatrists also might reach out to complementary and alternative medicine practitioners (e.g., acupuncturists) who are more familiar with local teaching networks. For clinicians interested in taking the time to make a specific referral, some questions for an instructor include the following: 1) Is the available instruction appropriate for the patient's physical condition? 2) Does the instructor have adequate experience in working with and adapting practices for patients with mental health issues? 3) How much individual attention do students receive?

After a patient initiates practice, the clinician should evaluate the effects of the program with continued monitoring. Possible inquiries for patients include the following:

- What are you doing in class?
- Are the practices suited to your needs and limitations?
- How do you feel about your teacher? (Is the teacher supportive and appropriate in his or her interactions?)
- Have you experienced any benefits from your practice?
- Have you noticed any changes in your condition?
- Have you had any negative reactions?

Clinicians should also monitor compliance. Noncompliant patients often need help to identify and overcome resistance to regular practice. Psychiatrists should actively support their patients' practices and inquire about experiences that occur during practice. If a patient experiences memories, images, or emotional release, it is important to address these in the therapeutic process. Patient feedback also can help clinicians in making referrals.

For patients inclined to practice alone at home, online programs and DVDs are available. We recommend a home DVD exercise tai chi program called *Tai Cheng* by Beachbody, LLC (Santa Monica, California). In addition, qigong master Robert Peng offers a series of qigong and meditation DVDs on his Web site (www.robertpeng.com). We also recommend that clinicians visit the Web site for the National Institutes of Health's National Center for Complementary and Integrative Health (https://nccih.nih.gov/health/taichi/introduction.htm), which has additional information and resources related to tai chi.

There has not been any research comparing different types of tai chi and qigong, although many tai chi RCTs use the Yang or Sun styles. Thus, we recommend that clinicians advise patients to practice the form of tai chi or qigong that they find to be helpful.

Conclusion

Tai chi and qigong have been used to improve mental and physical health for hundreds and thousands of years, respectively, but only recently has medical research begun validating their therapeutic potential. Although psychological benefits have been evaluated in only limited studies of select disorders, overall evidence indicates positive effects on symptoms and quality of life. Future research should focus on the mechanisms that contribute to therapeutic effects, efficacy in rigorously controlled trials, identification of fundamental practices found in diverse styles, and evaluation of effectiveness as complementary treatments. Twenty years ago, most psychiatrists would not refer patients to practice mind-body exercises. Now, as the scientific literature deepens our understanding, more clinicians are recommending tai chi and qigong as nonpharmacological, low-intensity exercises with physical and psychological benefits.

KEY POINTS

- A growing evidence base supports the use of tai chi and qigong to improve health outcomes, quality of life, and symptoms associated with mental health disorders.

- As low-risk interventions, tai chi and qigong are well suited to the needs of older patients.

- Tai chi and qigong are appropriate for patients who are motivated to practice a behavioral intervention and as complementary treatments for patients receiving pharmacotherapy.

- Tai chi and qigong should not be substituted for examination by a qualified mental health professional and, when indicated, conventional
medical treatment.

References

Abbott R, Lavretsky H: Tai chi and qigong for the treatment and prevention of mental disorders. Psychiatr Clin North Am 36(1):109–119, 2013 23538081

Abbott R, Hui KK, Hays RD, et al: A randomized controlled trial of tai chi for tension headaches: evidence-based complement. Altern Med 27(343):107–113, 2007 17342248

Barrow DE, Bedford A, Ives G, et al: An evaluation of the effects of tai chi chuan and chi kung
training in patients with symptomatic heart failure: a randomised controlled pilot study.
Postgrad Med J 83(985):717–721, 2007 17989272

Blake H, Batson M: Exercise intervention in brain injury: a pilot randomized study of tai chi qigong. Clin Rehabil 23(7):589–598, 2009 19237436

Bolton JM, Metge C, Lix L, et al: Fracture risk from psychotropic medications: a population-
based analysis. J Clin Psychopharmacol 28(4):384–391, 2008 18626264

Bond DS, Lyle RM, Tappe MK, et al: Moderate aerobic exercise, t'ai chi, and social problem-
solving ability in relation to psychological stress. Int J Stress Manag 9(4):329–343, 2002

Bower JE, Irwin MR: Mind-body therapies and control of inflammatory biology: a descriptive
review. Brain Behav Immun 51:1–11, 2016 26116436

Brown DR, Wang Y, Ward A, et al: Chronic psychological effects of exercise and exercise plus
cognitive strategies. Med Sci Sports Exerc 27(5):765–775, 1995 7674883

Bugg JM, Head D: Exercise moderates age-related atrophy of the medial temporal lobe. Neurobiol Aging 32(3):506–514, 2011 19386382

Cahn BR, Polich J: Meditation states and traits: EEG, ERP, and neuroimaging studies. Psychol
Bull 132(2):180–211, 2006 16536641

Charney DS, Nemeroff CB, Lewis L, et al: National Depressive and Manic-Depressive Association consensus statement on the use of placebo in clinical trials of mood disorders. Arch
Gen Psychiatry 59(3):262–270, 2002 11879164

Chen KW, Comerford A, Shinnick P, et al: Introducing qigong meditation into residential addiction treatment: a pilot study where gender makes a difference. J Altern Complement
Med 16(8):875–882, 2010 20649456

Chi I, Jordan-Marsh M, Guo M, et al: Tai chi and reduction of depressive symptoms for older
adults: a meta-analysis of randomized trials. Geriatr Gerontol Int 13(1):3–12, 2013 22680972

Choi HJ, Garber CE, Jun TW, et al: Therapeutic effects of tai chi in patients with Parkinson's
disease. ISRN Neuro 2013:548240, 2013

Chou KL, Lee PWH, Yu ECS, et al: Effect of tai chi on depressive symptoms amongst Chinese
older patients with depressive disorders: a randomized clinical trial. Int J Geriatr Psychiatry 19(11):1105–1107, 2004 15497192

Chow YW, Tsang HW: Biopsychosocial effects of qigong as a mindful exercise for people with
anxiety disorders: a speculative review. J Altern Complement Med 13(8):831–839, 2007
17983339

Deandrea S, Lucenteforte E, Bravi F, et al: Risk factors for falls in community-dwelling older people: a systematic review and meta-analysis. Epidemiology 21(5):658–668, 2010 20585256

Dechamps A, Gatta B, Bourdel-Marchasson I, et al: Pilot study of a 10-week multidisciplinary tai
chi intervention in sedentary obese women. Clin J Sport Med 19(1):49–53, 2009 19124984

Field T: Tai chi research review. Complement Ther Clin Pract 17(3):141–146, 2011 21742279

Field T, Diego M, Hernandez-Reif M: Tai chi/yoga effects on anxiety, heartrate, EEG and math
computations. Complement Ther Clin Pract 16(4):235–238, 2010 20920810

Fransen M, Nairn L, Winstanley J, et al: Physical activity for osteoarthritis management: a randomized controlled clinical trial evaluating hydrotherapy or tai chi classes. Arthritis Rheum 57(3):407–414, 2007 17443749

Frye B, Scheinthal S, Kemarskaya T, et al: Tai chi and low impact exercise: effects on the physical functioning and psychological well-being of older people. J Appl Gerontol 26(5):433–453, 2007

Galantino ML, Shepard K, Krafft L, et al: The effect of group aerobic exercise and t'ai chi on functional outcomes and quality of life for persons living with acquired immunodeficiency syndrome. J Altern Complement Med 11(6):1085–1092, 2005 16398601

Gemmell C, Leathem JM: A study investigating the effects of tai chi chuan: individuals with traumatic brain injury compared to controls. Brain Inj 20(2):151–156, 2006 16421063

Gillespie LD, Robertson MC, Gillespie WJ, et al: Interventions for preventing falls in older people living in the community. Cochrane Database Syst Rev 15(2):CD007146, 2009 19370674

Gladfelter BA: The Effect of Tai Chi Exercise on Balance and Falls in Persons With Parkinson's (Evidence-Based Practice Project Reports, Paper 2). Valparaiso, IN, Valparaiso University College of Nursing, 2011

Hackney ME, Earhart GM: Tai chi improves balance and mobility in people with Parkinson disease. Gait Posture 28(3):456–460, 2008 18378456

Hartman CA, Manos TM, Winter C, et al: Effects of t'ai chi training on function and quality of life indicators in older adults with osteoarthritis. J Am Geriatr Soc 48(12):1553–1559, 2000 11129742

Iaboni A, Flint AJ: The complex interplay of depression and falls in older adults: a clinical review. Am J Geriatr Psychiatry 21(5):484–492, 2013 23570891

Irwin MR, Olmstead R, Oxman MN: Augmenting immune responses to varicella zoster virus in older adults: a randomized, controlled trial of tai chi. J Am Geriatr Soc 55(4):511–517, 2007 17397428

Irwin MR, Olmstead R, Motivala SJ: Improving sleep quality in older adults with moderate sleep complaints: a randomized controlled trial of tai chi chih. Sleep 31(7):1001–1008, 2008 18652095

Jahnke R, Larkey L, Rogers C, et al: A comprehensive review of health benefits of qigong and tai chi. Am J Health Promot 24(6):e1–e25, 2010 20594090

Jevning R, Wallace RK, Beidebach M: The physiology of meditation: a review. A wakeful hypometabolic integrated response. Neurosci Biobehav Rev 16(3):415–424, 1992 1528528

Jin P: Efficacy of tai chi, brisk walking, meditation, and reading in reducing mental and emotional stress. J Psychosom Res 36(4):361–370, 1992 1593511

Kleim JA, Cooper NR, VandenBerg PM: Exercise induces angiogenesis but does not alter movement representations within rat motor cortex. Brain Res 934(1):1–6, 2002 11937064

Lam LC, Chau RC, Wong BM, et al: Interim follow-up of a randomized controlled trial comparing Chinese style mind body (tai chi) and stretching exercises on cognitive function in subjects at risk of progressive cognitive decline. Int J Geriatr Psychiatry 26(7):733–740, 2011 21495078

Lavretsky H, Alstein LL, Olmstead RE, et al: Complementary use of tai chi chih augments escitalopram treatment of geriatric depression: a randomized controlled trial. Am J Geriatr Psychiatry 19(10):839–850, 2011 21358389

Lee MS, Lee MS, Kim HJ, et al: Qigong reduced blood pressure and catecholamine levels of patients with essential hypertension. Int J Neurosci 113(12):1691–1701, 2003 14602541

Li F, Duncan TE, Duncan SC, et al: Enhancing the psychological well-being of elderly individuals through tai chi exercise: a latent growth curve analysis. Struct Equ Modeling 8(1):53–85, 2001

Li F, Fisher KJ, Harmer P, et al: Tai chi and self-rated quality of sleep and daytime sleepiness in older adults: a randomized controlled trial. J Am Geriatr Soc 52(6):892–900, 2004 15161452

Li F, Harmer P, Fitzgerald K, et al: Tai chi and postural stability in patients with Parkinson's disease. N Engl J Med 366(6):511–519, 2012 22316445

Li JY, Zhang YF, Smith GS, et al: Quality of reporting of randomized clinical trials in tai chi interventions: a systematic review. Evid Based Complement Alternat Med 2011:383245, 2011 19351709

Li M, Chen K, Mo Z: Use of qigong therapy in the detoxification of heroin addicts. Altern Ther Health Med 8(1):50–54, 56–59, 2002 11795622

Liu X, Clark J, Siskind D, et al: A systematic review and meta-analysis of the effects of qigong and tai chi for depressive symptoms. Complement Ther Med 23(4):516–534, 2015 26275645

Liu Y, Mimura K, Wang L, et al: Physiological benefits of 24-style taijiquan exercise in middle-aged women. J Physiol Anthropol Appl Human Sci 22(5):219–225, 2003 14519910

Logghe IH, Verhagen AP, Rademaker AC, et al: The effects of tai chi on fall prevention, fear of falling and balance in older people: a meta-analysis. Prev Med 51(3–4):222–227, 2010 20558197

McCain NL, Gray DP, Elswick RK, et al: A randomized clinical trial of alternative stress management interventions in persons with HIV infection. J Consult Clin Psychol 76(3):431–441, 2008 18540736

Miller SM, Taylor-Piliae RE: Effects of tai chi on cognitive function in community-dwelling older adults: a review. Geriatr Nurs 35(1):9–19, 2014 24252560

Motivala SJ, Sollers J, Thayer J, et al: Tai chi chih acutely decreases sympathetic nervous system activity in older adults. J Gerontol A Biol Sci Med Sci 61(11):1177–1180, 2006 17167159

Nguyen MH, Kruse A: A randomized controlled trial of tai chi for balance, sleep quality and cognitive performance in elderly Vietnamese. Clin Interv Aging 7:185–190, 2012 22807627

Rogers CE, Larkey LK, Keller C: A review of clinical trials of tai chi and qigong in older adults. West J Nurs Res 31(2):245–279, 2009 19179544

Ryu H, Lee HS, Shin YS, et al: Acute effect of qigong training on stress hormonal levels in man. Am J Chin Med 24(2):193–198, 1996 8874677

Sato S, Makita S, Uchida R, et al: Effect of tai chi training on baroreflex sensitivity and heart rate variability in patients with coronary heart disease. Int Heart J 51(4):238–241, 2010 20716839

Sun WY, Dosch M, Gilmore GD, et al: Effects of a tai chi chuan program on Hmong American older adults. Educ Gerontol 22(2):161–167, 1996

Taylor D, Hale L, Schluter P, et al: Effectiveness of tai chi as a community-based falls prevention intervention: a randomized controlled trial. J Am Geriatr Soc 60(5):841–848, 2012 22587850

Taylor-Piliae RE, Newell KA, Cherin R, et al: Effects of tai chi and Western exercise on physical and cognitive functioning in healthy community-dwelling older adults. J Aging Phys Act 18(3):261–279, 2010 20651414

Thase ME: Achieving remission and managing relapse in depression. J Clin Psychiatry 64 (suppl 18):3–7, 2003 14700448

Tsai JC, Wang WH, Chan P, et al: The beneficial effects of tai chi chuan on blood pressure and lipid profile and anxiety status in a randomized controlled trial. J Altern Complement Med 9(5):747–754, 2003 14629852

Vestergaard P, Rejnmark L, Mosekilde L: Selective serotonin reuptake inhibitors and other antidepressants and risk of fracture. Calcif Tissue Int 82(2):92–101, 2008 18219438

Wang C: Tai chi improves pain and functional status in adults with rheumatoid arthritis: results of a pilot single-blinded randomized controlled trial. Med Sport Sci 52:218–229, 2008 18487901

Wang C, Schmid CH, Hibberd PL, et al: Tai chi is effective in treating knee osteoarthritis: a randomized controlled trial. Arthritis Rheum 61(11):1545–1553, 2009 19877092

Wang C, Schmid CH, Rones R, et al: A randomized trial of tai chi for fibromyalgia. N Engl J Med 363(8):743–754, 2010a 20818876

Wang C, Bannuru R, Ramel J, et al: Tai chi on psychological well-being: systematic review and meta-analysis. BMC Complement Altern Med 10:23, 2010b 20492638

Wang W, Sawada M, Noriyama Y, et al: Tai chi exercise versus rehabilitation for the elderly with cerebral vascular disorder: a single-blinded randomized controlled trial. Psychogeriatrics 10(3):160–166, 2010 20860572

Wang WC, Zhang AL, Rasmussen B, et al: The effect of tai chi on psychosocial well-being: a systematic review of randomized controlled trials. J Acupunct Meridian Stud 2(3):171–181, 2009 20633489

Wayne PM, Walsh JN, Taylor-Piliae RE, et al: Effect of tai chi on cognitive performance in older adults: systematic review and meta-analysis. J Am Geriatr Soc 62(1):25–39, 2014 24383523

Wei GX, Xu T, Fan FM, et al: Can taichi reshape the brain? A brain morphometry study. PLoS One 8(4):e61038, 2013 23585869

Wei GX, Dong HM, Yang Z, et al: Tai chi chuan optimizes the functional organization of the intrinsic human brain architecture in older adults. Front Aging Neurosci 6:74, 2014 24860494

Woo J, Hong A, Lau E, et al: A randomised controlled trial of tai chi and resistance exercise on bone health, muscle strength and balance in community-living elderly people. Age Aging 36(3):262–268, 2007 17356003

Woolcott JC, Richardson KJ, Wiens MO, et al: Meta-analysis of the impact of 9 medication classes on falls in elderly persons. Arch Intern Med 169(21):1952–1960, 2009 19933955

Yeh GY, McCarthy EP, Wayne PM, et al: Tai chi exercise in patients with chronic heart failure: a randomized clinical trial. Arch Intern Med 171(8):750–757, 2011 21518942

Yost TL, Taylor AG: Qigong as a novel intervention for service members with mild traumatic brain injury. Explore (NY) 9(3):142–149, 2013 23643369

Zajecka JM: Treating depression to remission. J Clin Psychiatry 64 (suppl 1):7–22, 2003 14658985

Zheng G, Liu F, Li S, et al: Tai chi and the protection of cognitive ability: a systematic review of prospective studies in healthy adults. Am J Prev Med 49(1):89–97, 2015 26094229

CHAPTER 24

Mindfulness and Meditation in Psychiatric Practice

William R. Marchand, M.D.

Feelings come and go like clouds in a windy sky. Conscious breathing is my anchor.

Thích Nhất Hạnh, Stepping Into Freedom: Rules of Monastic Practice for Novices

Mindfulness and meditation-based interventions shown to be beneficial in the treatment of psychiatric conditions and substance use disorders include mindfulness-based stress reduction (MBSR), mindfulness-based cognitive therapy (MBCT), and mindfulness-based relapse prevention (MBRP). Acceptance and commitment therapy and dialectical behavior therapy, which incorporate components of mindfulness, are often referred to as mindfulness-based approaches. In this chapter, I focus on underlying mechanisms and research evidence for MBSR, MBCT, and MBRP.

Originating in Buddhist spiritual practices, modern mindfulness interventions are secular, clinically based group therapies that use manuals and standardized techniques. MBSR provides education about stress and coping strategies, as well as cultivation of the following attitudes: becoming an impartial witness to one's own experience; acceptance of reality as it is in the present moment; and observing one's thoughts as they come and go. Developed specifically to prevent relapse of depression, MBCT builds on MBSR and combines principles and techniques of cognitive therapy with those of mindfulness. MBCT teaches recognition of and disengagement from patterns of ruminative, negative thought that contribute to depressive symptoms. MBRP is similar to MBCT but focuses on relapse prevention of substance use disorders. The terms *mindfulness* and *meditation* are sometimes used interchangeably; however, they have distinct meanings.

Mindfulness

Mindfulness is a mental state in which one keeps attention focused on the present moment rather than allowing it to shift automatically. This includes awareness of visual and auditory stimuli as well as physical sensations, thoughts, and emotions as they occur. There are two fundamental differences between the mindful and the nonmindful states of mind. In the mindful state, attention is under conscious control and focused on the present moment. In the nonmindful state (i.e., *autopilot*), attention shifts from one thing to another without conscious control and is often focused on thinking about the past or future. Cognitive neuroscience would consider the nonmindful state to be one of automatic processing. Automatic mental processing includes stimulus-independent thought, which is commonly called *mind wandering*.

The practice of mindfulness entails avoidance of autopilot and the attentional focus on whatever is occurring at the moment: internal stimuli (thoughts, emotions, proprioception, pain, and interoception), external stimuli (auditory, olfactory, and visual stimuli, as well as general awareness of the environment), and current motor behaviors. For many people, this seemingly simple state of awareness is difficult to achieve. The key to developing a mindfulness practice is learning to recognize the autopilot state when it occurs and then shifting into mindful awareness.

Meditation

Meditation refers to numerous practices that can include mindfulness meditation. The word *meditation* stems from the Latin *meditari*, meaning to participate in contemplation or reflection. Many different meditation practices exist; however, most share the aim of bringing mental processes under voluntary control by intentionally focusing attention and awareness. The two general forms of meditation are *focused attention* and *open monitoring*. In focused attention, attention is typically focused on an anchor. In mindfulness training, attention is focused initially on the physical sensations of breathing or some other anchor for attention. In open monitoring meditation, an advanced mindfulness practice, attention is on open awareness and observation of external stimuli, thoughts, emotions, and physical sensations as they arise and as they pass. In open monitoring, an anchor generally is not used. However, focused attention and open monitoring are often combined during a single meditation session. Meditation can be practiced in a sitting posture, lying down, or during movement (e.g., walking meditation or yoga). In focused awareness during movement, the attention would be anchored on physical sensations as they occur with each step or pose.

The Practice of Mindfulness

Formal meditation, the process by which one trains the mind to practice mindfulness, is the foundation of an ongoing regular mindfulness meditation practice. Ideally, this is a daily practice and may include sitting meditation, walking meditation, or yoga. Although formal meditation is the foundational mindfulness practice, the overarching aim is to spend as much of one's life as possible in a state of mindful awareness. The goal of a mindfulness practice is not to completely avoid autopilot; rather, it is to become more skilled at recognizing when it occurs and to return to the present moment. The consistent practice of focused attention meditation facilitates development of mindfulness skills and over time the ability to practice mindfulness even when one is not engaged in formal meditation. Other practices used to develop mindfulness skills include simple activities, such as brushing one's teeth mindfully or eating a meal mindfully, with attention fully focused on the physical sensations of the activity.

Although mindfulness encourages accepting things as they are in the moment, the intent is not to become passive but rather to take appropriate, beneficial actions based on mindful awareness. For example, if one is experiencing symptoms of depression, mindfulness would facilitate acceptance of the emotion of sadness in the moment and taking appropriate action to decrease the symptoms, such as going for a walk, doing physical exercise, or engaging in an artistic activity. This is in contrast to autopilot-driven behaviors, such as self-medicating with substances of abuse, ruminating, or other negative behaviors.

Psychological Mechanisms of Mindfulness

A brief review of the origins of mindfulness will help explain neural and psychological mechanisms thought to underlie the benefits of mindfulness.

Origins of Mindfulness and the Concept of Resistance to Reality

Buddhism, a complex religion and philosophy encompassing many schools, is fundamentally a spiritual practice for the relief of suffering. Suffering is experienced through a range of mental states from vague dissatisfaction to persistent unhappiness as well as more intense physical or emotional pain. The Four Noble Truths, believed to represent the first instructions of the Buddha and the core teachings of Buddhism, explain the concept of relief of suffering.

The first truth says that all existence is characterized by suffering and dissatisfaction. In other words, unhappiness and suffering are a normal part of life for all people.

The second truth indicates that the causes of suffering are craving and desire—that is, we suffer because we want things to be different from the way they are. Desire also includes wanting to avoid situations that cause pain. In mindfulness language, the concept of *resistance* is that our resistance to aspects of reality that we dislike causes much of our suffering.

The third truth is that elimination of craving and desire (resistance) can result in the end of suffering. Resistance, or wanting things to be different, is often an autopilot process.

The fourth truth indicates that Buddhist practice can bring an end to suffering.

General Psychological Mechanisms of Mindfulness

Shapiro et al. (2006) suggested that a fundamental psychological mechanism of mindfulness is *reperceiving*, or shifting perspective, enabling us to step back from, and be less identified with, our thoughts and emotions. Mindfulness practitioners discover that they are greater than their thoughts and emotions (Shapiro et al. 2006). Becoming less identified with one's emotions and cognitions reduces their power. One cannot avoid physical and emotional pain; however, by becoming less identified with one's thoughts and feelings, it is possible to experience the pain and move on rather than being caught up in autopilot-driven suffering.

Resistance to physical and emotional pain increases pain and suffering. For example, if one is experiencing physical pain, the natural tendency of the mind is to wish that the pain would go away and to think about ways to eliminate the pain. This can be beneficial if it leads to adaptive behaviors, such as completing rehabilitative exercises. However, the mind's desire to be free of pain often increases suffering. This is, in part, because at the moment, the pain exists, and it is not possible to be free from it. The desire for it to be gone can result in increased frustration. Autopilot thinking is, by definition, focused on the past or the future rather than the present moment. When one is in pain, autopilot thinking often focuses on the future, with one perhaps worrying about how long the pain will last or how it will affect one's life.

Mindfulness helps practitioners better understand the workings of their minds by observing their mental processes. By paying very close attention to thoughts that come and go, practitioners may realize that autopilot thinking is almost always focused on the past or the future rather than the present moment. In the situation of chronic pain, thinking about the distress associated with past pain is not helpful, and worrying about future pain increases suffering. The ability to recognize when the mind is occupied with autopilot-driven thoughts allows practitioners to realize that, as indicated in the Second Noble Truth, suffering is a result of mental processes.

Another concept of mindfulness is that *thoughts are just thoughts*. This seems obvious, but the mind tends to perceive thoughts as representing truth and as being fundamental components of the self. Practitioners learn to "watch the mind," which allows them to observe the ephemeral nature of thoughts. Instructed to notice that thoughts and emotions come and go, practitioners see the transient nature of thoughts and recognize that thoughts are often irrational and unhelpful. This facilitates becoming less identified with thoughts and less likely to assume that they represent truth.

Watching one's mind may reveal that what one thinks of as self is a psychological construct made up of thoughts based on memories, beliefs, and ideas (Shapiro et al. 2006). Furthermore, this concept of self continuously changes as new memories are acquired and older ones are forgotten. This is perhaps the most insightful idea expressed by mindfulness. Our thinking patterns based on memories of our experiences and beliefs about ourselves define how we see ourselves and who we see ourselves to be. Many practitioners develop the realization that these memories and beliefs, too, are just ephemeral thoughts, often without deep meaning, that are sometimes irrational. This enables de-identification with the cognitive representation of self. Decreased identification with the idea of self also may diminish distress when the concept of self is threatened, whether the perceived threat is to the physical self, such as medical illness, or to the psyche, such as negative comments made by another person.

A reduced identification with the concept of self can broaden the perspective of reality such that one may more readily see the perspectives of others, even if one disagrees with their views. This shift of perception can facilitate increased compassion and concern for both self and others. Enhancing compassion is an important component of mindfulness and contributes to the benefits of this practice. Compassion specifically includes patience and kindness directed toward the self. Self-compassion is a predictor of psychological health, and increased caring for self contributes to the effectiveness of mindfulness.

Psychological Mechanisms of Mindfulness Relevant for Psychiatric Conditions

Aberrant self-referential thinking plays a key role in the etiology of many psychiatric disorders, particularly depression. For example, many studies indicate an association between low self-concept and negative self-schemas and depression.

In addition to the content of thought patterns, narrative thinking about the self plays a role in the cognitive aspects of depression. *Narrative thinking* includes generalized autobiographical memory, memories of the past, and intentions for the future. Narrative thinking is the basis for the sense of self. Narrative self-reference is composed of stimulus-independent thought-driven thinking patterns, which may take the form of self-referential rumination, an aspect of autopilot thinking. Narrative stimulus-independent thought, particularly when thinking analytically about self and depressive symptoms, is often maladaptive. Importantly, it is frequently associated with negative self-judgments and dysphoria. Excessive self-focus is associated with negative affect, and self-focused rumination is specifically associated with depression.

Depression is associated with the extent of self-referential thinking as well as the narrative stimulus–independent thought type of cognition. In mindfulness language, narrative stimulus-independent thought cognitions occur during autopilot. Mindfulness specifically targets the recognition and avoidance of this autopilot-based thinking. In contrast to self-referential thinking based on narrative stimulus-independent thought, mindful awareness is an adaptive and experiential sense of the self: the experience of self in the immediate moment without a story or theme. The literature suggests that mindfulness works, in part, by facilitating the ability to spend more time in an experiential state of mind rather than the self-focused, analytical autopilot state. Studies indicate that by reducing rumination, mindfulness practices have beneficial effects. Reperceiving and de-identification with self (Shapiro et al. 2006) may help individuals with psychiatric illness to be less focused on their symptoms and less likely to believe negative thoughts and schemas about the self.

Furthermore, research indicates that mindfulness is associated with enhanced emotional self-regulation and decreased emotional overreactivity. In mindful awareness, the ability to step back and observe rather than be controlled and carried away by emotions and thoughts improves self-regulation and adaptive coping skills while reducing maladaptive responses (Shapiro et al. 2006). Also, an increased ability to tolerate unpleasant emotions or sensations enables greater exposure to the discomfort and possibly eventual desensitization. The following case example illustrates some of these concepts.

> John is a 35-year-old man with a long history of depression and chronic back pain caused by a motorcycle accident. Over the course of 10 years, he received multiple antidepressant trials and intermittently engaged in supportive psychotherapy. Neither his depression nor his pain symptoms were ever in full remission. One year ago, he completed an 8-week MBCT class that I facilitated. By developing a meditation practice and the ability to observe his thinking patterns, John discovered that he tended to ruminate about his depressive and pain symptoms. He was also able to see that he was frequently carried away with ruminative thinking. In the MBCT class, he learned about gaining distance from negative thoughts and emotions and the use of positive coping strategies rather than simply reacting. An analogy provided in the class was standing on the bank of a flooded river watching the torrent (thoughts) flow by as opposed to falling in and being swept away with the current. Mindfulness facilitates recognition of being carried away by autopilot thinking and instead enables movement into mindful awareness.
>
> Another important effect of mindfulness practice for John was an increased ability to tolerate uncomfortable emotions and physical pain. In other words, he developed the ability to stay present with unpleasant sensations. This helped him avoid falling into negative and ruminative autopilot or stimulus-independent thought patterns that worsened both his pain and his depression. For example, he would think, "Oh no, another bout of depression. The last time this happened, it lasted for weeks." By watching his thoughts, he could see that these thinking patterns were not helpful and led to a vicious cycle of dysphoria leading to negative thoughts, which led to increased dysphoria, and so on. After completing the MBCT class, John still experienced chronic pain and intermittent depressive symptoms. However, he was able to better tolerate these symptom and engage in more adaptive behaviors, and as a result, he experienced significantly less distress from his symptoms.
>
> Although John benefited from MBCT, he experienced several challenges while trying to develop a mindfulness practice. One of these was his difficulty believing that mindfulness practice would actually be effective, because he had not found any previous treatments to be effective. Also, he thought of mindfulness and meditation as fads rather than evidence-based treatments. However, during the class, his belief gradually changed as he learned about the evidence that mindfulness is effective for pain and depression. Another obstacle was establishing a consistent daily meditation practice. The class focused on the need to establish a regular practice in order to experience benefits from MBCT, but like most mindfulness practitioners, John found that it was challenging to fit a daily meditation practice into his busy schedule. Students discussed their individual situations and solutions, and this helped John find ways to practice consistently.

Neural Mechanisms of Mindfulness

A growing literature is describing the neural mechanisms of mindfulness on the basis of human structural and functional neuroimaging studies. A recent review (Marchand 2014) noted that the heterogeneity of methodologies and diversity of populations studied limited interpretation, but nevertheless the studies provided convincing evidence that mindfulness and meditation practice are associated with changes in brain activation or connectivity of several regions.

Brain imaging studies of mindfulness implicate the frontal cortex (Marchand 2014). The strongest evidence is for medial frontal regions, including anterior cingulate cortex. Posterior medial regions are also involved, mostly in the posterior cingulate cortex and precuneus regions. Of the studies reviewed by Marchand (2014), a few indicated involvement of lateral frontal regions, including ventrolateral prefrontal cortex (PFC) and dorsolateral PFC. These studies provided very strong evidence that anterior and posterior cortical midline structures (CMS) play an important role in the neural mechanisms of mindfulness. The CMS are key components of the default mode network. In regard to noncortical regions, strong evidence indicates involvement of the insula and amygdala, and a few studies suggested involvement of the basal ganglia and thalamus.

Taken together, these studies provide convincing evidence that mindfulness mechanisms involve neural circuitry of the CMS/default mode network, insula, and amygdala (Marchand 2014), which is consistent with the psychological mechanisms outlined earlier. Mindfulness improves attention in general, which may involve CMS, parietal, and basal ganglia regions. Of note, mindfulness and meditation facilitate interoceptive attention, which is paying attention to visceral bodily sensations as they occur in the present moment. This probably involves CMS and insula regions. For example, one functional magnetic resonance imaging study found that mindfulness was associated with greater interoceptive attention–related activity in anterior insula regions as well as decreased recruitment of CMS (Farb et al. 2013). This suggests that mindfulness engages neuroplasticity such that interoceptive attention is enhanced and attention to self-referential thinking based in the CMS may be decreased. Neural mechanisms involving the default mode network may contribute to objectification of thoughts, which facilitates the interpretation of thoughts as "just thoughts." Enhancement of emotional regulation associated with mindfulness may entail modification of processing in lateral frontal regions, regions involved with interoception and the amygdala (Marchand 2014).

Review of Research Evidence

Although a large literature supports mindfulness-based interventions as being effective, substantial methodological problems limit the effect of many studies. Methodological concerns include lack of high-quality randomized controlled trials (RCTs) with adequate comparators, absence of follow-up measures, small sample sizes, reliance on self-report instruments, and differences across interventions. Methodological and conceptual challenges of mindfulness research were discussed in a recent review (Davidson and Kaszniak 2015). With these limitations in mind, a previous literature review (Marchand 2012) indicated that benefits associated with mindfulness practices and meditation may include better attention, enhanced self-compassion, decreased ruminative thinking, reduced cortisol levels, improved immune function, lower blood pressure, attenuated emotional reactivity, and enhanced cognition.

Mindfulness-Based Stress Reduction

A previous review of 35 studies of MBSR found evidence indicating effectiveness for depressive and anxiety symptoms, posttraumatic stress disorder, pain, insomnia, enhancing general mental health, and improving psychological functioning among individuals with a variety of medical disorders (Marchand 2012). Two rigorous randomized studies of a combined 240 participants, either healthy (MacCoon et al. 2012) or with fibromyalgia (Schmidt et al. 2011), that used an active control condition (for nonspecific effects of MBSR) found benefit equivalent to, but not better than, the active control condition. The active control condition was the Health Enhancement Program, which is structurally equivalent to MBSR. One meta-analysis of MBSR studies (Khoury et al. 2015) concluded that MBSR provides only relatively small effects on the reduction of depression, anxiety, and psychological distress in people with chronic medical illness. Effect sizes for MBSR were 0.26 for depression, 0.47 for anxiety, and 0.32 for psychological distress. For anxiety, quality of the studies was found to moderate the effect size, and when the studies of lower quality were excluded, an effect size of 0.24 was found. Khoury et al. (2015) concluded that MBSR was moderately effective in reducing stress, depression, anxiety, and distress and in improving the quality of life of healthy individuals. Finally, a systematic review and meta-analysis of systematic reviews of RCTs that used the standardized MBSR or MBCT programs concluded that evidence supports the use of MBSR and MBCT to alleviate psychiatric and physical symptoms in the adjunct treatment of cancer, cardiovascular disease, chronic pain, depression, and anxiety disorders (Gotink et al. 2015).

Mindfulness-Based Cognitive Therapy

Among the many studies of MBCT, the strongest evidence is for relapse prevention in major depression, particularly for individuals with three or more previous episodes (Chiesa and Serretti 2010). Several studies indicated that MBCT offers protection against relapse equal to that of maintenance antidepressant pharmacotherapy. However, one study found that adding MBCT to maintenance antidepressant medication did not further reduce the risk for relapse or residual depressive symptoms (Huijbers et al. 2015). Two studies, including one RCT, reported efficacy for acute depression. The first, a recent open, nonrandomized 8-week pilot study ($N=43$), compared MBCT monotherapy with sertraline monotherapy as a first-line intervention for acute major depressive disorder (Eisendrath et al. 2015). Findings indicated similar levels of symptom improvement on the primary measure (Hamilton Rating Scale for Depression). However, the MBCT group showed significantly ($P<0.0001$) greater improvement on a secondary measure (Quick Inventory of Depressive Symptomatology—Self-Report). The authors considered the results to suggest that an 8-week course of MBCT monotherapy may be effective in treating major depressive disorder and may offer a viable alternative to antidepressant medication. The second, a randomized study (N=45), reported MBCT to be as effective as cognitive-behavioral therapy in the treatment of acute depression (Manicavasgar et al. 2011). Finally, a recent randomized study (N=274) indicated that MBCT training can help to weaken the association between depressive symptoms and suicidal thinking (Barnhofer et al. 2015). A review of 23 studies indicated that this intervention also may be beneficial for anxiety associated with bipolar disorder, generalized anxiety disorder, panic disorder, hypochondriasis, and social phobia (Marchand 2012).

MBCT studies have had methodological shortcomings, including lack of adequate control groups. A recent randomized study of 43 patients (Chiesa et al. 2015) attempted to address this limitation by comparing MBCT with a psychoeducational control group designed to be structurally equivalent to the MBCT program but excluding mindfulness meditation practice for patients with major depression who did not achieve remission following at least 8 weeks of antidepressant treatment. Results suggested the superiority of MBCT over psychoeducation for nonremitted major depression. In contrast, a randomized study of 92 participants (Shallcross et al. 2015) comparing MBCT with an active control condition, which was structurally equivalent to MBCT, included instruction in physical activity, nutrition, and music therapy and controlled for nonspecific effects, including interaction with a facilitator, perceived social support, and treatment outcome expectations. Results indicated that MBCT did not differ from the active control condition on rates of depression relapse, symptom reduction, or life satisfaction.

Mindfulness-Based Relapse Prevention

Fifteen studies of MBRP have been published in regard to various aspects of this intervention. Some examined mechanisms of MBRP. However, five outcome studies indicated effectiveness for relapse prevention among individuals with substance use disorders. The strongest evidence was from a large RCT of 286 individuals that compared MBRP with treatment as usual (12-step programming and psychoeducation) and cognitive-behavioral relapse prevention (Bowen et al. 2014). Compared with treatment as usual, participants assigned to an 8-week MBRP and cognitive-behavioral relapse prevention reported significantly lower risk of relapse to substance use and heavy drinking and, among those who used substances, significantly fewer days of substance use and heavy drinking at 6-month follow-up. Cognitive-behavioral relapse prevention showed an advantage over MBRP in time to first drug use. At 12-month follow-up, MBRP participants reported significantly fewer days of substance use and significantly decreased heavy drinking compared with cognitive-behavioral relapse prevention and treatment as usual.

Risks and Contraindications

Mindfulness-based interventions are considered to be low risk, and potential risks have received little attention in the literature. Feelings of distress can be associated with mindfulness practice. I have observed MBCT participants experience short-term increases in anxiety during meditation exercises. Also, one study (Wilson et al. 2015) found that a potential unintended consequence of mindfulness meditation was that memories become less reliable. Contraindications and screening procedures for potential participants have not been well studied. However, common sense can serve as a guide such that individuals who have significant impairments of their cognitive function (e.g., psychosis) are not good candidates for mindfulness training. Patients who experience dissociation also may be at risk for increased symptoms when practicing mindfulness, but this has not been formally studied. Mindfulness requires dedication to the practice and thus is most appropriate for those who are highly motivated to practice regularly.

Clinical Guidelines for the Use of Mindfulness-Based Interventions

Although further research is needed, sufficient evidence exists to guide the use of MBCT, MBSR, and MBRP in clinical practice. MBCT can be strongly recommended as an adjunctive intervention or as monotherapy for maintenance treatment and relapse prevention in unipolar depression. It also should be considered as an adjunctive approach for acute and residual unipolar symptoms. MBCT also can be considered as an adjunctive intervention for anxiety associated with bipolar disorder, generalized anxiety disorder, panic disorder, hypochondriasis, and social phobia. MBSR is recommended as an adjunctive treatment for anxiety symptoms and pain management and for general psychological health and stress management among persons with medical or psychiatric illness and healthy individuals. Finally, MBRP is recommended for relapse prevention for persons with substance use disorders.

Evidence is currently limited in regard to patient characteristics that may be associated with a good response to these mindfulness-based interventions. Patient preference is always important, especially for mindfulness-based interventions. It is recommended to refer only patients who are enthusiastic about trying these approaches. Evidence suggests that meditation-associated changes in brain function may require extensive practice, and research indicates that greater meditation practice is associated with more improvement on some outcome measures. Thus, the most important considerations may be desire to try mindfulness and willingness to engage in a regular practice of meditation. However, the minimum effective doses of mindfulness are unknown. When teaching mindfulness, I recommend at least 15 minutes of practice for 6 of every 7 days.

Conclusion

Mindfulness-based interventions have been studied extensively in recent years. Although much of the literature has methodological limitations, recent studies have been more rigorous. Current evidence is adequate to recommend the use of MBCT,

MBSR, and MBRP. In addition to symptom management, these approaches have the potential to improve psychological well-being, compassion, and life satisfaction.

KEY POINTS

- Secular mindfulness-based interventions originated in Buddhist spiritual practices.

- Self-referential rumination contributes to the persistence of psychiatric symptoms.

- Mindfulness meditation is used to develop the skill to keep attention focused on the here and now and to avoid self-referential rumination.

- Focus on the present moment facilitates realization that thoughts and emotions come and go and have no real substance.

- Mindfulness-based cognitive therapy is effective for psychiatric symptoms and mindfulness-based relapse prevention for substance use disorders.

References

Barnhofer T, Crane C, Brennan K, et al: Mindfulness-based cognitive therapy (MBCT) reduces the association between depressive symptoms and suicidal cognitions in patients with a history of suicidal depression. J Consult Clin Psychol 83(6):1013–1020, 2015 26302249

Bowen S, Witkiewitz K, Clifasefi SL, et al: Relative efficacy of mindfulness-based relapse prevention, standard relapse prevention, and treatment as usual for substance use disorders: a randomized clinical trial. JAMA Psychiatry 71(5):547–556, 2014 24647726

Chiesa A, Serretti A: A systematic review of neurobiological and clinical features of mindfulness meditations. Psychol Med 40(8):1239–1252, 2010 19941676

Chiesa A, Castagner V, Andrisano C, et al: Mindfulness-based cognitive therapy vs. psychoeducation for patients with major depression who did not achieve remission following antidepressant treatment. Psychiatry Res 226(2–3):474–483, 2015 25744325

Davidson RJ, Kaszniak AW: Conceptual and methodological issues in research on mindfulness and meditation. Am Psychol 70(7):581–592, 2015 26436310

Eisendrath SJ, Gillung E, Delucchi K, et al: A preliminary study: efficacy of mindfulness-based cognitive therapy versus sertraline as first-line treatments for major depressive disorder. Mindfulness (N Y) 6(3):475–482, 2015 26085853

Farb NA, Segal ZV, Anderson AK: Mindfulness meditation training alters cortical representations of interoceptive attention. Soc Cogn Affect Neurosci 8(1):15–26, 2013 22689216

Gotink RA, Chu P, Busschbach JJ, et al: Standardised mindfulness-based interventions in healthcare: an overview of systematic reviews and meta-analyses of RCTs. PLoS One 10(4):e0124344, 2015 25881019

Huijbers MJ, Spinhoven P, Spijker J, et al: Adding mindfulness-based cognitive therapy to maintenance antidepressant medication for prevention of relapse/recurrence in major depressive disorder: randomised controlled trial. J Affect Disord 187:54–61, 2015 26318271

Khoury B, Sharma M, Rush SE, et al: Mindfulness-based stress reduction for healthy individuals: a meta-analysis. J Psychosom Res 78(6):519–528, 2015 25818837

MacCoon DG, Imel ZE, Rosenkranz MA, et al: The validation of an active control intervention for mindfulness based stress reduction (MBSR). Behav Res Ther 50(1):3–12, 2012 22137364

Manicavasgar V, Parker G, Perich T: Mindfulness-based cognitive therapy vs cognitive behaviour therapy as a treatment for non-melancholic depression. J Affect Disord 130(1–2):138–144, 2011 21093925

Marchand WR: Mindfulness-based stress reduction, mindfulness-based cognitive therapy, and Zen meditation for depression, anxiety, pain, and psychological distress. J Psychiatr Pract 18(4):233–252, 2012 22805898

Marchand WR: Neural mechanisms of mindfulness and meditation: evidence from neuroimaging studies. World J Radiol 6(7):471–479, 2014 25071887

Schmidt S, Grossman P, Schwarzer B, et al: Treating fibromyalgia with mindfulness-based stress reduction: results from a 3-armed randomized controlled trial. Pain 152(2):361–369, 2011 21146930

Shallcross AJ, Gross JJ, Visvanathan PD, et al: Relapse prevention in major depressive disorder: mindfulness-based cognitive therapy versus an active control condition. J Consult Clin Psychol 83(5):964–975, 2015 26371618

Shapiro SL, Carlson LE, Astin JA, et al: Mechanisms of mindfulness. J Clin Psychol 62(3):373–386, 2006 16385481

Wilson BM, Mickes L, Stolarz-Fantino S, et al: Increased false-memory susceptibility after mindfulness meditation. Psychol Sci 26(10):1567–1573, 2015 26341562

Open Focus Training for Stress, Pain, and Psychosomatic Illness

Lester G. Fehmi, Ph.D.

Edward T. Kenny, M.D.

Susan B. Shor, L.C.S.W.

The world is vast and wide. Why do you put on your robe at the sound of a bell?

Koan of Zen Master Ummon (Chan Master Yunmen Wenyan),
circa A.D. *862–949*

Portions of this chapter were condensed and paraphrased from *The Open-Focus Brain: Harnessing the Power of Attention to Heal Mind and Body*, copyright 2007 by Les Fehmi, Ph.D., and Jim Robbins, and *Dissolving Pain: Simple Brain-Training Exercises for Overcoming Chronic Pain*, copyright 2010 by Les Fehmi, Ph.D., and Jim Robbins, published by Trumpeter Books, an imprint of Shambhala Publications, Inc. By permission of Stuart Bernstein Representation for Artists, Bernstein Representation for Artists, New York, NY and protected by the Copyright Laws of the United States. All rights reserved. The printing, copying, redistribution, or retransmission of this Content without express permission is prohibited. The chapter was written with the lyrical and scholarly help of Jim Robbins; Patricia L. Gerbarg, M.D., contributed to contextualizing this chapter in light of recent research. We wish to thank them both. For Open Focus publications and workshops, see www.openfocus.com.

Open Focus is an attention training practice that enhances a sense of connectedness, which many people associate with spiritual development. However, it is a nonreligious discipline intended for clinical treatment of physical and mental symptoms.

Open Focus Versus Narrow Focus

The term *Open Focus* refers to a mental state of relaxed yet alert attention and to a method of training that fosters this mental state. Open Focus training develops the capacity to enter into awareness of all perceptions experienced simultaneously, including environmental stimuli and sensations of somatic or mental origin. The term *focus* usually means a constricted application of attention to a circumscribed activity, such as solving a math problem, while other perceptions are excluded, often with great effort. This type of attention is called *narrow focus* to distinguish it from the type cultivated in Open Focus. Narrow focus has great benefits, such as facilitating efficient task completion, but prolonged, excessive use can contribute to psychological and physical stress and exacerbate subjective experiences of pain. Different subjective mental states of attention correlate with measurable patterns of brain wave activity on electroencephalography; narrow focus attention tends to correlate with beta waves (13–40 Hz), whereas Open Focus attention correlates with alpha frequencies (8–12 Hz) (Fehmi 2007).

Many persons who seek Open Focus training have psychosomatic illnesses. If they are motivated to practice regularly, they can be trained to alter their global brain wave states by using neurofeedback equipment and guided exercises in specific methods of meditative imagery. The achievement of intentionally altered brain wave states is often associated with symptom relief and an enhanced sense of well-being. These methods are relatively simple, can be mastered by most people, and can be readily introduced in a range of treatment settings, either as the primary treatment modality or as an adjunct to other treatments. In this chapter, we describe the development of the Open Focus method, different attentional states, the use of Open Focus to alleviate pain, and an Open Focus exercise.

The Development of Open Focus and Alpha Synchrony

About 50 years ago, while studying brain wave states and visual perception in macaque monkeys, Fehmi discovered that synchrony—synchronization of the brain's electrical activity in one or more major areas—correlated with measurably improved performance in visual tasks (Fehmi et al. 1969). Early electroencephalogram studies of advanced Buddhist meditators identified a range from low-frequency waves (3–7 Hz) to higher-frequency waves (~40 Hz), with a significant cluster of individuals meditating in the alpha spectrum of 8–12 Hz (Benson et al. 1990; Kasamatsu and Hirai 1966).

Exploring whether induced synchrony in the human brain would result in improved performance in perceptual and processing systems, Fehmi tried to produce alpha frequencies voluntarily in all of the standard electrode positions using early neurofeedback equipment. His initial efforts to self-induce *alpha synchrony*, a global brain state requiring simultaneous production of in-phase alpha waves, were unsuccessful. Eventually, Fehmi found that alpha synchrony could be achieved by focusing on the feeling of space, both inside and outside the body. Immediately and afterward, he observed a heightened sense of well-being, vivid attention, reduced arthritic pain, and enhanced cognitive functioning at work. Clinical testing of this method showed that most patients learned it readily. However, not everyone attains a global state of alpha synchrony and its attendant benefits; many people quit prematurely because of frustration or lack of immediate results.

The process of training for alpha synchrony fosters *attentional flexibility*: the ability to consciously transition to different attentional states that are optimal for various activities. With training, the individual becomes less likely to get stuck rigidly in any one attentional state that may be associated with physical and mental stress.

Elaboration of Different Attentional States

Brain wave frequencies are classified from low to high: delta, theta, alpha, beta, and gamma. Modes of attention can be classified as narrow, diffuse, objective, and immersed. These modes correspond to ranges of brain wave frequencies, optimize performance of specific tasks, correlate with states of autonomic nervous system arousal, and play a role in emotion regulation. Attentional modes tend to exist in combinations (Table 25–1). Through training, one can learn to move consciously among these attentional styles.

Narrow attention is concentration on a very limited field of perception; attention may be focused on one portion of the visual field, on an aspect of the entire sensory field (vision, hearing, touch, smell, and taste), or on mental experiences. *Diffuse attention* tends to be panoramic rather than exclusive or single-pointed: "No particular target of attention stands out, and the distinctions between figure and ground are blurred or erased" (Fehmi and Robbins 2007, p. 49). *Objective attention* distances the observer from the object of attention, allowing for evaluation and control. If sustained, it can alienate the observer from experience. *Immersed attention* occurs when one enters into a union with an object of attention or a process requiring deep concentration to the point of complete unselfconsciousness.

Transitioning Among Modes of Attention

Open Focus training fosters transitions among attentional states so that the individual does not stay locked into one state as a pernicious habit (i.e., extreme attentional bias). Open Focus allows conscious control over the merging of attentional styles, such as using narrow focus while also admitting some awareness of space and other sense experiences, thus allowing attention to be more evenly distributed and thereby diffusing stress. The key to transitioning among different modes of attention is conscious attention to space. One can broaden attention to include space and all perceptible objects in it. This can be done with all sensory modalities. One also can exclude

TABLE 25–1. Modes of attention: effects on the central nervous system and electroencephalographic patterns

	Description and examples	Effects on the central nervous system	Electroencephalographic patterns
Diffuse-immersed mode	Panoramic attention distributed equally across figure and ground; unselfconsciousness, with body relaxed; capacity to rapidly regain homeostasis after stress (e.g., meditator in alpha synchrony)	Parasympathetic predominance; right brain predominance; low arousal, at the border of wakefulness and sleep	Low frequencies: delta and theta (<8 Hz); increased whole-brain synchrony
Diffuse-objective mode	Focus on objective sensations with simultaneous diffuse awareness of space (e.g., player of an instrument in a band who is also able to hear and respond to the other instruments)	Relative sympathetic and parasympathetic balance; relative right-left brain balance; moderate arousal; relaxed alertness	Middle frequencies: alpha and low beta (~8–15 Hz); moderate whole-brain synchrony
Narrow-immersed mode	Immersed attention in a limited activity; enjoyment amplified by narrow focus so as to intensify and savor the selected experiences (e.g., professional wine taster or avid television football watcher)	Relative sympathetic and parasympathetic balance; relative right-left brain balance; moderate arousal; relaxed alertness	Middle frequencies: alpha and low beta (~8–15 Hz); moderate whole-brain synchrony
Narrow-objective focus	Focused narrowly on one object to the exclusion of other stimuli in the total perceptual field; high stress state; preoccupied with work-related problem to the exclusion of emotional and physical responses	Sympathetic predominance; left brain predominance; high arousal (fight-flight response)	High frequencies: high beta and gamma (~15–40 Hz); reduced amplitude waves and reduced whole-brain synchrony

Source. Adapted from Table 1 in Fehmi LG, Shor SB: "Open Focus Attention Training." *Psychiatric Clinics of North America* 36(1):153–162, 2013.

space from awareness, narrowing and objectifying attention to one or a few objects. One can immerse attention into space and objects. Conversely, one can create distance from space and objects. In Open Focus, it is possible to attend to aspects of all these attentional modes simultaneously and equally.

Levels of Arousal

An individual whose arousal is chronically low may feel fatigued, lethargic, and depressed. Conversely, if arousal is chronically elevated, the individual may be hypervigilant, stressed, anxious, or angry. Arousal levels in the mid-range, associated with alpha synchrony, are often optimal for a variety of tasks. Conscious control of arousal through manipulation of awareness of space can enable transient shifts to different levels of arousal when necessary. Open Focus inclusion of sensory information in concert with awareness of space promotes awareness of how we are attending and cultivates capacities for decisions regarding the appropriate style to use in a given context.

Pain Theories and the Open Focus Approach

Pain Theories

René Descartes (2003) theorized a *pain pathway* whereby signals generated from the periphery of the body in response to injury travel along nerves to the brain, where they stimulate perceptual responses. This specificity model saw perceived pain as proportional to the tissue damage. In the eighteenth century, Franz Mesmer, using a technique later called hypnosis, claimed that altered mental states could influence perception of pain, regardless of the injury (Crabtree 1993). Hypnosis involves a shift in attention *away* from feelings of pain and toward other thoughts or images. Recent research confirms that hypnosis can ameliorate the subjective experience of pain (Del Casale et al. 2015). The gate-control theory of pain proposes that pain-conducting neurons open a neurological "gate" for propagation of pain-related impulses, and pain-inhibiting neurons close the gate, reducing pain perception (Melzack and Wall 1965). Emotions profoundly influence the balance of activation between these two pathways. In this departure from specificity theory, the mind can influence the experience of pain. Similarly, Fredrick Lenz theorized that pain is experienced through the influence of neuromodules, "programs" that bind together perceptual montages of moods, sensory data, and memory from separate regions of the brain (Lenz et al. 1995). These networks of neurons are unstable and can be triggered by factors other than pain impulses, such as moods, memories, and psychological distress. In this model, at the root of pain perception is a hypersensitive, unstable brain.

The Open Focus Model of Pain

In the Open Focus model, it is not emotions themselves that cause pain but rather resistance to fully experiencing emotions that destabilizes the mind and brain, causing malfunction of pain regulatory systems. When physical tissue damage is significant or functional dysregulation occurs at specific anatomical sites, pain signals are produced distally; however, the experience of pain is mediated by the central nervous system. Although any effective treatment targeting pain in the periphery should be administered, intervention at the level of the brain is often necessary. In many cases of chronic pain, the Open Focus model postulates a negative feedback loop involving pain signals generated at a specific somatic site, a maladaptive attentional pattern at the level of the mind-brain, with subsequent negative neural feedback to the bodily sites of injury, resulting in ongoing dysfunction (e.g., signals from the stressed brain may promote muscle tension, constriction of blood flow, or immune dysregulation). The attentional mode that contributes to the propagation of chronic pain is narrow-objective attention, employed so as to focus away from the painful perception. The attempt to keep pain distant from consciousness results in a state of hyperarousal, maintaining neural patterns conducive to chronic pain. A painful perception, feeling, or stimulus can be a seemingly limited physical sensation from residual physical damage, or it can be compounded by emotional overlay. "Physical" pain and "emotional" pain are approached similarly in Open Focus.

Of course, the meaningful contents of emotions are important for the clinician to explore. Psychotherapy can help identify emotional issues, work through them, and reduce distress, but it may not address dimensions of emotional pain experienced somatically. When Open Focus is used to address the bodily manifestations of emotional distress, the emphasis is on the way emotions are attended to. This shifts the way the patient pays attention to the body, to emotions, and to the surrounding world.

Rather than seeking to distract the patient from pain, Open Focus teaches the patient first to localize the pain, immerse attention directly into the pain, and then use diffuse attention to the body and space surrounding the pain. The conscious deployment of attentional modes, using a narrow-immersed focus on the pain that is then transitioned to a more encompassing diffuse-immersed focus, can resolve chronic pain syndromes.

Anecdotally, in our clinical experience, cultivating immersion in the feelings of pain while maintaining diffuse attention to the total perceptual field, including space, results in dissolution of the pain. The proposed Open Focus model partially explains how the subjective experience of pain can be so radically altered: attentional modes directed toward the experiencing of space that surrounds and permeates the "objects" of attention foster the production of synchronous alpha waves. The subjectively experienced separation of subject and object is partly mediated by asynchronous activity among different brain regions. When brain wave activity in the occipital cortex is out of phase with activity in the frontal cortex, this facilitates the perception of an "object" that is different from the "subject." In order to objectify something, the phase relationship between different parts of the brain must be out of sync so that the part mediating perception of the constructed object is in one phase while the constructed subject of experience is in another. During whole-brain phase synchrony, the neural "program" for separating subject and object is altered. By shifting to the diffuse-immersed attentional mode characterized by whole-brain alpha synchrony, the disparate mental worlds of the pain-experiencing subject and the "objective" pain are merged, resulting in dissolution of perceived pain as a separate entity (Fehmi and Shor 2013).

Open Focus Exercise: Experiencing Space While Reading

The following is an abbreviated combination of sequences used in clinical practice (adapted from "Expanding Your Awareness of Visual Space," in Fehmi and Robbins 2007). In shortening it, we risk not immersing the reader sufficiently in the method to allow for a noticeable shift in attentional mode. However, we offer it as a brief exposure to Open Focus training. Ideally, you would make an audio recording of the first part of the exercise, including 15-second breaks between each question, so that you can hear the instructions in your own voice and maintain an inward focus rather than having to read. Alternatively, you can open your eyes when necessary to read the questions, pausing at least 15 seconds between each question to allow time to realize the experience.

Expanding Your Awareness of Visual Space (Adapted)

- *Close your eyes* for the first portion of this exercise.
- Can you imagine feeling the space between your eyes?
- Can you imagine feeling the space inside your throat as you inhale and exhale naturally?
- Can you imagine feeling the space inside your abdomen as you breathe?
- Can you imagine feeling the volume of your upper legs, lower legs, feet, and toes and the feeling of space between your toes?
- Can you imagine feeling the volume of your thumbs?
- Can you imagine feeling the volume of your forefingers?
- Can you imagine feeling the space between your thumbs and your forefingers?
- Can you imagine feeling your whole hands and all your fingers, as well as the spaces between your fingers?
- Now *open your eyes* for the remainder of this exercise.
- As you continue to read this page, allow yourself to become aware of the three-dimensional physical space between your eyes and the words printed on the page. Allow this to occur gradually as you continue reading. Once you become aware of this space, pause for a few seconds as you gently maintain this awareness.
- Now, without shifting the direction of your gaze from the page, gradually begin to sense the space to the right and to the left of the page. Let this awareness of your peripheral field of vision widen spontaneously. Once you develop this expanded perceptual field, pause to experience it for a few moments.
- Up until now, these words have been your foreground, and everything visible in the periphery has been the background. Now let that back-

ground become equally as important as the foreground in your awareness. Allow the whole page, the boundaries of the book, and everything
in your peripheral vision to have equal attention. As this happens gradually, sit for some seconds in the awareness of this new, expanded visual field.

- As you continue reading, also begin to include in your awareness the
  appearance of space surrounding your entire body. Allow time for this
  to take place as your awareness opens and broadens.

- Now permit yourself to become aware of the space between the lines of
  this page, as you continue to read.

- Next, bring your awareness to the spaces between the words, then the
  spaces between the letters.

- You also may bring to your awareness other sensations of the absence
  we call space—feeling space, tasting and smelling space, hearing silence, and experiencing the space and silence in your mind from which
  visual images and internal dialogues emerge.

- As you continue to allow your awareness to expand and become more in-
  clusive, you may notice subtle changes in your reading experience. Perhaps your eyes feel less strained, or perhaps thoughts seemingly
  unrelated to what you are reading may float through your mind. Many
  kinds of changes are possible. Perhaps you also may experience the rising
  up of some unpleasant feelings that have been repressed by a previously
  sustained state of narrow focus. (These unpleasant feelings can be worked
  through with other Open Focus exercises not included in this chapter.)

Our goal in this exercise is to cultivate a lightly held narrow-objective attention to
reading, amid a diffuse-immersed attention to the background of empty space that
can be experienced through many senses. We suggest that you practice the exercise
again in the course of reading other chapters in this volume.

Clinical Case: Open Focus for Anxiety, Depression, and Pain Following Trauma

When physical trauma occurs, concomitant emotional trauma develops. The following case illustrates how Open Focus can be used to alleviate physical and emotional
pain following a serious trauma.

> Janie was already anxious and depressed when she had an accident: A truck snagged a
> power line and pulled down a telephone pole, crushing the top of her car. The truck
> driver fled, leaving her pinned in the car for more than an hour. Despite multiple sur-
> geries, she experienced chronic neck, back, and shoulder pain. Anxiety and depression
> worsened, and she developed lethargy, insomnia, nightmares, and chronic anger to-
> ward the truck driver. Psychotherapy and pharmacological treatment were ineffective,
> so her psychologist recommended Open Focus training.

Janie's anxiety was addressed first because it was exacerbating the depressive symptoms and physical pain. She was directed to feel the space in the room and to maintain attention to this throughout the initial exercises because the feeling of space can foster awareness of repressed emotions. She was then asked to scan her body for the most intense physical sensations of anxiety. By the sixth session, she became able to dissolve anxiety in the office and at home. Janie also used Open Focus to alleviate severe upper back, spine, and shoulder pain. After 10 sessions, she reported feeling happier and resumed doing chores at home. Although treatment focused mainly on anxiety and depression, much of her physical pain improved. Neurovegetative symptoms also diminished. (Adapted from Fehmi and Robbins 2010, p. 129)

Clinical Guidelines

Open Focus attention training has no strict inclusion or exclusion criteria. Commitment to learning the system, to attending a sufficient number of office sessions, and to practicing consistently at home has led to satisfactory outcomes. Patients with pain unresponsive to standard treatment tend to be highly motivated. Also, patients who wish to avoid prescription analgesics or opioids are good candidates. Military veterans or cancer patients may particularly benefit from the training.

Good clinical judgment should be used. A patient in full-blown mania, suicidal depression, or a psychotic episode should be stabilized psychiatrically before attempting Open Focus. Patients with severe personality disorders should first receive specific psychotherapy for their conditions, because they are unlikely to make good use of training until they attain greater object integration. In our clinical experience, a few patients with stable schizophrenia who pursued Open Focus training had improvements. Dissociation in posttraumatic stress disorder and related problems can be improved with attention training. Those with this type of mental illness may feel overwhelmed at first. The guided exercises can be modified so that these patients begin by working in areas of the body that feel comfortable to them until they feel safe enough to venture further. Open Focus can be a useful tool because it encourages merging with feelings and other sensory experiences. This movement toward union can ameliorate feelings of separation in dissociative disorders.

Open Focus training fosters a type of attention that aids the psychotherapist in becoming aware simultaneously of the patient's conscious and unconscious communications and of the therapist's own responses within the multilayered therapeutic encounter. Open Focus can be integrated into the psychotherapeutic session or administered by an outside trainer who collaborates with the psychotherapist. It also can be integrated with other treatment approaches by clinicians who are trained in the method. Adding the dimensions of working with attention to the body and to space can augment the benefits of psychotherapeutic treatment.

KEY POINTS

- Open Focus attention training is a therapeutic method that addresses pain and stress-related problems.

- Training involves guided imaginal exercises that systematically develop the subjective experience of *space*, both inside and outside the body.

- Open Focus training is facilitated through neurofeedback equipment; the goal is attainment of objectively measurable whole-brain alpha synchrony.

- The ultimate aim is to develop attentional flexibility: the ability to consciously choose and employ different attentional styles needed for specific tasks.

References

Benson H, Malhotra MS, Goldman RF, et al: Three case reports of the metabolic and electroencephalographic changes during advanced Buddhist meditation techniques. Behav Med 16(2):90–95, 1990 2194593

Crabtree A: From Mesmer to Freud. New Haven, CT, Yale University Press, 1993

Del Casale A, Ferracuti S, Rapinesi C, et al: Pain perception and hypnosis: findings from recent functional neuroimaging studies. Int J Clin Exp Hypn 63(2):144–170, 2015 25719519

Descartes R: Treatise of Man (1664). Amherst, NY, Prometheus Books, 2003

Fehmi LG: Multichannel EEG phase synchrony training and verbally guided attention training for disorders of attention, in Handbook of Neurofeedback. Edited by Evans JR. Binghamton, NY, Haworth, 2007, pp 301–320

Fehmi L, Robbins J: The Open-Focus Brain: Harnessing the Power of Attention to Heal Mind and Body. Boston, MA, Trumpeter Books, 2007

Fehmi L, Robbins J: Dissolving Pain: Simple Brain-Training Exercises for Overcoming Chronic Pain. Boston, MA, Trumpeter Books, 2010

Fehmi LG, Shor SB: Open focus attention training. Psychiatr Clin North Am 36(1):153–162, 2013 23538084

Fehmi LG, Adkins JW, Lindsley DB: Electrophysiological correlates of visual perceptual masking in monkeys. Exp Brain Res 7(4):299–316, 1969 4308046

Kasamatsu A, Hirai T: An electroencephalographic study on the Zen meditation (Zazen). Folia Psychiatr Neurol Jpn 20(4):315–336, 1966 6013341

Lenz FA, Gracely RH, Romanoski AJ, et al: Stimulation in the human somatosensory thalamus can reproduce both the affective and sensory dimensions of previously experienced pain. Nat Med 1(9):910–913, 1995 7585216

Melzack R, Wall PD: Pain mechanisms: a new theory. Science 150(3699):971–979, 1965 5320816

SECTION VI

Technologies

CHAPTER 26

Neurofeedback Therapy in Clinical Practice

David V. Nelson, Ph.D.

Mary Lee Esty, Ph.D.

Benjamin Barone, M.A.

Neurofeedback is applied neuroscience—it is a new frontier in helping innumerable people who up until now have been condemned to just make the best of feeling chronically fearful, unfocused and disengaged.

Bessel A. van der Kolk, M.D. (in Fisher 2014, p. xvii)

Neurofeedback, also known as electroencephalogram (EEG) biofeedback or neurotherapy, is a brain wave–based emerging technology used to treat neurodevelopmental disorders, anxiety and mood disorders, addictions, posttraumatic stress disorder (PTSD), traumatic brain injury (TBI), and chronic pain. In addition, neurofeedback has applications for enhancing sports participation and peak performance. In this chapter, we provide historical and technical background, summarize key neurofeedback models, distill salient research findings, highlight selected evidence-based clinical applications, and offer a perspective on future directions. All of the techniques discussed invoke the notion of neuroplasticity, with the goal of improved self-regulation and cognitive function.

A Brief History

The first description of the human EEG by Hans Berger in the early twentieth century was followed by investigations confirming that classical Pavlovian conditioning could be applied to the EEG in regard to the alpha brain wave band–blocking response. Patients could learn voluntary control over this response (Knott and Henry 1941). Kamiya (1968) applied learning theory to demonstrate voluntary control via operant conditioning (reward or reinforcement) of the alpha frequency range, 8–12 Hz (Skinner 1953), and the ability of patients to voluntarily control the contingent negative variation or slow cortical potential was confirmed (McAdam et al. 1966). Sterman, applying operant conditioning of the EEG sensorimotor rhythm (12–15 Hz) to alter sleep spindle density and sleep quality, serendipitously discovered an anticonvulsant effect (Sterman et al. 1970; Wyrwicka and Sterman 1968). Sterman's largely unrecognized work eventually led to studies confirming the effectiveness of EEG biofeedback for treating seizure disorders and the recent surge of research interest.

Models of Neurofeedback

Traditional Frequency Band Training

Neurofeedback therapy is brain wave–based biofeedback that uses the EEG as the signal to control the feedback. The electrical activity of the brain is recorded via non-invasive sensors (electrodes) attached to the scalp as active, reference, and ground sites. This makes it possible for other sources of ambient stray signals to be separated from the EEG signal. The electrical potentials are digitized and further processed to reflect various characteristics (e.g., frequency, amplitude) that may be used to produce and present feedback information regarding brain activity to patients via auditory, visual, tactile, or other modalities. The objective is to change patterns of brain wave functioning, presumably through learning processes that influence brain activity associated with subjective states and observable symptoms or behaviors. In the earliest days of neurofeedback, this feedback was as simple as a single tone or flashing light that indicated change had occurred. More modern applications use tones, music, movies, other visual displays, and even video games to train people in more engaging and sophisticated ways. Targeted changes in the various displays correspond to targeted changes in aspects of the EEG. The goal is for the brain to learn more adaptive ways of responding.

Early neurofeedback interventions relied on single-channel or single active site recordings and focused primarily on changes in amplitudes of various frequencies. This is accomplished by setting thresholds for reinforcements, either for achieving a certain amplitude level or for remaining below a certain amplitude level. In this manner, increased production of the desired brain wave activity may be "rewarded" at a certain rate to increase further production. Alternatively, specified brain wave frequencies may be "inhibited" by withholding reward if the threshold is exceeded or providing reward when activity goes below threshold. Combinations of reward and inhibit thresholds may be used. The reward/inhibit paradigm remains in widespread use.

Connectivity-Based Developments

The development of multiple-channel site recordings paved the way for brain region connectivity feedback measures. These measures incorporate aspects such as the amount of information shared between sites at a given time (coherence), speed of information transfer at a given time (phase), similarities in amplitudes across times (comodulation), and extent to which phase and amplitude match (synchrony). These aspects are neither inherently desirable nor undesirable; their utility depends on the nature of the brain activity and the desired goals for brain functioning (Collura 2014).

Quantitative Electroencephalography

The complexity and flexibility of neurofeedback have been enhanced by the quantitative EEG (qEEG), in which multiple simultaneous site recordings are made (using the entire standard international 10–20 system or more sites) and processed into highly diverse metrics for use in the feedback process. A qEEG typically generates a colored brain map of relative EEG activity; a normative database is used to compare how the patient's EEG varies from what is expected for a well-functioning brain. The practitioner uses this database to choose a protocol for training, which may be modified over time depending on subjective report and objective data obtained.

Various training paradigms using qEEG information have been devised; some rely on the static image and associated frequency and amplitude information of the EEG, and others are more interactive in real time, such as live z-score training (grounded in normative databases) of any number of EEG metrics in the feedback mechanism. This approach capitalizes on the inherent variability in EEG metrics, as represented in the standard deviation, with presumed greater flexibility for changing the particular patient's EEG metrics in the desired direction (Collura 2014). Another paradigm of particular interest is low-resolution electromagnetic tomographic analysis (LORETA; Pascual-Marqui et al. 2002). Using sophisticated mathematical operations, LORETA analyzes scalp recordings from a full-head EEG; transforms these into three-dimensional voxels, which combine into regions of interest; enables visualization of brain activity images over time that cannot be appreciated in static images; and allows more specific neurofeedback targeting of these regions of interest compared with single specific scalp sites. Advances in technology and software have made this approach more accessible to practitioners.

Slow Cortical Potentials

Further developments influencing neurofeedback approaches involve slow cortical potentials. Traditional frequency-band training techniques focus largely on distinctions among the various frequency wave bands: delta, 0.5–4 cycles/oscillations/second or Hz; theta, 4–8 Hz; alpha, 8–12 Hz; sensorimotor rhythm, sometimes also referred to as low beta, 12–15 Hz; beta, 15–20 Hz; high beta, 20–30 Hz; and gamma, 35–45 Hz. The slow cortical potentials are generally within the 0.01- to 2-Hz range. They typically do not demonstrate the kind of rhythmic oscillation seen in the more standard wave bands. Accordingly, they are not as amenable to training with standard reward and inhibit protocols.

Very slow activity involving a negative shift in the EEG in anticipation of an expected event, known as *contingent negative variation*, was first reported (Walter et al. 1964) and shown to be potentially under voluntary control (McAdam et al. 1966) in the 1960s. Variations in the slow cortical potential signal occur with activation or deactivation, thereby permitting training in a given direction. In the 1990s, clinical investigations identified the potential for treating a variety of challenging conditions, such as paralyzed or "locked-in" syndromes. This approach enabled patients with amyotrophic lateral sclerosis to express themselves with an electronic spelling device. Subsequently, benefits were shown in attention-deficit/hyperactivity disorder (ADHD), epilepsy, and migraine (Birbaumer 1999; Strehl 2009).

Infralow-Frequency Training

Infralow-frequency (ILF) training is related to slow cortical potential training in that very slow frequency (below 0.1 Hz) monitoring is involved. At this level, amplitude training and setting thresholds within an operant conditioning (reward or reinforcement) paradigm are not possible. Information about higher frequencies is typically removed from the feedback, and only subtle shifts or fluctuations over time, not rhythmic oscillations per se, in the ultralow range are presented. With such feedback, once the connection between the external signal and the internal signal is established, "the brain takes responsibility for the signal and tries to steer it. This is a natural process, like the brain taking charge of the…steering wheel of the car even while the driver's thoughts are directed elsewhere" (Othmer 2015).

Training entails recording from two channel sites, which are associated with electrode placements corresponding to presumed nodes of resting state networks—specifically, the default mode network, dorsal attention network, and central executive network. By targeting the nodes of these networks, it is conjectured that ILF training reorganizes brain network connectivity (Othmer et al. 2013). Treatment is highly individualized and less able to be captured in standard protocols. Consequently, the overall conceptualization and rapid positive responses reported, even with quite severe psychopathology, are not without controversy (Collura 2014). ILF training also has been advocated to address pediatric problems such as autism spectrum disorder, early childhood emotional and physical trauma, migraine, sleep disturbances, feeding and eating disorders, and drug dependencies before dysfunctional network connectivity has crystallized into more difficult and refractory conditions (Othmer et al. 2013).

Real-Time Functional Magnetic Resonance Imaging

Soon after the inception of functional magnetic resonance imaging (fMRI), it became apparent that the technology lent itself to applications involving real-time information about changes in blood oxygen level–dependent (BOLD) signal (Weiskopf 2012). Confidence in the BOLD response as an indirect measure of brain activity, the potential for enhanced spatial resolution of specific regions of interest, and the strong association of the BOLD signal with brain electrical signals gave impetus for studying real-time fMRI responses with conditioning principles to change brain activation patterns. This provides another avenue for influencing the connectivity of brain networks (Ruiz et al. 2014). One major drawback is the expense associated with imaging equipment. ILF training has been offered as a more economical alternative, given that fluctuations posited in ILF training also correspond to activation of core networks.

Standard Protocols

Collura (2014) described standard protocols that have been modified over three decades of clinical practice. Table 26–1 presents an example of the key components of protocols derived from Collura's work and their clinical applications. Numerous other systems and protocols have been developed and are being used effectively (see Chapter 3, "Complementary and Integrative Medicine in Child and Adolescent Psychiatric Disorders").

It is important to remember that standard protocols can have modifications with combinations of multiple inhibits, multiple thresholds, overlapping bands, or other features. Variations also occur with multiple channels and even multiple persons involved in the same training protocol. Furthermore, a myriad of applications use neurofeedback for optimal or peak performance, such as for the enhancement of athletic or musical performances, sharpened clarity and concentration in business decisions, and other aspects of emotional control and stability under pressure. These protocols commonly use elements of sensorimotor rhythm, alpha, and/or Squash protocol training with other procedures. The potential for so many applications is accelerating neurofeedback research.

Evidence Base and Clinical Applications

In order to understand the breadth of neurofeedback applications, it is important to keep in mind that the EEG is an epiphenomenon of neurochemical brain activity that correlates with (but does not necessarily cause) regulation and dysregulation of brain function. Consistent with the conceptualization in the proposed National Institute of Mental Health Research Domain Criteria for mental disorders, certain neurophysiological (and other, such as psychosocial) domains may cut across (and interact reciprocally with) current diagnostic categories and the broad range of human experience (Lilienfeld 2014). The fundamental principles of neuroplasticity support the potential for change in brain function. Increasingly sophisticated conceptualizations of the interrelations and mutual integration of brain regulatory networks (e.g., default mode, dorsal attention, central executive) are incorporated into the current zeitgeist for understanding the complexity of brain function (Othmer et al. 2013). The EEG provides a method to view this activity. Shaping the EEG into alternative patterns may be a vehicle through which change can occur. In the following subsections, we review evidence on neurofeedback for selected clinical conditions, some of which have been studied far more than others.

TABLE 26–1.   Standard neurofeedback protocols and clinical applications

Protocol	Description	Clinical conditions and benefits	Risks
Alert	Specific activation paradigm: increasing beta is rewarded; theta and high beta are inhibited. Designed for beta deficits. Recorded from international 10–20 system left hemisphere C3 or central vertex Cz sites.	Counter hypoarousal states (e.g., sometimes seen in ADHD); reduced fatigue; improved mood, information-processing speed, and clarity.	Overactivation; may need to be countered by focus procedures.
Focus	Relaxed, but focused, internal sense; SMR is rewarded. Trained primarily at right hemisphere C4 or Cz sites.	Motoric and mental calming with focused attention; ADHD; anxiety disorders.	Excessive underactivation; may be countered with brief beta training.
Peak	Two-channel setup combining aspects of alert (left hemisphere C3 or Cz) and focus (right hemisphere C4 or Cz) protocols.	Optimal/peak performance (e.g., sports, music, business, or other decision making; enhanced emotional control; and stability under pressure).	Imbalance of overactivation and underactivation; may require relative titration.
Squash	"Family of designs" to reduce amplitude. Down-training via reward when specified band amplitude is below set value. "Bench press" workout analogy: repetitive process of modest effort exerted to make signal go down, which is rewarded, then followed by brief relaxation. Variable sensor placements depending on desired effect.	Optimal mental fitness/sharpness and improved mood.	Working too hard to achieve desired effect may backfire and require reorientation to enhance sense of flow with attentiveness or sense of release and letting go.
Relax	Specific alpha training with theta and high beta inhibition. Posterior sensor placements often preferred.	Lower hyperarousal; relaxation; improved mood; reduced headaches, insomnia, anxiety, and depression.	Adverse mood reactions (more common with frontal placements).

TABLE 26–1. Standard neurofeedback protocols and clinical applications *(continued)*

Protocol	Description	Clinical conditions and benefits	Risks
Deep	Specific kind of alpha/theta training. Alpha initially rewarded with transition to increased theta reward. Augmented with therapeutic suggestions, imagery, or visualization. "Crossover" eventually occurs with transition from alpha-dominant to theta-dominant; concomitant hypnagogic state facilitates "deep" processing of issues or other personal exploration. Strong therapeutic abreactions can occur. Posterior sensor placements are typical.	Relief from posttraumatic stress responses; reduction of substance abuse; personal exploration.	Abreactions require careful therapeutic monitoring.

Note. Protocols derived from work by Collura (2014). Many other neurofeedback protocols are effective. ADHD=attention-deficit/hyperactivity disorder; SMR=sensorimotor rhythm.

Attention-Deficit/Hyperactivity Disorder

ADHD has been the condition for which the greatest amount of investigation in regard to neurofeedback has been conducted. Monastra et al. (2005) presented the first review of case and controlled group studies examining the effects of EEG biofeedback on ADHD symptom dimensions and related measures. They determined EEG biofeedback to be "probably efficacious" on the basis of guidelines jointly established by the Association for Applied Psychophysiology and Biofeedback (AAPB) and the Society for Neuronal Regulation (now the International Society for Neurofeedback and Research [ISNR]) and in effect at the time. Subsequently, Arns et al. (2009) provided meta-analytic data (10 prospective controlled studies, total $N=476$; 5 studies with pretest and posttest designs, $N=718$) that showed large effect sizes for neurofeedback on impulsivity and inattention and a medium effect size for hyperactivity. When Arns and colleagues used AAPB and ISNR guidelines for rating treatment efficacy, they considered neurofeedback for ADHD to be "efficacious and specific."

Sonuga-Barke et al. (2013), in their review of eight randomized controlled trials (RCTs; total $N=273$), used criteria some believe to be more stringent and considered the findings to be less conclusive, despite evidence for some reductions in core ADHD symptoms. They made the case for more methodologically sound studies before assigning the highest level of evidence as a first-line treatment for ADHD. A recent meta-analytic update (Micoulaud-Franchi et al. 2014) in which very stringent criteria were applied, including five randomized semiactive or sham-control neurofeedback studies (total $N=263$), found the strength of effects likely to be dependent on the nature of the outcome rater (e.g., blinded or unblinded). They highlighted particularly notable improvements in the inattentive dimension of ADHD symptoms. Taken together, a consensus emerges that neurofeedback is efficacious to different degrees for dysregulation associated with ADHD, that neurofeedback fits well within an integrative model of treatment for ADHD, and that neurofeedback may enhance response to other concurrent interventions. The conclusion that for ADHD, neurofeedback is probably efficacious and appropriate for integration into more comprehensive treatment has been echoed by other reviews (Gevensleben et al. 2012; Holtmann et al. 2014; Hurt et al. 2014; Lofthouse et al. 2012; Moriyama et al. 2012).

Substance Use Disorders

Substance use disorders (SUDs) are remarkably difficult to treat. Various substances of abuse affect the EEG and evoked response potentials differently. EEG alterations are further influenced by the extensive comorbidity (e.g., ADHD, depression, anxiety, neurotoxicity, posttraumatic stress, TBI) associated with SUDs. Within the neurofeedback literature on SUDs, one particular protocol (and a specific modification of it) has garnered a notable degree of qualified support. This approach includes a key element of alpha/theta ("deep") training that was originally reported by Green et al. (1974). It was further developed and popularized by Peniston in a series of reports on incorporating alpha/theta training into more comprehensive treatment packages (Peniston and Kulkosky 1989, 1990).

The basic "Peniston protocol" involves a preconditioning relaxation process comprising at least five initial sessions of thermal (autonomic) biofeedback training augmented with autogenic phrases and abdominal breathing to induce relaxation and quieting of the mind, and an induction script is read at the beginning of each session. After patients are able to consistently sustain hand warming to at least 94 degrees, they are instructed in the EEG biofeedback aspects of the intervention. EEG activity is recorded from occipital sites (typically O1), and with the patient's eyes closed, the therapist gives suggestions for relaxation and sometimes instructions to construct visualizations of specific personally relevant scenes and ultimately to "sink down" into a (theta) state of reverie as the mind is kept quiet and alert and the body calm. A quiet command, "Do it," initiates the process. As threshold criteria are met for alpha production, a tone sounds, and the patient becomes progressively more relaxed as he or she produces more of this brain wave activity. When threshold criteria for the theta amplitude are met, another tone sounds as the patient becomes more relaxed and enters a hypnagogic state of more freely accessible memories and reverie. The transition in reduction of alpha to greater preponderance of theta may signify "crossover" reactions, including strong therapeutic abreactions. Subsequently, in the relaxed and suggestible (or abreactive) state, the experience is discussed with the therapist. This can be even more beneficial when the clinical picture includes comorbid posttraumatic stress features.

Although several studies have supported the efficacy of this integrated approach with specific alpha/theta training, individuals addicted to certain substances, particularly the stimulants (e.g., methamphetamine, cocaine), may have neurophysiological effects that preclude effective use of the prototypical Peniston protocol. This may be exacerbated if comorbid ADHD features are present. Accordingly, Scott and Kaiser (1998) proposed a modification of the Peniston protocol with an initial course of attentional training—beta or sensorimotor rhythm augmentation with theta suppression—before proceeding to alpha/theta training. Their own research and subsequent research by others (Burkett et al. 2005) with homeless crack cocaine users have supported the utility of this modification.

Given the complex comorbidity associated with SUDs, the role of qEEG in guiding more specifically targeted neurofeedback modifications also has been suggested (Sokhadze et al. 2008). Alpha/theta training is likely to be most effective when integrated into more comprehensive treatment programs that could include motivational interviewing, cognitive-behavioral therapy, medication management, and diet modifications. The most thorough review to date of published clinical studies evaluated with the efficacy criteria of the AAPB and ISNR concluded that "alpha theta training—either alone for alcoholism or in combination with beta training for stimulant and mixed substance abuse and combined with residential treatment programs, is probably efficacious" (Sokhadze et al. 2008, p. 1). Slow cortical potential neurofeedback also has been reported to be potentially as efficacious as alpha/theta training in individuals with alcoholism (Schneider et al. 1993). Simple reliance on a routine protocol is ill advised. As in all fields of medicine, clinical judgment is critical at each step along the treatment trajectory, and alterations in approach may be required to optimize outcomes.

Posttraumatic Stress Disorder

The literature on neurofeedback treatment of posttraumatic stress has unfolded in tandem with that for SUDs. The pioneering work of Peniston with alpha/theta training for addictions was conducted with Vietnam War veterans who often presented with comorbid alcoholism and PTSD. The procedures adopted for these cases mirrored those described earlier for SUDs (Peniston et al. 1993). The crossover effect, associated reverie, and frequent abreactions experienced by veterans undergoing this neurofeedback training suggested that this kind of "deep" protocol could be potentially advantageous. It is important to keep in mind that the reexperiencing of posttraumatic memories and the associated intense affective-emotional responses and processing with the therapist are reminiscent of other evidence-based therapies such as cognitive processing therapies for PTSD. Accordingly, alpha/theta training may have a role as an adjunctive, if not always first-line, treatment. Additional comorbidities may complicate the picture and require clinical judgment regarding further modifications.

Traumatic Brain Injury

The diverse sequelae of TBI, including attentional and memory difficulties, executive control dysfunctions, headaches, fatigue, sleep disturbances, and emotional overreactivity, suggest the need for specifically targeted neurophysiological interventions. Various EEG-based approaches have been explored (Thornton and Carmody 2008), including a standard qEEG approach that incorporates aspects of protocols that have been used with ADHD and involve increasing beta and decreasing theta along the sensorimotor strip (central active sites of C3, Cz, and C4). Customized procedures also can be used to compare the patient's resting eyes-closed qEEG with a reference database. An activation database–guided qEEG biofeedback approach also may be used while patients actively engage in specific cognitive tasks. With an empirically derived normative database from individuals with no known history of TBI, a variety of metrics can be used, often including a combination of variables relevant to a specific cognitive task, and thereby can address the many bothersome symptoms within a broader rehabilitation program. For example, the most substantiated benefits were observed in tasks involving auditory memory. A review (May et al. 2013) of a broader range of neurofeedback approaches contained in 14 case reports (single or series) and 8 well-designed prospective cohort investigations found consistent evidence for statistically and clinically significant subjective and objective improvements, especially in attention, impulse control, executive functioning, processing speed, and general cognition. Hence, neurofeedback is a "promising treatment" that "warrants further investigation" as an adjunctive treatment for TBI (May et al. 2013, pp. 289, 295).

Chronic Pain

Several studies have used neurofeedback for chronic pain syndromes; for example, Blanchard et al. (1997) found biofeedback to suppress EEG alpha activity to be as effective for significantly reducing headaches as temperature (hand-warming) biofeedback. Open-label studies in children and adults for treatment of migraine have been encouraging (Siniatchkin et al. 2000; Walker 2011).

In an RCT of patients with fibromyalgia syndrome, Kayiran et al. (2010) found significant improvements in pain, psychological symptoms, and quality of life among the group receiving neurofeedback. Caro and Winter (2011) reported that among patients with fibromyalgia, those receiving neurofeedback showed improvements in visual attention parameters, tenderness, pain, and fatigue. Given that reviews have found inconsistent results, research is needed to identify the most beneficial neurofeedback protocols for treating fibromyalgia (Glombiewski et al. 2013; Lauche et al. 2015).

Neurofeedback also has been explored for treatment of spinal cord injury–related and other neuropathic pain. Hassan et al. (2015) found immediate and longer-term reduction of central neuropathic pain corresponding to measurable short- and long-term modulation of cortical activity in a small case series of patients with paraplegia with central neuropathic pain. Jensen et al. (2013) have taken a systematic approach toward developing potential EEG biofeedback treatments for chronic pain. They used different neurofeedback protocols in a small series of individuals with spinal cord injury pain and found similar reductions in pain intensity that continued at 3-month follow-up. Further investigations of the efficacy and mechanisms of noninvasive neuromodulatory treatments suggest that neurofeedback can reduce the severity of chronic pain to a moderate extent but with uncertain durability and potential variability across heterogeneous pain conditions (Jensen et al. 2013). However, Jensen et al. (2013) suggested that neurofeedback may act synergistically by priming the central nervous system to be more responsive to other neuromodulatory or psychosocial treatments.

Further developments may be enhanced by capitalizing on evidence that neuropathic and musculoskeletal pain are associated with substantial reorganization of various brain regions, that this reorganization increases with chronicity, and that it is associated with the magnitude of pain experienced (Moseley and Flor 2012). Accordingly, cortical plasticity may be targeted for neurotherapeutic approaches. This may be even more effective when applied in new paradigms based on real-time fMRI, which allows for more fine-grained effect on functional connectivity and spatiotemporal patterns of brain activity (Ruiz et al. 2014). Initial investigations have been promising but are not economically feasible at present in most clinical settings (Chapin et al. 2012). Alternative, less expensive methods of brain imaging, such as near-infrared spectroscopy, could facilitate translation of these principles into practice (Chapin et al. 2012). Moreover, real-time fMRI and other brain imaging techniques are applicable to neuropsychiatric disorders and symptoms other than pain (Weiskopf 2012).

Neurofeedback Treatments in Other Disorders or Conditions

Reviews of other clinical conditions suggest potential benefits with neurofeedback, but these are often amalgams of single case studies, case series, or comparison groups. Overall, the findings provide encouragement to adapt neurofeedback interventions to anxiety disorders, obsessive-compulsive phenomena, depressive disorders, learning disabilities, autism spectrum disorder, epilepsy or seizure disorders, and others (Hurt et al. 2014; Simkin et al. 2014; Tan et al. 2009). Therapeutic benefits for some of the most challenging and severe presentations (e.g., bipolar disorder, nightmares, night terrors, sleepwalking, restless legs syndrome, pain medication dependency) are being reported for newly emerging ILF training, which, unfortunately, does not lend itself readily to investigation with standardized clinical trial protocols (Othmer et al. 2013).

Voluntary Versus Involuntary or Passive Control

In addition to neurofeedback techniques in which the patient exerts volitional control while learning to change the EEG patterns, other approaches involve the patient remaining relatively passive while the EEG signal controls the feedback, such that the therapeutic effects occur without volitional effort. For example, studies of audio and visual (e.g., photic) stimulation of the EEG date back as far as the more operant-based learning procedures discussed earlier (Collura 2014). Involuntary or passive approaches use the properties of the EEG to determine the nature of the feedback signal on a continuously interactive basis as the EEG is sampled; essentially, then, these are EEG-driven procedures that incite changes to aid in altering dysfunctions reflected in the EEG. Our own work (D.V.N. and M.L.E.) includes EEG-driven (photic and minutely pulsed, subliminal electromagnetic) stimulation to treat fibromyalgia symptoms, mixed TBI and PTSD, headaches, and attentional problems (Mueller et al. 2001; Nelson and Esty 2011, 2012, 2015a, 2015b; Nelson et al. 2010; Schoenberger et al. 2001). Our impression is that these procedures sometimes work well as stand-alone interventions but may work even better when integrated into a more comprehensive treatment package. They also may work in conjunction with techniques that involve voluntary control. Moreover, consistent with some of the findings for operant-based procedures noted previously, these more passive or involuntary techniques prime the nervous system to be more responsive to other interventions, including those to which patients' symptoms were previously refractory, such as psychotherapy, cognitive-behavioral therapy, and cognitive rehabilitation. Also, our impression is that these techniques fit well within the concept of neurofeedback affecting connectivity of brain networks. Only more rigorous controlled clinical trials involving sequencing of multiple interventions will more definitively determine their relative utility and the validity of effects produced by underlying mechanisms.

Clinical Case: Neurofeedback for Traumatic Brain Injury, Posttraumatic Stress Disorder, and Substance Abuse in an Afghanistan/Iraq War Veteran

David served 6 years in the army, with three deployments in combat zones in Afghanistan and a fourth in Iraq. Three concussions plus numerous blasts caused TBI, with frequent severe headaches and hypersensitivity to light and noise. Multiple shrapnel wounds and other injuries caused chronic pain. David developed PTSD with insomnia, flashbacks to scenes of his buddies bleeding to death, hypervigilance, and intense anxiety, which made it impossible for him to be in crowds, on busy streets, or on public transportation. Heavy drinking and prescription drug abuse contributed to explosive behavior and four assault charges. During a panic attack on the firing range, David could not pull the trigger. This led to admission to a medical center. After a suicide attempt there, he transferred to the inpatient psychiatric ward at a tertiary care center, where his diagnoses included mild TBI; adjustment disorder with mixed anxiety and depressed mood; PTSD; major depressive disorder, recurrent, with psychotic features; bipolar disorder, manic, with psychotic features; borderline personality disorder; alcohol use disorder, in remission; and prescription drug abuse. He had no history of mental illness prior to the second deployment. David was placed in an intensive substance abuse track and was given PTSD treatments. Medications generally made him feel worse. Trials of paroxetine, venlafaxine, trazodone, lorazepam, diphenhydramine, zolpidem, and quetiapine were ineffective. David was maintained on nortriptyline and hydroxyzine, even though he experienced only minimal benefit.

David recalled, "All traditional treatments failed. To call my prognosis unhopeful was an understatement. I was aggressive, paranoid, angry, depressed, and nihilistic, unable to focus enough to take part in conversations, unable to read more than a few sentences. Sleep was an hour or two in 48 hours. I left my room only when forced to for appointments, or (rarely) for food. Drug abuse and violent behavior continued, and I was still suicidal."

David was referred for neurofeedback. A modification of the Flexyx Neurotherapy System (FNS; Flexyx LLC, Walnut Creek, California) was used. FNS involves monitoring the EEG with a two-channel module that has on-board feedback-generating power; it uses proprietary software to link the digital brain wave recording module through the computer, which then sets the parameters for the module to emit pulsed electromagnetic stimulation. The system returns a signal to the participant via conduction from the module, varying as a function of the detectable peak EEG frequency (but offset from it), thereby permitting strategic distortion of the EEG. The amount of electromagnetic stimulation was standardized, with the feedback frequency being offset from the dominant EEG frequency at +20 Hz. Pulses of electromagnetic energy operated at a duty cycle of 1% of the maximum permissible on-time for each pulse; they were powered no more than 1% of the time (e.g., the maximum on-time for 1% for 1-Hz pulse was 0.01 seconds). Testing indicated a power level of 100 pW through the sensor cable.

David attended approximately two or three neurofeedback sessions per week. He sat comfortably, eyes closed, engaged in no specific activity. Electrodes were placed over all areas of the cortex over the course of 25 half-hour sessions. Each session included a total of 4-second stimulation spaced over 4 minutes. Stimulation was not immediately discernible. No adverse reactions occurred. David was not asked to discuss past traumas as part of the procedure. After six sessions, his headaches, anxiety, and explosive behaviors subsided. Hydroxyzine was discontinued. Ongoing treatment led to substantial improvements in insomnia, nightmares, anger, suicidal thoughts, fatigue, hypersensitivities, flashbacks, and abuse of cigarettes, alcohol, and drugs. After 25 neurofeedback treatments, David said, "Now I remember so much. I'm not numb. I have a life. Now I can just brush things off. I'm not angry anymore. It still hurts, but not the searing pain and anger. It feels good to talk." Before neurofeedback, he had no idea what he wanted to do after discharge. After neurofeedback, he wrote, "I want to help other veterans who find themselves in situations similar to mine." David enrolled in college, graduated with honors, and is now in a doctoral program.

How to Find a Qualified Neurofeedback Therapist

Neurofeedback is not the province of any one discipline. Sophisticated practice of qEEG requires some specialist training. The practice of neurofeedback requires understanding of brain function and the autonomic nervous system and specific training in neurofeedback techniques. Basic understanding and training can be obtained by physicians, psychiatrists, psychologists, nurses, social workers, and other counselors or therapists who practice within the scope of their education and licensure. Neurofeedback may be the primary focus of a clinician's practice or an adjunct to it. Various certifications are available through professional organizations that provide information about training, literature, practitioner support, and professional meetings. Clinicians wishing to find local practitioners may consult organizations devoted to neurofeedback: the AAPB (www.aapb.org), the Biofeedback Certification International Alliance (http://bcia.org), and ISNR (www.isnr.org).

Summary and Conclusion

Dysfunction in attentional, affective, and executive control networks, and their integration, is reflected in the EEG. Such dysfunctions may be amenable to differentially targeted neurofeedback interventions that give the brain the opportunity to establish or reestablish more optimal levels of functioning. The potential of neurofeedback as a stand-alone or adjunctive treatment will develop through clinical trials, refinement of protocols, and other research.

KEY POINTS

- Neurofeedback therapy is brain wave–based biofeedback that enables patients to alter their own electroencephalogram (EEG) signal on the basis of real-time feedback.

- Feedback about brain wave activity is typically provided via one or more sensory modalities and is based on operant and classical conditioning learning theories.

- The EEG signal can be used to set parameters for electromagnetic and other sources of stimulation to alter brain wave functioning while patients remain relatively passive.

- The current evidence base suggests broad transdiagnostic applicability of existing and emerging neurofeedback treatment paradigms and protocols.

References

Arns M, de Ridder S, Strehl U, et al: Efficacy of neurofeedback treatment in ADHD: the effects on inattention, impulsivity and hyperactivity: a meta-analysis. Clin EEG Neurosci 40(3)180–189, 2009 19715181
Birbaumer N: Slow cortical potentials: plasticity, operant control, and behavior effects. Neuroscientist 5(2):74–78, 1999

Blanchard EB, Peters ML, Hermann C, et al: Direction of temperature control in the thermal bio-feedback treatment of vascular headache. Appl Psychophysiol Biofeedback 22(4):227–245, 1997 9595177

Burkett SV, Cummins JM, Dickson R, et al: An open clinical trial utilizing real-time EEG oper-ant conditioning as an adjunctive therapy in the treatment of crack cocaine dependence. J Neurother 9(2):27–47, 2005

Caro XJ, Winter EF: EEG biofeedback treatment improves certain attention and somatic symp-toms in fibromyalgia: a pilot study. Appl Psychophysiol Biofeedback 36(3):193–200, 2011 21656150

Chapin H, Bagarinao E, Mackey S: Real-time fMRI applied to pain management. Neurosci Lett 520(2):174–181, 2012 22414861

Collura TF: Technical Foundations of Neurofeedback. New York, Routledge, 2014

Fisher SF: Neurofeedback in the Treatment of Developmental Trauma: Calming the Fear-Driven Brain. New York, WW Norton, 2014

Gevensleben H, Rothenberger A, Moll GH, et al: Neurofeedback in children with ADHD: val-idation and challenges. Expert Rev Neurother 12(4):447–460, 2012 22449216

Glombiewski JA, Bernardy K, Häuser W: Efficacy of EMG- and EEG-biofeedback in fibromyal-gia syndrome: a meta-analysis and a systematic review of randomized controlled trials. Evid Based Complement Alternat Med 2013:962741, 2013 24082911

Green EE, Green AM, Walters ED: Alpha-theta biofeedback training. Journal of Biofeedback 2:7–13, 1974

Hassan MA, Fraser M, Conway BA, et al: The mechanism of neurofeedback training for treatment of central neuropathic pain in paraplegia: a pilot study. BMC Neurol 15:200, 2015 26462651

Holtmann M, Sonuga-Barke E, Cortese S, et al: Neurofeedback for ADHD: a review of current evidence. Child Adolesc Psychiatr Clin N Am 23(4):789–806, 2014 25220087

Hurt E, Arnold LE, Lofthouse N: Quantitative EEG neurofeedback for the treatment of pediat-ric attention-deficit/hyperactivity disorder, autism spectrum disorders, learning disor-ders, and epilepsy. Child Adolesc Psychiatr Clin N Am 23(3):465–486, 2014 24975622

Jensen MP, Gertz KJ, Kupper AE, et al: Steps toward developing an EEG biofeedback treatment for chronic pain. Appl Psychophysiol Biofeedback 38(2):101–108, 2013 23532434

Kamiya I: Conscious control of brain waves. Psychol Today 1:56–60, 1968

Kayiran S, Dursun E, Dursun N, et al: Neurofeedback intervention in fibromyalgia syndrome; a randomized, controlled, rater blind clinical trial. Appl Psychophysiol Biofeedback 35(4):293–302, 2010 20614235

Knott JR, Henry CE: The conditioning of the blocking of the alpha rhythm of the human en-cephalogram. J Exp Psychol 28(2):134–144, 1941

Lauche R, Cramer H, Häuser W, et al: A systematic overview of reviews for complementary and alternative therapies in the treatment of the fibromyalgia syndrome. Evid Based Com-plement Alternat Med 2015:610615, 2015 26246841

Lillienfeld SO: The Research Domain Criteria (RDoC): an analysis of methodological and con-ceptual challenges. Behav Res Ther 62:129–139, 2014 25156396

Lofthouse N, Arnold LE, Hersch S, et al: A review of neurofeedback treatment for pediatric ADHD. J Atten Disord 16(5):351–372, 2012 22090396

May G, Benson R, Balon R, et al: Neurofeedback and traumatic brain injury: a literature review. Ann Clin Psychiatry 25(4):289–296, 2013 24199220

McAdam DW, Irwin DA, Rebert CS, et al: Conative control of the contingent negative varia-tion. Electroencephalogr Clin Neurophysiol 21(2):194–195, 1966 4162012

Micoulaud-Franchi J-A, Geoffroy PA, Fond G, et al: EEG neurofeedback treatments in children with ADHD: an updated meta-analysis of randomized controlled trials. Front Hum Neu-rosci 8:906, 2014 25431555

Monastra VJ, Lynn S, Linden M, et al: Electroencephalographic biofeedback in the treatment of attention-deficit/hyperactivity disorder. Appl Psychophysiol Biofeedback 30(2):95–114, 2005 16013783

Moriyama TS, Polanczyk G, Caye A, et al: Evidence-based information on the clinical use of neurofeedback for ADHD. Neurotherapeutics 9(3):588–598, 2012 22930416

Moseley GL, Flor H: Targeting cortical representations in the treatment of chronic pain: a review. Neurorehabil Neural Repair 26(6):646–652, 2012 22331213

Mueller HH, Donaldson CCS, Nelson DV, et al: Treatment of fibromyalgia incorporating EEG-driven stimulation: a clinical outcomes study. J Clin Psychol 57(7):933–952, 2001 11406805

Nelson D, Esty M: Neurotherapy of attention deficit/hyperactivity symptoms. J Neuropsychiatry Clin Neurosci 23(2):14, 2011

Nelson DV, Esty ML: Neurotherapy of traumatic brain injury/posttraumatic stress symptoms in OEF/OIF veterans. J Neuropsychiatry Clin Neurosci 24(2):237–240, 2012 22772672

Nelson DV, Esty ML: Neurotherapy for chronic headache following traumatic brain injury. Mil Med Res 2:22, 2015a 26328060

Nelson DV, Esty ML: Neurotherapy of traumatic brain injury/post-traumatic stress symptoms in Vietnam veterans. Mil Med 180(10):e1111–e1114, 2015b 26444476

Nelson DV, Bennett RM, Barkhuizen A, et al: Neurotherapy of fibromyalgia? Pain Med 11(6):912–919, 2010 20624243

Othmer S: A rationale and model for infra-low frequency neurofeedback training. Available at: https://www.eeginfo.com/research/researchpapers/A-Rationale-for-InfraLow-Frequency-Neurofeedback-Training.pdf. Accessed November 27, 2015.

Othmer S, Othmer SF, Kaiser DA, et al: Endogenous neuromodulation at infralow frequencies. Semin Pediatr Neurol 20(4):246–257, 2013 24365573

Pascual-Marqui RD, Esslen M, Kochi K, et al: Functional imaging with low-resolution brain electromagnetic tomography (LORETA): a review. Methods Find Exp Clin Pharmacol 24 (suppl C):91–95, 2002 12575492

Peniston EG, Kulkosky PJ: Alpha-theta brainwave training and beta-endorphin levels in alcoholics. Alcohol Clin Exp Res 13(2):271–279, 1989 2524976

Peniston EG, Kulkosky PJ: Alcoholic personality and alpha-theta brainwave training. Medical Psychotherapy 3:37–55, 1990

Peniston EG, Marrinan DA, Deming WA, et al: EEG alpha-theta brainwave synchronization in Vietnam theater veterans with combat-related post-traumatic stress disorder and alcohol abuse. Advances in Medical Psychotherapy 6:37–50, 1993

Ruiz S, Buyukturkoglu K, Rana M, et al: Real-time fMRI brain computer interfaces: self-regulation of single brain regions to networks. Biol Psychol 95:4–20, 2014 23643926

Schneider F, Elbert T, Heimann H, et al: Self-regulation of slow cortical potentials in psychiatric patients: alcohol dependency. Biofeedback Self Regul 18(1):23–32, 1993 8448237

Schoenberger NE, Shif SC, Esty ML, et al: Flexyx Neurotherapy System in the treatment of traumatic brain injury: an initial evaluation. J Head Trauma Rehabil 16(3):260–274, 2001 11346448

Scott W, Kaiser D: Augmenting chemical dependency treatment with neurofeedback training. J Neurother 3(1):66, 1998

Simkin DR, Thatcher RW, Lubar J: Quantitative EEG and neurofeedback in children and adolescents: anxiety disorders, depressive disorders, comorbid addiction and attention-deficit/hyperactivity disorder, and brain injury. Child Adolesc Psychiatr Clin N Am 23(3):427–464, 2014 24975621

Siniatchkin M, Hierundar A, Kropp P, et al: Self-regulation of slow cortical potentials in children with migraine: an exploratory study. Appl Psychophysiol Biofeedback 25(1):13–32, 2000 10832507

Skinner BF: Science and Human Behavior. New York, Simon & Schuster, 1953

Sokhadze TM, Cannon RL, Trudeau DL: EEG biofeedback as a treatment for substance use disorders: review, rating of efficacy, and recommendations for further research. Appl Psychophysiol Biofeedback 33(1):1–28, 2008 18214670

Sonuga-Barke EJS, Brandeis D, Cortese S, et al: Nonpharmacological interventions for ADHD: systematic review and meta-analyses of randomized controlled trials of dietary and psychological treatments. Am J Psychiatry 170(3):275–289, 2013 23360949

Sterman MB, Howe RC, Macdonald LR: Facilitation of spindle-burst sleep by conditioning of electroencephalographic activity while awake. Science 167(3921):1146–1148, 1970 5411633

Strehl U: Slow cortical potentials neurofeedback. J Neurother 13:117–126, 2009

Tan G, Thornby J, Hammond DC, et al: Meta-analysis of EEG biofeedback in treating epilepsy. Clin EEG Neurosci 40(3):173–179, 2009 19715180

Thornton KE, Carmody DP: Efficacy of traumatic brain injury rehabilitation: interventions of QEEG-guided biofeedback, computers, strategies, and medications. Appl Psychophysiol Biofeedback 33(2):101–124, 2008 18551365

Walker JE: QEEG-guided neurofeedback for recurrent migraine headaches. Clin EEG Neurosci 42(1):59–61, 2011 21309444

Walter WG, Cooper R, Aldridge VJ, et al: Contingent negative variation: an electric sign of sensorimotor association and expectancy in the human brain. Nature 203:380–384, 1964 14197376

Weiskopf N: Real-time fMRI and its application to neurofeedback. Neuroimage 62(2):682–692, 2012 22019880

Wyrwicka W, Sterman MB: Instrumental conditioning of sensorimotor cortex EEG spindles in the waking cat. Physiol Behav 3(5):703–707, 1968

CHAPTER 27

Cranial Electrotherapy Stimulation in the Psychiatric Setting

Jeff Marksberry, M.D.

Michel Woodbury-Farina, M.D.

Timothy Barclay, Ph.D.

Daniel L. Kirsch, Ph.D.

The real voyage of discovery consists not in seeking new landscapes but in having new eyes.

Marcel Proust

The Advent of Cranial Electrotherapy Stimulation

Cranial electrotherapy stimulation (CES) is a noninvasive, U.S. Food and Drug Administration (FDA)–approved prescriptive medical treatment for anxiety, insomnia, and depression. About the size of a smartphone, a CES device uses electrodes typically placed on both earlobes or on the scalp to transmit low-level (<1 mA) pulsed electrical current transcranially to the brain (Kirsch 2009).

The modern era of electromedicine started in 1902, when French physiologist Stéphane Leduc produced sleep in rabbits by the transcranial delivery of 35 V at 110 Hz.

When he administered a similar current to himself, he remained conscious with blunted sensations but could neither move nor speak. After administering a series of 50-V pulses in the milliampere range, he described the experience as similar to "a dream but I was conscious of the absence of power to move and an inability to communicate with my colleagues; I felt the contact, the pinches, striking of pins in my forearm, but the sensations were dulled" (Leduc et al. 1903, p. 403). Despite Leduc's success, his findings failed to arouse much interest outside of France and the former Soviet Union.

In 1914, Louise Robinovitch distinguished between electrically induced sleep and electroanalgesia when she produced sleep in patients with insomnia by applying a negative electrode to the forehead and a positive electrode to the hand. Patients fell asleep within the 1-hour treatment period and continued to sleep after the current stopped (Robinovitch 1914). Researchers have used a variety of frequencies, current levels, waveforms, and electrode configurations. Older CES devices used frequencies ranging from 100 to 4,000 Hz and current intensity up to 8 mA, whereas more recent devices use frequencies as low as 0.5 Hz and current as low as 100 μA (Kirsch 2009).

When CES was introduced in the United States in the 1960s, fewer pharmaceutical treatments were available. Consequently, intense interest was generated by the possibility that CES could provide new treatments for difficult psychiatric disorders. Studies were conducted in university laboratories to identify the mechanisms of action responsible for the clinical responses beginning to be observed.

Researchers documented that CES ensured sound, restful sleep for patients with insomnia and, on the basis of standardized psychological measures, was effective for stress-related symptoms. Psychophysiological measures, including sleep patterns, improved regardless of whether the patient slept during the treatment (Magora et al. 1965). Consequently, the term *electrosleep* was dropped in the United States, although it remained in use in Europe. In 1978, the FDA Neurology Panel renamed the procedure *cranial electrotherapy* and determined that CES would require a prescription, making the United States one of the few countries in which an order from a licensed health care practitioner must be obtained for its use.

In an editorial on psychiatry's future, Henry Nasrallah predicted that "neurostimulation for brain repair" would be one of the top six trends in clinical practice. He pointed out that repetitive transcranial magnetic stimulation, vagal nerve stimulation, and deep-brain stimulation are invasive, costly medical procedures with numerous potential side effects (Nasrallah 2009). In comparison, CES is a noninvasive neurostimulation modality that can be used safely by patients at home as an adjunct to medication or psychotherapy or as stand-alone treatment. The cost of an FDA-cleared CES device in the United States ranges from $700 to $1,200. The only contraindication is the presence of an implanted electrical device, such as a defibrillator. Safety in pregnancy has not been established. The FDA recognizes CES devices for treatment of anxiety, insomnia, and depression (U.S. Food and Drug Administration 2013). Current CES devices deliver frequencies from 0.5 to 15,000 Hz with an intensity of 50 μA to 4 mA.

Mechanisms of Action

Several mechanisms of action of CES have been postulated, involving a direct mode of action on the brain's electrical activity, neurotransmitters, and neurohormones. Animal studies indicated two possible effects: postsynaptic hyperpolarization and alterations in neurotransmitters. Early research identified increased inhibitory processes resulting in analgesia and sleep (Pozos et al. 1968, 1969). A pilot study with nondepressed and depressed patients receiving CES documented increased blood concentrations of serotonin after a single 20-minute session and following 2 weeks of daily 20-minute sessions (Shealy et al. 1989). In a double-blind, randomized placebo-controlled trial (DBRPCT), 20 patients with substance abuse who received 30-minute sessions of CES per day for 4 weeks had increased blood concentrations of monoamine oxidase B ($P<0.05$) and γ-aminobutyric acid (GABA) ($P<0.05$), with corresponding improvements in symptoms, in comparison with the control subjects (Krupitsky et al. 1991).

A small study of five healthy adults reported an increase in cerebrospinal fluid concentrations of serotonin and β-endorphin following 20 minutes of CES. The average increase for β-endorphin was 50% from baseline, although one participant had a 219% increase (Liss and Liss 1996). The generalizability of these data is limited because of the small sample size. Nevertheless, these biochemical changes—increased GABA and β-endorphins—are consistent with clinical findings that CES exerts sedative, anxiolytic, and analgesic effects (Shealy et al. 1998). Increased concentrations of GABA, a major inhibitory neurotransmitter, are associated with reducing anxiety, and sedation is one result of μ opioid receptor stimulation. Several studies reported decreased opioid requirements and increased potency of nitrous oxide in surgical patients receiving CES; increases in β-endorphin were postulated to be the likely mechanism (Mignon et al. 1996; Stanley 1982a, 1982b).

Siegesmund et al. (1967) found that electrical stimulation of the brain tended to force presynaptic vesicles to release their contents into the synaptic space while causing the development of many more presynaptic vesicles. Once the stimulus was terminated, the system tended to return toward normal. These findings strongly suggest that CES is capable of inducing neurotransmitter release and resynthesis, a process known as *turnover*.

Imaging studies and other technologies have been used to explore the physiological processes that occur during CES. One functional magnetic resonance imaging (fMRI) study found that CES causes cortical deactivation in the midline frontal and parietal regions after one 20-minute treatment (Feusner et al. 2012). Another fMRI study reported decreased activity in the pain processing regions of the brain in fibromyalgia patients (Taylor et al. 2013b).

Electroencephalogram (EEG) analysis of patients who received one 20-minute CES treatment showed significant increases in alpha activity (increased relaxation) and decreases in delta activity (increased alertness) and theta activity (increased ability to focus) (Kennerly 2004). The changes in brain wave patterns are thought to represent a calm, relaxed, alert state. These imaging changes coupled with the available neurochemical research help to explain the positive clinical responses reported with CES.

Physiological and Psychological Effects of Cranial Electrotherapy Stimulation on Anxiety

The effects of CES are thought to be mediated through the limbic system, reticular activating system, and hypothalamus (Gilula and Barach 2004). The fMRI research indicates that CES causes cortical brain deactivation and alters connectivity within the default mode network, specifically in the midline prefrontal and parietal regions.

Physiological effects of CES can be attributed to the psychoneuroimmunology response, the interaction between thoughts and behaviors in the central nervous system. Anxiety, depression, and sleep disturbances are associated with dysregulation of the hypothalamic-pituitary-adrenal axis and sympathetic-adrenal-medullary axis. The chronic activation of these interacting systems is thought to influence the production and availability of serotonin, norepinephrine, and dopamine (Rose et al. 2009). A recent DBRPCT ($N=115$) in patients with anxiety and comorbid depression found that 5 weeks of daily CES treatment resulted in a significant change in mean Hamilton Anxiety Scale (Ham-A) scores from a baseline of 29.51 (severe) to 13.37 ($P=0.001$) (Barclay and Barclay 2014). The mean Ham-A end score was 13.37, lower than the mild score range (14–17), indicating reduction to a normal anxiety range. This reduction in anxiety is consistent with results of a previous DBRPCT, which treated mixed anxiety ($P<0.01$) and depressive disorder ($P<0.01$) in children (Chen et al. 2007), and an open clinical trial for generalized anxiety disorder ($P=0.01$) (Bystritsky et al. 2008).

CES can be used as a solo treatment or combined with psychotherapy, as the following case illustrates.

> L.J., a middle-aged single mother with generalized anxiety disorder with obsessive-compulsive tendencies, was seen for evaluation. She had a history of psychotherapy and pharmacotherapy with various selective serotonin reuptake inhibitors, but she was no longer taking medication and remained symptomatic. Her current Ham-A score was 24 (high-moderate). L.J. was concerned about continuing psychotherapy because of limited income and time conflicts with work and child care. Considering L.J.'s concerns and availability, the psychiatrist scheduled her for a 50-minute session, during which he reinforced her previously learned cognitive-behavioral therapy (CBT) skills and taught her the Alpha-Stim AID (anxiety, insomnia, depression; Electromedical Products International, Mineral Wells, Texas) CES protocol for home use, with instructions to use the device 1 hour/day for 5 weeks. L.J. was scheduled for a 15-minute follow-up 2 weeks later and was told to call if she had any problems or questions. At 2-week follow-up, her Ham-A score decreased from 24 to 15 (mild), a 37.5% decrease. After 5 weeks of Alpha-Stim treatment, her Ham-A score was 10, a 58.3% reduction.

The model used in clinical settings can include home CES use, medication, or, as in L.J.'s case, reinforcement of CBT. When used routinely, CES may decrease or obviate the need for medication to treat anxiety or insomnia.

Physiological and Psychological Effects of Cranial Electrotherapy Stimulation on Pain

A body of research exists on the physiological effects of CES on pain management, muscle tension, pulse rate, finger temperature, and electromyography (Donaldson et al. 2001; Kirsch 2009; Lande and Gragnani 2013; Rose et al. 2009; Taylor et al. 2013a). Treatment of chronic pain, particularly from the spine, is often insufficiently effective, and the patient's quality of life is compromised (Tan et al. 2006). In a DBRPCT, CES reduced short-term pain intensity ($n=38$; $P<0.05$) and mitigated long-term pain ($n=24$; $P<0.001$) (Tan et al. 2011). Another DBRPCT ($N=43$) found that patients with fibromyalgia who used an active CES device reported a significant decrease in average pain (McGill Pain Questionnaire, $P=0.023$) and sleep disturbance (General Sleep Disturbance Scale, $P=0.001$) compared with control subjects (Taylor et al. 2013a).

Stress, anxiety, and muscle tension can exacerbate pain and amplify the subjective experience of pain. CES studies also indicate improvements in psychophysiological stress responses such as muscle tension, pulse rate, and finger temperature. Stress, particularly chronic stress, increases muscle tension (electromyogram) and pulse rate and can reduce blood flow to the hands and feet, which lowers the temperature in the extremities. After CES treatment, participants showed reduced muscle tension as seen in electromyogram and pulse rate as well as increased finger temperature as a result of increased blood flow compared with control subjects (Heffernan 1996; Overcash 1999).

Effects of Cranial Electrotherapy Stimulation on Insomnia

In a study by Pearson et al. (2006), of the 18.9% of adults who reported experiencing insomnia, 7% used a complementary and alternative medicine treatment for the following reasons: conventional treatment was not helpful (40.7%); conventional treatment was too expensive (24.8%); or they thought that complementary and alternative interventions were worth a try (66.6%). In one early DBRPCT sleep study, EEG data indicated that after 24 days of 15-minute electrosleep treatments (Electrodorm, manufactured by Electrodorm, France), the treatment group had a statistically significant ($P<0.001$) faster onset of sleep, less time awake, less time in stage 1 sleep, and increased time in delta sleep (including stage 4 sleep) (Weiss 1973). At 14-day follow-up, the treatment group maintained these improvements. No improvements occurred in the sham treatment group. Of note, the largest improvement was in the group whose participants stated that they had quite a bit of difficulty sleeping. A meta-analysis (Kirsch and Gilula 2007a) of 21 published studies of CES for insomnia associated with other conditions (Jadad scores=0–5) included 7 double-blind, randomized controlled trials (RCTs), 3 single-blind RCTs, 4 open-label studies, 4 crossover studies, and 3 survey designs. The mean effect size was 0.64 (large) with a 0.36 standard deviation (Kirsch and Gilula 2007a).

Another meta-analysis (Smith 2007) of 16 studies of CES treatment of insomnia (total $N=648$ patients) included 7 double-blind RCTs, 3 single-blind RCTs, 3 open-label studies, and 3 crossover designs. In these studies, 25% of the patients presented with fibromyalgia, and 25% had drug withdrawal syndrome. However, in most of the studies, insomnia was the presenting diagnosis. Analysis of the pooled studies showed an *r* value (correlation) of 62% (large).

In a double-blind, randomized controlled pilot study (Lande and Gragnani 2013), 57 military service members who scored higher than 21 on the Pittsburgh Insomnia Rating Scale were administered Alpha-Stim SCS (manufactured by Eletromedical Products International) at its lowest effective intensity, 100 μA, which is subsensory. Each group was exposed to daily 60-minute sessions of either Alpha-Stim SCS at 100 μA or sham Alpha-Stim at 0 μA (device has a nonconductive component to prevent treatment) for 5 consecutive days. By the third session, participants had a significant change in total time slept: the treatment group slept 43 minutes more than at baseline; the control subjects averaged 19 minutes less sleep than at baseline. In 3- and 10-day follow-ups, the changes had not endured. A definite trend of the Alpha-Stim was toward increasing time slept when compared with sham; however, it did not reach statistical significance. These encouraging results warrant further study with a larger sample size. Higher levels of intensity (e.g., 300 μA), as are used clinically, should be tested as treatment for insomnia.

Effects of Cranial Electrotherapy Stimulation on Depression

Clinicians routinely treat depressive symptoms that do not meet DSM-5 (American Psychiatric Association 2013) criteria for major depressive disorder (MDD); patients with these symptoms are generally excluded from medication trials or, if included, do not respond well to prescription antidepressants. Nonpharmacological approaches, including CES, are particularly helpful in such cases. Alpha-Stim CES was studied in an RCT of 21 sheriffs who did not meet criteria for a clinical diagnosis of MDD but had signs of depression and anxiety akin to ICD-10 (World Health Organization 1992) mixed anxiety and depressive disorder (Mellen and Mackey 2009). The patients were randomly assigned to Alpha-Stim CES either "on" or "off." After 20 daily sessions, the active CES subjects showed significant improvements in pretreatment and posttreatment Beck Depression Inventory scores ($P<0.01$) compared with those given sham treatment.

One meta-analysis of CES trials for depression (Kirsch and Gilula 2007b) included 20 studies (total $N=937$). Analysis of these 20 studies showed a strong effect size (0.50). A second meta-analysis of 18 trials (total $N=853$) (Smith 2007) found an effect size of 0.47. Few of the studies in this second meta-analysis were of major depression, but most were of depressive symptoms in numerous psychiatric conditions, and they showed positive responses to CES. The heterogeneity of subjects in these studies was a limitation.

Clinicians have limited treatments for subthreshold anxiety and depression in children. In China, a DBRCT of 30 children 8–16 years old diagnosed with mixed anxiety and depressive disorder (Zung Self-Rating Depression Scale and Zung Self-Rating Anxiety Scale) were randomly assigned to two groups that were exposed to Alpha-

Stim CES either "on" or "off." The Alpha-Stim SCS device generates bipolar, asymmetric, rectangular waves with a variable frequency averaging 0.5 Hz. The investigators used the technique of increasing the current until a slight tingling was felt. In the treatment group, the current was decreased to the level at which no sensation was felt, and in the sham group, the current was decreased to "off," which results in no current. Following three cycles of treatment for 15 minutes once a day for 5 consecutive days and then 2 days off for 3 weeks, significant improvements in anxiety ($P<0.01$) and depression ($P<0.01$) occurred in the treatment group compared with the control group. Brain electrical activity mapping showed statistically significant decreases in high baseline alpha 1 and alpha 2 frequencies of the left ($P<0.05$ and $P<0.05$) and right ($P<0.01$ and $P<0.05$) occipital lobes' power measures. These decreases in frequencies indicate that the alpha 1 and alpha 2 became lower, smoother, and slower, a more efficient alpha state that is associated with relaxation (Chen et al. 2007).

In an RCT of anxiety with comorbid depression, 116 patients with a treatment-resistant anxiety disorder with concomitant depression received 5 weeks of active CES or sham (Barclay and Barclay 2014). The Ham-A and Hamilton Rating Scale for Depression (Ham-D) scores were obtained at baseline and at the end of weeks 1, 3, and 5. At the end of the study, when compared with baseline, anxiety and depression scores decreased significantly in the treatment group but not in the sham group. The CES treatment group scores decreased by 50% in 83% of the initial anxiety scores ($P=0.001$) and in 82% of the initial depression scores ($P=0.001$). In the CES treatment group, the decrease in anxiety scores was more than 3 times that in the sham group, and the decrease in depression scores was more than 12 times that in the sham control group.

A recent negative RCT investigated 30 patients with treatment-resistant depression taking antidepressant medications and using a Fisher Wallace CES device (FW-100, manufactured by Fishwer Wallace Industries, New York) (Mischoulon et al. 2015). The mean baseline Ham-D scores reflected moderate depression (18.1 ± 1.5). The patients were given one daily 20-minute active or sham CES treatment 5 days a week for 3 weeks. FW-100 emits three synchronous waveform frequencies: 15 Hz, 500 Hz, and 15,000 Hz, with current ranges from 0 to 4 mA. Neither arm showed any improvements in sleep, but both treatments showed a Ham-D score decrease of three to five points, a significant improvement ($P<0.05$). However, a larger than expected number of side effects occurred, so it is possible that the setting used was not optimal for this population. The current level used was not noted in the article. Participants receiving active treatment complained of poor concentration (59%), decreased energy (35%), fatigue (29%), general malaise (29%), and anxiety (29%); only poor concentration ($P=0.019$) and malaise ($P=0.043$) showed a significant separation from the sham group.

McClure et al. (2015) used the Fisher Wallace CES to study bipolar II depression in 16 patients taking medication. Entry criteria included being diagnosed by the Structured Clinical Interview for DSM-5, being in a depressive episode (Ham-D score=17–28), and not having treatment-resistant depression. The 12-week study had three phases. For the first 2 weeks, patients were randomly assigned double-blind to

CES treatment either "on" or "off." In the second 2-week phase, the nonresponders (Ham-D score≥7) were given active CES in an open protocol (the study did not list the number of patients who qualified for this phase). In the final 8-week phase, participants were given five 20-minute CES sessions per week. The protocol used involved increasing the current until a sensation of tingling was felt and then turning it off for sham treatment or lowering it to the first moment of imperceptibility for active treatment. The investigators found no significant differences between the two groups in any of the mood scales. A further analysis indicated that both groups improved Ham-D scores equally and maintained the gains throughout the study. Clinical Global Impression Scale–Severity and Quality of Life Enjoyment and Satisfaction Questionnaire scores significantly improved ($P=0.023$) in the active treatment group between baseline and week 1. A confounding variable was that patients were undergoing medication changes during the study.

Military Service Member and Veteran Survey

Since the early 2000s, U.S. Department of Defense and Department of Veterans Affairs practitioners have prescribed CES for the treatment of anxiety, posttraumatic stress disorder (PTSD), insomnia, depression, pain, and headaches (Bracciano et al. 2012; Tan et al. 2011). CES is classed as a tier II modality for pain by the Office of the Army Surgeon General's (2010) Pain Management Task Force. When CES is used to treat central pain syndrome, it can also reduce anxiety, insomnia, and depression, common comorbidities of pain. Tan et al. (2010) compared service members' and veterans' preferences for five different therapeutic modalities for decreasing stress, anxiety, insomnia, and pain at a veterans' outpatient pain management clinic. Participants could choose the device they wanted to use and could use a different device if they chose to at future clinic visits. CES was preferred 73% of the time ($N=144$), whereas the other four stress-reducing modalities (StressEraser, manufactured by Helicor Inc., New York; EmWave, manufactured by HeartMath LLC, Boulder Creek, California; RESPeRATE, manufactured by Intercure, Minden, Nevada; and DAVID PaL, manufactured by Mind Alive Inc., Edmonton, Alberta, Canada) were chosen 4%–11% of the time.

As part of a postmarketing surveillance report for the FDA, the manufacturers of the Alpha-Stim CES device conducted a service member and veteran survey to evaluate perceptions of the effectiveness and safety of CES for treatment of anxiety, PTSD, insomnia, depression, pain, and headaches. The survey was sent to a total of 1,514 active duty and veteran service members, and veterans were given an Alpha-Stim device through the Department of Defense at Veterans Affairs Medical Centers from 2006 to 2011. There were 152 surveys returned, for a total response rate of 10%. Respondents were asked to rate their improvement since beginning CES treatments on a seven-point Likert clinical improvement scale. Moderate improvement (50%–74%), marked improvement (75%–99%), and complete improvement (100%) categories were collapsed into one category defined as substantial clinical improvement (≥50%

improvement). The fair clinical improvement category (25%–49%) was designated moderate clinical improvement (Dworkin et al. 2008). Participants in the CES-only group had consistently higher improvement ratings than did those in the CES plus medication group. For example, 100% of the participants in the CES-only group reported either substantial clinical improvement (≥50%) or moderate clinical improvement (25%–49%) in headaches. The CES plus medication group possibly had more serious injuries or medical problems than did the CES-only group, which could account for those findings. Figure 27–1 illustrates the reported improvements for each condition: anxiety, PTSD, insomnia, depression, pain, and headache (Kirsch et al. 2014, 2015). The major limitation of this survey was that it included data only from service members and veterans who chose to complete the survey. Subjects with positive responses to CES could have been more likely to complete the survey than those who did not respond well to CES.

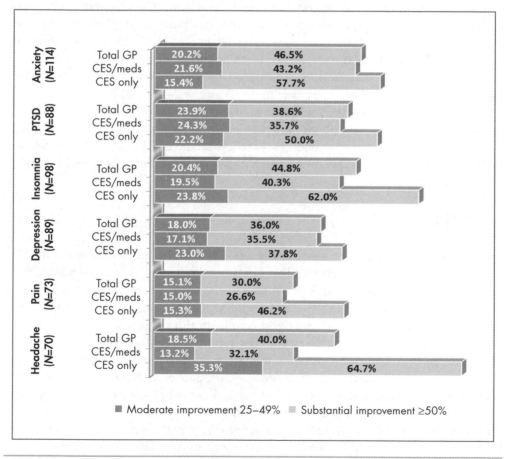

FIGURE 27–1. Response to cranial electrotherapy stimulation (CES) by service members and veterans (*n* =152), 2006–2011.

Note. CES only=CES-alone group; CES/meds=CES plus medication group; PTSD=posttraumatic stress disorder; Total GP=total group.

Clinical Issues

CES can be easily integrated into clinical settings to help alleviate commonly encountered conditions. If used before or during individual or group psychotherapy, CBT, or hypnotherapy, it can decrease anxiety, enabling the patient to engage in therapy and better tolerate working on distressing issues. Clinicians can either refer patients to CES providers or learn how to administer CES devices themselves by using the following resources:

* The American Institute of Stress: www.stress.org/ces-research
* *Bioelectromagnetic and Subtle Energy Medicine*, 2nd Edition, by Paul J. Rosch
* *Cranial Electrotherapy Stimulation: Its First Fifty Years, Plus Three: A Monograph* by Ray B. Smith

Once the clinician decides that a patient might benefit from a trial of CES, the next steps are to educate the patient and then initiate treatment. The physician may obtain a demonstration device for office use. Many patients, particularly those with anxiety disorders or PTSD, are afraid to consider electrostimulation. However, when the physician shows patients the device, which is small and benign looking, they have less fear. Patients also are much more willing to try the device in the office with their trusted physician first than to try it at home alone. Once the patient agrees to treatment, the physician sends the prescription, and the patient orders the device online. For many technologies, compliance is a problem because patients have difficulty taking time out from their busy schedules. One advantage of CES is that it can be used while the patient is engaged in routine activities such as reading, walking, or working on a computer.

Safety

The FDA cleared CES for the treatment of anxiety, depression, and insomnia in 1979. CES is noninvasive and has an excellent safety profile. The FDA, reclassifying CES to a Class II device in the *Federal Register*, stated: "In terms of safety, there is little evidence of device risk" and "In general, CES devices appear to have a favorable long-term safety profile" (U.S. Food and Drug Administration 2016).

No serious adverse effects have ever been reported from using CES (Kirsch 2009). Adverse effects of CES occur infrequently, are mild, and are self-limiting. These include vertigo, skin irritation at electrode sites, headaches, dizziness, decreased concentration, and malaise. Headaches and vertigo are usually experienced when the current is set too high for a particular individual. These effects resolve when the current is reduced or within minutes to hours following treatment. Irritation at the electrode site can be avoided by moving electrodes around slightly during treatments. The only precautions to CES are pregnancy and having a pacemaker or other implanted electrical device (U.S. Food and Drug Administration 2013).

In the Alpha-Stim survey described earlier (Kirsch et al. 2014), 99% of the service members and veterans ($n=152$) considered CES technology to be safe. An important safety benefit of CES is that it leaves the user alert and relaxed after treatment, in contrast to drugs that can have adverse effects on service members' ability to function on missions that require intense focus and attention (Tilgman and McGerry 2013).

Conclusion

CES is being used and studied for anxiety, insomnia, depression, PTSD, pain, substance abuse, and other conditions. Protocols are being tailored for specific conditions and individual sensitivities. Clinician access to information and basic training in CES are essential for this versatile, safe treatment to become fully integrated into psychiatric and medical practice.

KEY POINTS

- Cranial electrotherapy stimulation (CES) is a U.S. Food and Drug Administration–approved medical device for the treatment of anxiety, insomnia, and depression, as prescribed by a licensed health care practitioner in the United States.

- CES uses low-amplitude frequencies to influence brain activity. Functional magnetic resonance imaging studies show cortical deactivation and reduced pain processing; electroencephalograms show increased alpha activity.

- CES has been proven safe; side effects occur in less than 1% of patients. The most common side effects are mild transient headaches, vertigo, and skin irritation at the site of the electrode.

References

American Psychiatric Association: Diagnostic and Statistical Manual of Mental Disorders, 5th Edition. Arlington, VA, American Psychiatric Association, 2013, pp 663–666

Barclay TH, Barclay RD: A clinical trial of cranial electrotherapy stimulation for anxiety and co-morbid depression. J Affect Disord 164:171–177, 2014 24856571

Bracciano AG, Chang WP, Kokesh S, et al: Cranial electrotherapy stimulation in the treatment of posttraumatic stress disorder: a pilot study of two military veterans. J Neurother 16(1):60–69, 2012

Bystritsky A, Kerwin L, Feusner J: A pilot study of safety and efficacy of cranial electrotherapy stimulation in treatment of bipolar II depression. J Clin Psychiatry 69(3):412–417, 2008 18348596

Chen Y, Yu L, Zhang J, et al: Results of cranial electrotherapy stimulation to children with mixed anxiety and depressive disorder. Shanghai Arch Psychiatry 19(4):203–205, 2007

Donaldson CCS, Sella GE, Mueller HH: The neural plasticity model of fibromyalgia. Pract Pain Manag 1(6):25–29, 2001

Dworkin RH, Turk DC, Wyrwich KW, et al: Interpreting the clinical importance of treatment outcomes in chronic pain clinical trials: IMMPACT recommendations. J Pain 9(2):105–121, 2008 18055266

Feusner JD, Madsen JA, Moody TD, et al: Effects of cranial electrotherapy stimulation on resting state brain activity. Brain Behav 2(3):211–220, 2012 22741094

Gilula MF, Barach PR: Cranial electrotherapy stimulation: a safe neuromedical treatment for anxiety, depression, or insomnia. South Med J 97(12):1269–1270, 2004 15646771

Hefferman MS: Comparative effects of microcurrent stimulation on EEG spectrum and correlation dimension. Integr Physiol Behav Sci 31(3):202–209, 1996 8894721

Kennerly RC: QEEG analysis of cranial electrotherapy: a pilot study. J Neurother 8:112–113, 2004

Kirsch DL: The Science Behind Cranial Electrotherapy Stimulation, 2nd Edition. Edmonton, AB, Canada, Medical Scope Publishing, 2009

Kirsch DL, Gilula M: CES in the treatment of insomnia: a review and meta-analysis. Pract Pain Manag 7(7):28–39, 2007a

Kirsch DL, Gilula M: Cranial electrotherapy stimulation in the treatment of depression: part 1. Pract Pain Manag 7(4):33–41, 2007b

Kirsch DL, Price LR, Nichols F, et al: Military service member and veteran self reports of efficacy of cranial electrotherapy stimulation for anxiety, posttraumatic stress disorder, insomnia, and depression. US Army Med Dep J Oct–Dec:46–54, 2014 25830798

Kirsch DL, Marksberry JA, Price LR, et al: Cranial electrotherapy stimulation: treatment of pain and headache in military population. Pract Pain Manag 15(8):57–64, 2015

Krupitsky EM, Burakov AM, Karandashova GF, et al: The administration of transcranial electric treatment for affective disturbances therapy in alcoholic patients. Drug Alcohol Depend 27(1):1–6, 1991 2029855

Lande GR, Gragnani C: Efficacy of cranial electric stimulation for the treatment of insomnia: a randomized pilot study. Complement Ther Med 21(1):8–13, 2013 23374200

Leduc S: La narcose electrique. Zeitschrift fuer Electrotherapie 11(1):374–381, 403–410, 1903

Liss S, Liss B: Physiological and therapeutic effects of high frequency electrical pulses. Integr Physiol Behav Sci 31(2):88–95, 1996 8809593

Magora F, Beller A, Aladjemoff L, et al: Observations on electrically induced sleep in man. Br J Anaesth 37(7):480–491, 1965 5318569

McClure D, Greenman SC, Koppolu SS, et al: A pilot study of safety and efficacy of cranial electrotherapy stimulation in treatment of bipolar II depression. J Nerv Ment Dis 203(11):827–835, 2015 26414234

Mellen RR, Mackey W: Reducing sheriff's officers' symptoms of depression using cranial electrotherapy stimulation (CES): a control experimental study. The Correctional Psychologist 41(1):9–15, 2009

Mignon A, Laudenbach V, Guischard F, et al: Transcutaneous cranial electrical stimulation (Limoge's currents) decreases early buprenorphine analgesic requirements after abdominal surgery. Anaesth Analg 83(4):771–775, 1996 8831319

Mischoulon D, De Jong MF, Vitolo OV, et al: Efficacy and safety of a form of cranial electrical stimulation (CES) as an add-on intervention for treatment-resistant major depressive disorder: a three week double blind pilot study. J Psychiatr Res 70:98–105, 2015 26424428

Nasrallah HA: Psychiatry's future is here: 6 trends to watch that will affect your practice. Current Psychiatry 8(2):16–18, 2009

Office of the Army Surgeon General: Pain Management Task Force Final Report. Washington, DC, Department of the Army, Office of the Surgeon General, May 2010, p 44. Available at: http://www.armymedicine.army.mil/reports/Pain_Management_Task_Force.pdf. Accessed August 2, 2012.

Overcash SL: Cranial electrotherapy stimulation in patients suffering from acute anxiety disorders. American Journal of Electromedicine 16(1):49–51, 1999

Pearson NJ, Johnson LL, Nahin RL: Insomnia, trouble sleeping, and complementary and alternative medicine: analysis of the 2002 National Health Interview Survey data. Arch Intern Med 166(16):1775–1782, 2006 16983058

Pozos RS, Richardson AW, Kaplan HM: Low wattage electroanesthesia in dogs: modification by synaptic drugs. Anesth Analg 47(4):342–344, 1968 5690522

Pozos RS, Richardson AW, Kaplan HM: Mode of production and locus of action of electroanesthesia in dogs. Anesth Analg 48(3):342–345, 1969 5815095

Robinovitch LG: Electrical analgesia, sleep, and resuscitation, in Anesthesia. New York, Appleton, 1914, pp 628–643

Rose KM, Taylor AG, Bourguignon C: Effects of cranial electrical stimulation on sleep disturbances, depressive symptoms, and caregiving appraisal in spousal caregivers of persons with Alzheimer's disease. Appl Nurs Res 22(2):119–125, 2009 19427574

Shealy C, Cady R, Wilkie R, et al: Depression: A diagnostic neurochemical profile and therapy with cranial electrotherapy stimulation. Journal of Neurological and Orthopaedic Medicine and Surgery 10(1):319–321, 1989

Shealy C, Cady R, Culver-Veehoff D, et al: Cerebrospinal fluid and plasma neurochemicals: response to cranial electrostimulation. Journal of Neurological and Orthopaedic Medicine and Surgery 18(2):94–97, 1998

Siegesmund KA, Sances A, Larson SJ: The Effects of Electrical Currents on Synaptic Vesicles in Monkey Cortex. New York, Excerpta Medica Foundation, 1967

Smith, RB: Cranial Electrotherapy Stimulation: Its First Fifty Years, Plus Three: A Monograph. Mustang, OK, Tate, 2007

Stanley TH, Cazalaa JA, Limoge A, Louville Y: Transcutaneous cranial electrical stimulation increases the potency of nitrous oxide in humans. Anesthesiology 57(4):293–297, 1982a 6982009

Stanley TH, Cazalaa JA, Altinault A, et al: Transcutaneous cranial electrical stimulation decreases narcotic requirements during neurolept anesthesia and operation in man. Anesth Analg 61(10):863–866, 1982b 7125252

Tan G, Rintala DH, Thornby JI, et al: Using cranial electrotherapy stimulation to treat pain associated with spinal cord injury. J Rehabil Res Dev 43(4):461–474, 2006 17123186

Tan G, Dao TK, Smith DL, et al: Incorporating complementary and alternative medicine (CAM) therapies to expand psychological services to veterans suffering from chronic pain. Psychol Serv 7(3):148–161, 2010

Tan G, Rintala DH, Jensen MP, et al: Efficacy of cranial electrotherapy stimulation for neuropathic pain following spinal cord injury: a multi-site randomized controlled trial with a secondary 6-month open-label phase. J Spinal Cord Med 34(3):285–296, 2011 21756567

Taylor AG, Anderson JG, Riedel SL, et al: Cranial electrical stimulation improves symptoms and functional status in individuals with fibromyalgia. Pain Manag Nurs 14(4):327–335, 2013a 24315255

Taylor AG, Anderson JG, Riedel SL, et al: A randomized, controlled, double-blind pilot study of the effects of cranial electrical stimulation on activity in brain pain processing regions in individuals with fibromyalgia. Explore (NY) 9(1):32–40, 2013b 23294818

Tilgman A, McGerry B: Medicating the military—use of psychiatric drugs has spiked; concerns surface about suicide, other dangers. Army Times, March 29, 2013. Available at: http://www.militarytimes.com/story/military/archives/2013/03/29/medicating-the-military-use-of-psychiatric-drugs-has-spiked-concerns/78534358. Accessed August 2, 2012.

U.S. Food and Drug Administration: Cranial electrotherapy stimulator. Code of Federal Regulations, Title 21, Vol 8, Sec. 882.5800. Silver Spring, MD, U.S. Food and Drug Administration, 2013

U.S. Food and Drug Administration: 81 FR 3751: Neurological Devices; Reclassification of Cranial Electrotherapy Stimulator Intended to Treat Insomnia and/or Anxiety; Effective Date of Requirement for Premarket Approval for Cranial Electrotherapy Stimulator Intended to Treat Depression. Fed Regist 81(14):3751–3762, 2016

Weiss MF: The treatment of insomnia through the use of electrosleep: an EEG study. J Nerv Ment Dis 157(2):108–120, 1973 4146811

World Health Organization: The ICD-10 Classification of Mental and Behavioural Disorders: Clinical Descriptions and Diagnostic Guidelines. Geneva, World Health Organization, 1992

CHAPTER 28

Integrating Visual Processing Systems in Mental Health Care

Melvin Kaplan, O.D.

Human vision is an extremely powerful information processing system that facilitates our interaction with the surrounding world. Nearly half of our cerebral cortex is busy with processing visual information. From an interactive perspective, the human organism is a spatial action system.

David Marr (Marr 1982)

The Interactive Role of Vision: Psychological and Perceptual Performance

We do not usually think of symptoms that occur in disorders of emotion, cognition, learning, and behavior as involving visual processing dysfunctions, but we should. Visual perceptual deficits can translate into emotion dysregulation, learning disabilities, impaired social skills, poor language skills, motor problems, and a host of other neuropsychiatric symptoms, even in individuals with normal visual acuity.

Studies suggest that delays of infant development are best understood in terms of the interaction of multiple factors of mind-body and world. A child with delayed developmental control in the brain area that governs visual saccade may be seen toe walking as a result of moving too fast to get from point A to B. (For definitions of saccade and other eye movements, see sidebar below.) Visual processing disorders entail an impaired ability to make sense of information taken in through the eyes. Visual processing goes beyond refractive disorders involving sight or clarity of objects. The question often asked by individuals with visual processing disorders is "If I see so well, why do I perform so poorly?"

Four Basic Eye Movements: Saccades, Vergence, Smooth Pursuit, and Vestibulo-ocular

- A *saccade* (French for "jerk") is a quick, spontaneous movement of both eyes between two phases of fixation in the same direction. It can be associated with a shift in frequency of an emitted signal or movement of a body part. Normal saccades are accurate, high-velocity, darting movements, most easily observed during reading or while scanning a scene. Saccades provide brief high-resolution "samples" of the world. Abnormal saccadic eye movements can be observed with eye tracking or by moving a wand. Impaired saccadic eye movements have been associated with schizophrenia. When saccadic eye movements are hypo or hyper—under effort or over effort—the eyes make excessive movements to compensate, which can cause suppressions or compressions during visual processing, thus interfering with visual selective attention. Visuospatial attention is an important mechanism in generating voluntary saccadic eye movements (Hoffman and Subramaniam 1995). Visual perceptual training strongly improves visual motion perception in studies of schizophrenia (Norton et al. 2011).

- *Vergence* is the simultaneous converging of movement from both eyes, which allows the person to maintain a single object in space. The *vergence system* conjugates the movement of the eyes. *Vergence movement* occurs when a target is moved toward the person's eyes along the midline, requiring him or her to converge (bring the eyes toward each other) on the target. Near point of convergence is measured by bringing an object toward the nose and observing at what point the patient sees double.

- *Smooth pursuit movements* are much slower tracking movements of the eyes designed to track a moving object by keeping the visual stimulus on the fovea.

- *Vestibulo-ocular movements* are reflexes that stabilize images on the retinas during head movement by producing eye movements in the direction opposite to head movement, thus preserving the image on the center of the visual field.

Visual processing disorders generate emotional distress. Anxiety stems from the inability to answer the questions "Where am I?" and "Where is it?" Consider how anxious you might be if you could see clearly while driving a car but you had no depth perception. What happens when an individual must visually compress the spatial world in order to maintain some form of homeostasis? This adaptation can impair the ability to distinguish figure from ground and lead to a secondary depression.

Jean Piaget viewed stages of development as a blueprint for normal cognitive development from infancy through adulthood (Piaget et al. 2001). He acknowledged that some children pass through the stages at different ages, some children show characteristics of more than one stage at a given time, stages cannot be "skipped," and each stage is marked by new intellectual abilities and a more complex understanding of the world. Missed developmental steps are a source of visual perceptual difficulties that are associated with and contribute to emotional, cognitive, and behavioral problems. Missing steps during development can contribute to the emergence of learning disabilities. Missed steps in visual information processing may be factors in autistic eye contact and visual attention impairments, schizophrenic problems with visual organization of space, and anxiety issues in many other conditions. Visual processing can be divided into three major developmental stages:

Stage 1: The action-specific child (birth to 10 years)
Stage 2: The adaptive adolescent (11–17 years)
Stage 3: The thought-oriented adult (18 years and older)

In accord with Piaget, some children pass through stages at different ages, and some characteristics of early stages may appear even in the adult learning stage. These complex phenomena can be best understood in terms of the complete interaction of multiple factors: bodily growth, environmental factors, brain maturation, and learning. The ultimate goal is homeostasis with the world in which one lives. Homeostasis entails self-regulation and the ability to maintain a steady state. The purpose of visual intervention is related to the mind's control system. When visually transformed light encounters delays in information processing, the effects include negation of feedback, alterations in perception and performance, and deviation from the expected initiated action. The deviations we may see result in either compression or suppression of visual fields. The goal of a vision specialist is to restore homeostatic control—biologically, emotionally, and socially.

Missing steps leads to the substitution of performance mechanisms according to the functional needs related to the missed steps and their survival importance. Unfortunately, missing steps invariably affects both performance and perceptual adaptation. Missed milestones and compensatory developmental adaptations interfere with attainment of full intellectual potential and underlie many emotional disorders.

Body Schema, Spatial Orientation, and Spatial Organization

To orient ourselves in space, we need to develop a mental model of our body that allows us to organize the information we get from our senses in order to constantly update our position. This mental model or representation is called the *body schema*. Observe a young baby developing her body schema as she discovers herself by moving parts of her body and using her eyes: "Where is my hand?" "What are my fingers doing in space?" "Where does my hand stop and the outside world begin?" Three systems work together to create awareness of our position and movement in space: the *visual* system, the *proprioceptive* system (which provides feedback from muscles, tendons, and skin), and the *vestibular* system. This awareness develops slowly as we age and makes a sudden big leap between ages 7 and 8 years. As children refine their body schema, they master new skills, including rolling over, sitting up, crawling, standing, walking, and running. Most children can achieve these skills fairly easily because the *eyes are leading the mind*. In other words, these children's brains are smoothly and unconsciously processing information from their eyes, allowing them to orient themselves as they move through space.

Spatial orientation refers to our internal development of a body schema. *Spatial organization* refers to the ability to organize the objects and events in our world in relation to one another, ourselves, and other people. Good spatial organization allows us to hit a baseball (because we know our location and can swing accurately toward the location of the ball) or to drive safely in traffic (because we know the position of our own car, the cars around us, and the cars parked to the side). Spatial organization originates with the body schema, which provides a three-dimensional reference point of self. Once we know where we are in space, we can begin to tell left from right and ascertain what is above or below us. We can determine which direction an animal is moving and how quickly it is moving toward or away from us.

Spatial constancy is the ability of the visual system to account for self-motion. The brain determines what the eyes look for, how we process visual information, and the response to environmental demands. The goal of this mind game is spatial constancy. In processing signals from the retina, the brain must compensate for movements of the eyes, head, and body to maintain an accurate image of an object and its location in space—object constancy—and requires an updating of internal representations in response to these movements. Such updating is critically important when remembering spatial information about form movements and events.

The Visual Processing System: A Perceptual Model of Vision

The eyes are optical transformers that create images on the retina. The optic nerve carries visual information from the retina to four brain nuclei: the lateral geniculate nucleus in the thalamus (visual perception), superior colliculus in the midbrain (control of eye movements), pretectum in the midbrain (pupillary light reflex), and suprachiasmatic nucleus in the hypothalamus (diurnal rhythms and hormone regulation). Most lateral geniculate nucleus axons terminate in level V1 of the striate cortex, the primary visual cortex in the occipital lobe, where cortical processing of visual information begins.

From the visual cortex, the information follows two pathways: the *dorsal pathway* and the *ventral pathway* (Figure 28–1). The dorsal pathway tells us where we and other objects are in space, allowing us to respond with a wide range of behaviors, such as walking, touching, or reading. The ventral pathway enables us to recognize specific aspects such that we can identify objects and is involved in judging their significance. The ventral and dorsal pathways are interconnected but act independently. In order to construct an accurate internal model of the world, a foundation for appropriate behaviors, the two systems must complement each other. Failures of complementarity can contribute to problems in learning, mood, and behavior (Kaplan 2015).

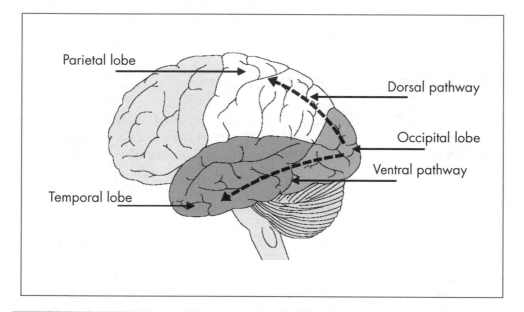

FIGURE 28–1. Visual pathways.

The dorsal pathway runs from the primary visual cortex (V1) in the occipital lobe forward to the parietal lobe, where it is involved in spatial awareness functions. It is responsible for spatial orientation; binocular fusion; depth perception; and determining location, movement, direction, and velocity of objects in space. The ventral pathway runs from the visual cortex (V1) downward into the temporal lobe, where it is affected by attention, working memory, and stimulus salience.

In formulating conceptual models of neural organization for the adaptive interaction of a complex system with its environment, the following general principles have been proposed (Szentágothai and Arbib 1974):

1. The system must be action oriented.
2. The system must perceive not only *what* but also *where*.
3. The adaptive system must be able to correlate sensory data and actions in such a manner as to update its internal model of the world and to modify this internal model to accommodate aspects of the environment not initially provided for in the model.
4. Organization must be hierarchical, with adequate feedback loops to coordinate subsystems. Advantages of this principle include the following: more time is

available for creative problem solving, more space is available for working memory, and new tasks (or similar tasks) are more easily and rapidly learned.

Applying these principles to a visual model of information processing favors a neurological model in which the eyes lead the mind, enabling individuals to perceive, process, and perform optimally. Conversely, when the mind leads the eyes, interferences occur, which impairs perception, processing, and performance. Vision is an emergence of the mind-body world. When the eyes lead the mind through developmental stages, adaptive changes are possible. When developmental stages in visual processing have been skipped, as in patients with attention-deficit/hyperactivity disorder (ADHD), depression, mood disorders, autism spectrum disorder, and schizophrenia, diagnosis and treatment with visual management strategies can be very beneficial.

Visual Processing Disorders

Visual processing disorders are characterized by an impaired ability to make sense of information taken in through the eyes. These disorders differ from refractive problems involving sight or clarity of objects. Disorders of visual processing entail a loss of congruence between the central nervous system and the peripheral nervous system, conscious and preconscious, space and self. This may include a loss of constancy. In cases of developmental delay, the mode of attention is constantly changing, resulting sometimes in reduced responses and at other times exaggerated responses. An example of failure of response is seen in someone who shows no physical reaction to the visual stimulus of a ball when it is thrown to him. Another example is the patient who does not look at a video but instead listens to the sound. In clinical practice, we observe that a developmental delay can lead to the switching on and switching off of peripheral nervous system responses to visual stimuli. In a sense, the mind chooses a different path for interacting with its world. When visual processing malfunctions and fails to negotiate the demands of the environment, the mind may substitute another sensory function, such as touch, sound, smell, or taste, to maintain homeostasis in the world.

Visual processing anomalies have a strong influence on learning disorders, anxiety, mood disorders, autism spectrum disorder, and schizophrenia; however, controversies exist among visual and psychology researchers who study reading disorders. The joint technical report "Learning Disabilities, Dyslexia, and Vision" (Handler et al. 2011) recognized that etiologies are multiple and reflect influences and dysfunction of the brain stem. However, the researchers denied the role of vision and instead considered learning disabilities to be primarily language based. Furthermore, they concluded that evidence was insufficient to support the use of visual therapies such as prisms. They noted that the studies reviewed used diverse practices, protocols, and populations, complicating the analysis.

In contrast, Margaret Livingstone, professor of neurobiology at Harvard Medical School, defined developmental dyslexia as the selective impairment of reading skills despite normal intelligence, sensory acuity, and instruction. Her research showed that visual abnormalities were reported in more than 75% of the children with reading disorders who were tested (Galaburda and Livingstone 1993). It is critical that testing for reading disorder (dyslexia) be multidisciplinary and include thorough testing of the child's sensory function and integration. In the *Optometric Clinical Practice Guideline*, the American Optometric Association Consensus Panel on Care of the Patient With Learning Related Vision Problems supported the position that it is critical that testing for dyslexia be multidisciplinary and that it should include thorough testing of the child's sensory function and integration. The guideline also includes prisms as a valuable treatment (Garzia et al. 2008).

Most studies that fail to show a relation between vision and emotion view refraction as a top-down treatment approach. Conventional treatments that use a top-down model with conscious intention, cognitive control, ocular alignment, and forced attention on focal task may fail to reach individuals in whom visual processing problems underlie learning disabilities.

Autism Spectrum Disorder

Autism spectrum disorder and other learning, neurodevelopmental, and emotional disorders have been shown to be characterized by disruption in autonomic nervous system processing, specifically, increased activity in the sympathetic branch (responsible for how the body functions under stress) and decreased activity in the parasympathetic branches (which counters the sympathetic activity through rest and repose). Therefore, gastrointestinal, cardiovascular, and respiratory symptoms are of concern in individuals with autism spectrum disorder. The study "Effects of Ambient Prism Lenses and Visual-Motor Training on Heart Rate Variability and Behavioral Outcomes in Autism" (Dombroski et al. 2014) supported the hypothesis that prism lenses in combination with standard therapy improves heart-rate variability, hyperactivity, and repetitive behaviors.

Stages of Development

The Action-Specific Child

Developmentally, *action-specific* refers to learning directed toward the control of movement in general and in specific body actions (e.g., balance, walking, eye movements). This includes development and establishment of body schema and orientation to the spatial world. In "ordered" (typical) development, the action-specific child shows attentional preference for right-brain hemisphere dominance. As the child matures, he or she enters the adaptive adolescence stage of development. During this stage, world demands require the mind to shift attention, hence a neurological crossover from visual thinking (right brain) to communicating with others using verbal thinking (left brain) activities. This shift is further driven by changing academic demands as children move from the first six grades to seventh grade. As reading assignments become more difficult, the child must use more complex verbal processing to comprehend what he or she reads.

Adaptive Adolescence and Relaxed Attention

The child who reaches the stage of adaptive adolescence, having successfully shifted attention to bridge the right and the left brain organizations, displays *relaxed attention*. Relaxation is staying loose, and attention involves focusing energy and finding excitement in discovery. A healthy balance allows for focused attention while maintaining varying degrees of relaxation. Individuals who are unable to experience relaxed attention have excess body tension, divert attention, restrict their space, waste energy, lose body awareness, and restrict thought processes. These dysfunctions can distort the body schema (a necessary building block for orienting the mind) and impair awareness of where the body is and where objects are in the world.

We think with our whole being. The ability to maintain relaxed attention is extremely important to brain intelligence. Forced attention can be associated with excessive eye tension, which interferes with eye movements, visual span, and visual organization. Conversely, relaxed attention enhances creativity, imagination, and speed of performance. There are other forms of attention, some undesirable. For instance, individuals who use forced attention cannot sustain attention because of the need for constant reinforcement. They show symptoms of fatigue, loss of depth perception, slowing down to keep their place when reading, and various controlling behaviors. In order to succeed, they are tenacious, focused, and, in many cases, arbitrary.

In the adaptive adolescent, ADHD and other learning difficulties often become more pronounced. During this stage, optimal decision making based in the preconscious senses starts to be overridden by the frontal lobe. Information processing continues to develop as the adolescent grows into the thought-oriented adult in whom conscious cognition becomes dominant. At this stage, disorders of visual processing are related more to selective attention.

Visual Processing Evaluation and Treatment With Yoked Prisms

> The fastest way to change behavior is through a lens.
>
> *A.M. Skeffington*

All optical lenses are light transformers. Conventional optical lenses are designed to correct errors in refraction and positional displacement. Structural problems, such as myopia, hyperopia, and astigmatism, are inherited or acquired problems of visual clarity. The plus or minus and astigmatic corrections alter the flow of information into the central nervous system.

Single-prism lenses are three-sided transparent pyramids, rather than traditional refractive lenses, that are positioned to bend light and affect perception of depth and space. They are used to correct displacement by establishing fusion of the patient's visual field. Prism lenses can differ in strength (diopter). Single prisms are usually prescribed in cases of double vision to achieve single vision. These prisms affect the frontal reference plane, which is perpendicular to the ground and divides the body into dorsal (posterior) and frontal (anterior), supplying two dimensions of information.

Yoked prisms are binocular prism lenses of equal length and strength oriented with the pyramid bases in the same direction. Beyond fusion of the visual field, they lead to establishment of depth perception. Yoked prisms can be used to move the world in a particular direction (up, down, right, or left), depending on the orientation of the prisms. They are prescribed to alter action (performance) and perceptual information of the spatial environment. They affect the sagittal plane, which is perpendicular to the ground and divides the body into right and left halves. The sagittal axis passes from posterior to anterior, whereas the frontal axis passes from left to right. Yoked prisms affect degrees of freedom or motor equivalence in motor control for how we organize movement and orient the interaction of mind, body, and world.

Yoked prism lenses are used during in-office vision therapy and may be prescribed for full- or part-time wear outside the office. In the past 40 years, behavioral optometrists have gone beyond using single prisms for displacement by using yoked prisms of the same magnitude with their bases aligned in the same direction to modify perception, change performance, and improve behavioral adaptation, as is shown in the following clinical examples.

- A child who presented as a toe walker was fitted with large-magnitude yoked prisms oriented base down. He then began to walk with feet flat on the floor instead of on his toes.
- The left shoulder of a scoliosis patient was lower than the right. When the patient was given yoked prisms facing leftward, the left shoulder moved upward to match the level of the right shoulder.
- Many patients with dyslexia or other reading problems respond to yoked prisms added to their current prescription by reading faster with greater comprehension.

Yoked prisms can help identify the underlying mechanism through which neurological systems mediate behavior. During the initial evaluation and trial of yoked prisms, the intent is that spatial rearrangement begin immediately (visual capture) and improve further with ongoing therapy. When properly administered, this treatment has no adverse effects. Once the adaptation has become permanent, the changes have been documented, and the patient no longer notices differences with the lenses on or off, the prisms can be removed. The effects of yoked prisms are outlined in Table 28–1.

Diagnosing Disorders of the Visual Processing System

A comprehensive eye and vision examination includes patient history, visual acuity refraction, eye focusing, eye teaming, eye movement tests, eye examination, and vi-

TABLE 28–1.   Effects of yoked prism alignments

Alignment	Effects
Bases down	This alignment affects rotation about the horizontal axis in space, rotating visual level of attention higher and further away. It leads to slight upward expansion of the field of vision. There is a corresponding effect on vergence movements, improving spatial organization, sense of timing, and awareness of depth.
Bases left	This alignment rotates visual energy input about the vertical axis, moving attention toward the right field of view. It affects orientation, posture, transport (walking), and vergence eye movements.
Bases right	This alignment rotates visual energy input about the vertical axis, moving attention toward the left field of view. It affects orientation, transport (walking), and vergence eye movements.
Bases up	This alignment affects rotation about the horizontal axis in space, rotating visual level of attention to lower, closer field of view. It leads to slight downward tunneling or focusing of field of vision. There is a corresponding effect on vergence movements, improving spatial organization, sense of timing, and awareness of depth.

sual behavioral assessment. A conventional eye examination primarily addresses the "hardware" of the visual system at the level of the eyes rather than the "software" of the visual system at the level of the central and peripheral nervous systems. The hardware examination evaluates what the patient sees. The goal is to make vision clearer using lenses to correct errors in refraction related to the lens or the shape of the eyeball. In contrast, the software examination entails searching for how the patient's brain and body process, respond to, and adapt behaviorally to visual information. Prisms, as used in visual therapy, can alter the mind's processing of visual information according to the principles for adaptation of a complex system to its environment as described in the previous section. The organization of the adaptive system must be hierarchical.

The visual behavioral assessment includes testing measures and observations of behaviors before and after prisms are applied. For example, balance, eye movement, and depth perception can be assessed by observing the performance of an activity, such as catching a ball before and after placement of prisms. The Kaplan Star Test, a test of ambient space perception and parasympathetic nervous system function, is a measure of internal projected action of guided hand movement whose measurements reflect orientation, organization, stability of eye movements, and attention to perceptual illusions formed by "ordered" and "disordered" processing (Figure 28–2) (Kaplan 2015).

The Kaplan Nonverbal Battery, also based on pre- and postprism testing, evaluates performance without the need for verbalization (Kaplan 2015). It assesses three major factors: 1) posture (orientation), the sense of "Where am I?"; 2) levels of atten-

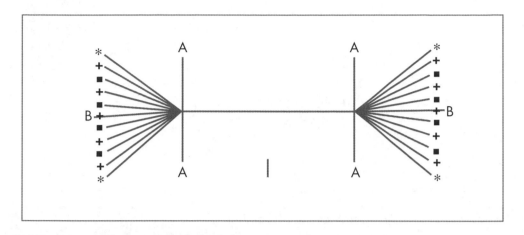

FIGURE 28–2.   Normal Kaplan Star pattern.
Source.   Kaplan M: *Seeing Through New Eyes: Changing the Lives of Children With Autism, Asperger Syndrome and Other Developmental Disabilities Through Vision Therapy.* London, Jessica Kinglsey, 2006, p. 188. Reproduced with permission of Jessica Kingsley Publishers Limited via PLSClear.

tion (organization) and stability of eye movements; and 3) disposition—how the patient responds to action challenges, such as head posture or eye movements.

Interpreting Kaplan Star Patterns

Figure 28–2 shows a normal Kaplan Star pattern. The vertical "A" lines create an illusion of a frontal plane. The horizontal "B" line creates an illusion of the sagittal plane. The A's are associated with postural alignment of the body. The B's are associated with depth perception of the world.

Execution of a normal Kaplan Star pattern requires rapid and accurate interpretation of what the individual sees, generation of a motor response, and maintenance of attention throughout. The appearance of this star pattern is a predictor of spatial behavior, showing the way the person responds to internal and external constraints and depicts his or her version of homeostasis.

Figure 28–3 was drawn by a 13-year-old boy who was at the top of his class academically. He was referred for a visual perceptual analysis because of anxiety, impaired attention, and incoordination. His Kaplan Star Test indicated a visual perceptual disorder characterized by dysfunctions in spatial orientation and spatial organization. Visually, his motor response was to alternately suppress his visual field and his attention. High anxiety, inability to sustain long-term attention, inaccurate sense of body position, and poor control of movements are to be expected. Fortunately, he responded well to yoked prisms oriented bases up, which superimposed his visual field and reduced the number of saccadic eye movements necessary for processing.

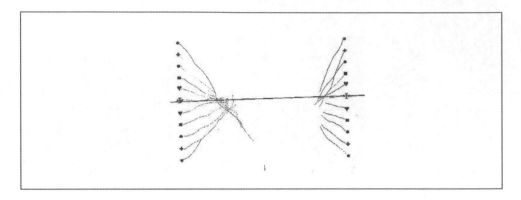

FIGURE 28–3.   Near-point testing in real time.

Interpreting the Skills Test

The skills test is a modified Gesell Battery of the Keystone Skills (Gesell et al. 1970). It provides information about how a disorder of the visual system can generate and operate in a reduced two-dimensional world (Kaplan 2015). Before and after perceptual and performance tests use the kinesthetic and visual senses simultaneously. Kinesthetic sense is the sense of body position and of the movement of body parts relative to one another. The wearing of yoked prisms during the postexamination captures the following neural changes that affect performance:

1. Keeping track of body parts relative to one another
2. Providing constant sensory feedback from muscles in the body during motion
3. Knowing what types of body movement are needed and how to adjust the body in different situations
4. Engaging in a process whereby a stimulus is received, transduced, and conducted as impulses to be interpreted by the brain

The following case exemplifies a visual transformation with yoked prisms.

A 32-year-old stockbroker became nauseated, highly anxious, and emotional when watching the moving news ticker on a screen. During visual testing, when he was asked to look at himself in a mirror from across the room while walking to the mirror, he turned pale and vomited. As soon as yoked prisms, bases up, were placed over his eyes, a smile broke out, and the color in his face returned to normal. He was then able to look in the mirror while walking without any nausea. The bases-up yoked prisms altered his sensory environment, superimposed his visual field, and reduced the number of saccadic eye movements necessary for processing.

Visual Management Therapy

The goal of visual management therapy is to enable individuals to accurately process information about the environment more rapidly, reduce stress, enrich perceptual awareness, and enhance performance. Yoked prisms initiate changes immediately; however, these are fleeting (visual capture), and adaptation is not possible if perceptual rearrangements change radically from moment to moment. Therefore, vision therapy sessions are necessary to stabilize the gains. The changes are tied to movements of the eyes and body parts—the interaction of mind, body, and world. Visual clinical intervention involves three steps: awareness, attention, and automaticity. Specific interventions make the patient consciously aware of visual processing problems. Yoked prisms and visual therapy can reduce the amount of forced or effortful attention a task requires such that attention is commensurate to the task. New developments in visual processing with properly adjusted prisms, over time and with training, replace the previous dysfunctional processes such that self-organization at a higher level of control becomes automatic.

Practice in shifting attention by expanding the visual field of view while maintaining awareness of central field information increases the ability to process more information in less time through relaxed attention. These changes are accompanied by a feeling of well-being, improved short-term memory, and conscious empathy. Changes in attentional focus also have been used to treat physical and psychological pain, as discussed in Chapter 25, "Open Focus Training for Stress, Pain, and Psychosomatic Illness."

Visual management therapy is a global processing program, directed toward establishing the relationship between "figure" and "ground" and further providing context within the perceptual individual's construction of mind and world. Individuals with developmental delays present with major constraints in the ambient visual system's processing capacity and the ability to detect vital information in the complex outer world. In an attempt to cope with these limitations, the processing of ground, the aspect of space in the perceptual field, is reduced. These individuals process figure, a representation of the focal visual tract, at the expense of ground. One consequence is an inability to adjust flexibly to the environment. We can observe that posture, attention, and emotions are modulated to form and improve the relationships between figure and ground in order to reduce or resolve the behavioral characteristics stemming from the developmental delays. When the visual system is overlooked as an etiology contributing to the diagnosis, an integral tool for change is lost. Visual processing of the complex spatial world we live in gives humans more information in less time than any other modality, as the following case illustrates.

Clinical Case: A Two-Dimensional Person Illustrates a Three-Dimensional World

Stephen, a 30-year-old gifted artist, was offered a one-man show at a prestigious New York City gallery. He called my office in a quandary. His inability to sustain visual attention long enough to finish the portfolio of his work for the upcoming show had thrown him into a state of depression. As an artist, Stephen must "capture" the viewer's attention, bring the viewer into the canvas, and move him or her visually around the canvas, creating the illusion of ambiguous depth. Ambiguous depth allows the mind's eye to see phenomena characteristically related to distance and to go one step further to map and read them as being distant. However, Stephen's visual perceptual analysis indicated that he had missed steps in developing depth perception (dorsal pathway information processing of spatial awareness and guidance of movement). He had adapted to his inability to see depth by alternating attention to right and left visual fields by compression and suppression, a strategy that consumed most of his visual energy.

Stephen's visual anomaly was inability to see depth. Yet he created the illusion of depth unambiguously on the basis of geometric principles in the same manner that a surveyor builds roads. Stephen created a unique method to convey the illusion of unambiguous depth. Rather than look directly at the subject he was painting, he would set his line of sight by looking into a mirror to see the reflection of his subject. Stephen used the geometric principle that the angle of incidence equals the angle of reflection to construct the illusion of depth.

Stephen had 20/20 acuity and was free of ocular pathology. Eye movement evaluation found that he was able to track smoothly when standing; however, when he was seated, his tracking was saccadic and jumpy. The implication was that he needed to force his attention when standing and exert greater energy; when seated with his attention relaxed and with exertion, it was harder to stabilize the image on the retina. Stephen's near point of convergence was 10 cm away from his nose, indicating a convergence insufficiency. He also had difficulty releasing his attention from the target object, suggesting that he was using forced attention and alternate suppression.

Stephen's performance on the Kaplan Star Test (Figure 28–4) is a representation of the spatial organization of his world, which was formed inside out by an exhaustive number of alternating saccadic eye movements. This was the etiology of his fatigue and depression. Stephen's visual therapy program used a bottom-up approach. Treatment began with preconscious enlargement of spatial organization, establishing relaxed attention through movement awareness (which is controlled by the peripheral nervous system) and the emergence of sensory integration leading to perceptual adaptation. Both the Kaplan Star Test and analytical testing indicated the need for yoked prisms oriented bases up.

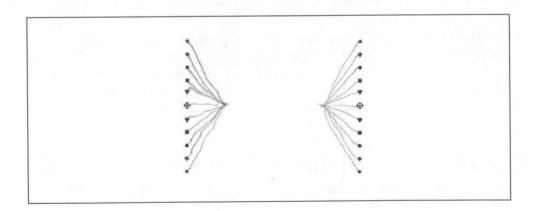

FIGURE 28–4.   Stephen: performance on Kaplan Star Test.

Qualitative observations, before and after the testing sequence with the yoked prisms, were as follows. First was the Disruption Walk and Sit test, a task that required Stephen to walk and sit wearing 20-diopter yoked prisms placed in a sequence: bases down—bases right—bases up—bases left. This was followed by balancing on one foot and then mirror walking wearing 2-diopter bases-up yoked prisms. Stephen showed positive behavioral performance responses to both tasks, as well as to ball bunting, pre and post, seated and standing. Finally, positive behavioral responses occurred in reading with kinesthesiology (motor testing) before and after 2-diopter bases-up prisms posttask. Stephen felt stronger, read faster, and had greater comprehension. See sidebar below for an example of a common treatment sequence using pursuits with disruptive method.

Pursuits With Disruptive Method: Common Treatment Sequence

- Step 1: Patient is seated and asked to track a white Wiffle ball on a string at chest height. The ball passes like a pendulum (note that the patient will exhibit symptoms such as saccadic eye movements, stress, and possibly high blinking rate).

- Step 2: Step 1 is repeated with the patient wearing 20-diopter prisms with bases down in the right eye and bases up in the left with red and green filters underneath.

- Patient becomes aware of suppression and starts to attend to two balls: one red and one green at different heights with smooth eye movement. The lenses are then removed, and patients typically respond by saying, "The room looks bigger; I feel relaxed."

- During step 1, the patient is not consciously aware, but in step 2, the patient is consciously aware. If asked to read a paragraph, the patient is aware of smoother eye movements, increased speed, and greater comprehension of the content.

Stephen's program of visual management entailed wearing a full-time prescription of 2-diopter bases-up prisms and participation in an office- and home-based visual management therapy. He was prescribed a bottom-up visual management program. This type of program begins by stressing the reorganization of saccadic eye movements, the ability to move and breathe simultaneously, and the enrichment of figure and ground organization. These procedures were then integrated with somatic sensory orientation—a developmental process that Stephen had missed—to maintain a semblance of homeostasis with his environment. At the end of the year, his progress in examination measures and observed behaviors showed improved organization, which was apparent in his improved ability to look directly at his subjects and portray depth in his paintings. Stephen no longer felt depressed, and he had considerable reduction in anxiety, insomnia, and fatigue. He was able to read faster with better comprehension and no longer needed to reread. He received many new commissions for murals in restaurants and other businesses.

KEY POINTS

- Dysfunctions in visual processing systems contribute to learning disabilities and may underlie symptoms of attention-deficit/hyperactivity disorder, coordination disorders, anxiety, depression, obsessive-compulsive disorder, autism spectrum disorder, and schizophrenia.

- Evaluation by a behavioral optometrist and visual management therapy can be very beneficial.

- Controlled studies are needed to validate the benefits of various visual therapy approaches, such as eye training and yoked prisms.

References

Dombroski B, Kaplan M, Kotsamanidis-Burg B, et al: Effects of ambient prism lenses and visual-motor training on heart rate variability and behavioral outcomes in autism, in Cutting Edge Therapies for Autism, 4th Edition. Edited by Siri K. New York, Skyhorse, 2014, pp 138–150

Galaburda A, Livingstone M: Evidence for a magnocellular defect in developmental dyslexia. Ann N Y Acad Sci 682:70–82, 1993 8323161

Garzia RP, Borsting EJ, Nicholson SB, et al: Care of the patient with learning related vision problems. Optometric Clinical Practice Guideline. St. Louis, MO, American Optometric Association Consensus Panel on Care of the Patient With Learning Related Vision Problems, 2008. Available at: http://www.aoa.org/documents/optometrists/CPG-20.pdf. Accessed January 12, 2016.

Gesell A, Ilg FL, Bullis G: Vision: Its Development in Infant and Child. Darien, CT, Hafner, 1970

Handler SM, Fierson WM, Section on Ophthalmology, et al: Learning disabilities, dyslexia, and vision. Pediatrics 127(3):e818–e856, 2011 21357342

Hoffman JE, Subramaniam B: The role of visual attention in saccadic eye movements. Percept Psychophys 57(6):787–795, 1995 7651803

Kaplan M: The Secrets in Their Eyes. London, Jessica Kingsley, 2015

Marr D: Vision: A Computational Investigation Into the Human Representation and Processing of Visual Information. New York, Freeman, 1982

Norton DJ, McBain RK, Ongür D, et al: Perceptual training strongly improves visual motion perception in schizophrenia. Brain Cogn 77(2):248–256, 2011 21872380

Piaget J, Piercy M, Berlyne DE: The Psychology of Intelligence. London, Routledge, 2001

Szentágothai J, Arbib MA: Conceptual models of neural organization. Neurosci Res Program Bull 12(3):305–510, 1974 4437759

CHAPTER 29

Using Technology-Based Mind-Body Tools in Clinical Practice

Frederick Muench, Ph.D.

Danusha Selva Kumar, B.A.

Embedded in nearly all health technologies is the opportunity to connect individuals and groups with each other.

Anonymous

Substantial empirical evidence indicates that digital health technologies (DHTs) have tremendous potential to enhance care and deliver stand-alone remote services to individuals seeking to engage in mind-body practices such as meditation, mindfulness, and breathing for stress-related problems, either under the guidance of a health care practitioner or on their own. Scientists and entrepreneurs are now using technology to facilitate mind-body practices. In the broader health care arena, DHTs are transforming how health professionals assess, prevent, and treat physical and mental health problems by delivering interventions via computer, Internet, mobile phone, and wireless or wearable devices.

The technology-based movement for well-being, productivity, and health behavior is a rapidly emerging field with its roots in the early 1960s biofeedback movement, which used technology to enhance awareness of the mind-body connection. Today, countless applications (apps) and new groups are focused on the intersection between technology and meditative practices, such as Consciousness Hacking, Buddhist Geeks, Essential Self, and Positive Technology (Mossbridge 2015). The two main types of mind-body-based feedback systems are biofeedback, which focuses on physiological feedback (e.g., heart rate, skin conductance), and neurofeedback, which uses brain waves and brain activity for feedback. Both have been used as diagnostic and assessment tools for meditative states. For more information on biofeedback, see Chapter 26, "Neurofeedback Therapy in Clinical Practice," and Chapter 3, "Complementary and Integrative Medicine in Child and Adolescent Psychiatric Disorders."

In this chapter, we provide a general review of some of the most common types of technology-based tools for guided meditation, mindfulness, cognitive restructuring, breath retraining, physiological assessment and feedback, and entrainment. Of the thousands of apps, we offer examples of each type, their purported mechanisms of action, and outcomes from the available published controlled studies. We discuss studies of smartphone apps.

Operationalizing the mechanisms of in-person or self-guided meditation and well-being interventions is quite difficult because many practices integrate several interventions (e.g., breath and movement), and most technology-based apps incorporate multiple targets into a single app. Overall, most technology-based apps appear to target the most commonly cited mechanisms of meditation and well-being, such as nonjudgment, connection, autonomy, relatedness, meaning, focus, breath retraining, intentionality, gratitude, empathy, mind and body awareness, and embodiment. However, it is often unclear whether these tools can deliver on the promised goals. Table 29–1 offers a basic overview of the types of technologies, sensors, and data analytic strategies used to foster well-being and help determine which technologies may be optimal for enhancing care. This is followed by a broad overview of basic technologies to enhance well-being.

Technology and Guided Meditation Practice

Meditation Applications

Most meditation apps use technology simply to deliver guided instruction through text, audio, and visual cues on any device. These programs vary in the type of education or guidance they provide but often focus on breathing, body scanning, sitting meditation, walking meditation, loving kindness meditation, thought and emotion regulation retraining, and specific guided meditations (e.g., mountain meditation) (Mani et al. 2015). Some of the apps also contain special features, such as breath detection, holographic theming (i.e., background graphics), ability to support single or multiple users, questions about the users' feelings and emotions, and difficulty levels (Plaza et al. 2013). Most of the apps come with timer and reminder features and include text and videos that explain the concept of mindfulness and meditation to users.

Despite the proliferation of apps, there is a dearth of empirical research, and the existing research is rarely generalizable to real-world settings, where long-term user engagement is uncommon without human support (Mani et al. 2015). Research has found that guided audio and video training can assist users in improving well-being with older tools such as compact discs (Crane et al. 2014). Two small studies have extended this literature to generalize to Web-based and mobile interventions. An app with relaxation training videos outperformed neutral videos by reducing state anxiety

TABLE 29–1. Application of technology components to foster well-being

Component	Potential applications to foster well-being
Text	Reminders, alerts, natural language processing, narratives
Visual display	Any application design, dashboards, visual feedback, guidance, video instruction, virtual reality, augmented reality
Sound	Music, binaural beats, guidance
Camera	Telecounseling, self- and other guidance and modeling, environmental monitoring, physiological monitoring (camera sensors)
Accelerometers and gyroscope	Activity monitoring, behavioral activation, movement, sleep monitoring
Geolocation	Location-based experiences, mapping, activity scheduling
Ambient light and sound sensing	Improved understanding of environment around patient— environmental light and noise, speech prosody, light and sound scanning of physiology
Proximity sensors	Other phones, social gathering, mutual behaviors, crowds
Connection	Social meditation, norms, peer support
General analytics	Phone use, specific application use, social network engagement
Wearables: heart rate, HRV, GSR, EEG	Biofeedback or neurofeedback, arousal assessment, autonomic balance, stress reactions, circadian rhythms
Entrainment or stimulation	Light, sound (e.g., binaural beats), vibration, electrical stimulation, movement, pressure
Other	Nanotechnology to understand physiological symptoms, implants

Note. EEG=electroencephalogram; GSR=galvanic skin response; HRV=heart rate variability.

and increasing coping skills at 4-week follow-up (Villani and Riva 2012). Another randomized controlled trial (RCT) found that listening to a 20-minute self-compassion meditation podcast significantly increased self-compassion and body appreciation compared with a wait-list control (Albertson et al. 2015). Participants from the intervention group also had a significant decrease in body shame, body dissatisfaction, and contingent self-worth based on appearance. Other less rigorous or shorter-term studies have found that computer-based meditation interventions and apps can improve happiness and positive affect (Howells et al. 2014), as well as reduce stress and depression levels (Carissoli et al. 2015; Cavanagh et al. 2013), compared with wait-list or no-treatment control groups.

In an RCT, Ly et al. (2014) compared the effects of an 8-week behavioral activation smartphone app and a mindfulness smartphone app on reducing depressive symptoms. The mindfulness app, which included guided and unguided meditations, audio tracks, and psychoeducation on meditation, was more effective than the behavioral activation app for participants with lower self-reported severity of depression, whereas the behavioral activation app was slightly better for those with more severe depression. In another study, the use of a mindfulness-based decentering app was associated with greater thought distancing than were traditional mindfulness techniques. The app used in this study is a good example of nontraditional uses of technology to foster mechanisms of mindfulness. Users enter negative thoughts into the app and "swipe them away" to distance themselves from the thoughts (Chittaro and Vianello 2014). Interestingly, participants in this study reported preferring the app-based distancing technique to traditional nontechnology-related distancing techniques.

Although research is still in its infancy, apps such as Headspace, Calm, buddhify, The Mindfulness App, and Personal Zen have millions of downloads, indicating an enormous demand for guided meditations. Part of the promise of these apps is that they offer a wide range of practices to the user. For example, Headspace has approximately 350 hours of guided meditation lessons. Mobile apps also are being developed for specific groups or tailored to needs based on an assessment. For example, a mindfulness app called Smiling Mind has a 10-week program tailored to different age groups. Other apps attempt to focus on outcomes through self-report. Buddhify has a mood-tracking component that asks users for mood ratings to track their mood and observe how meditation affects their mood, and users then receive recommendations for certain exercises based on their mood (Mossbridge 2015).

Cognitive-Restructuring Applications

Although positive psychology and cognitive-restructuring apps are more intentional and goal directed, they have significant overlap with meditation apps (Riva et al. 2012). For example, Happify attempts to tailor to individual needs by asking users about their life goals and then recommending specific cognitive-restructuring tracks based on the answers. Some mobile apps also encourage caring and sympathetic behavior (Hughes 2014). One app, Compassion, reports that it facilitates sponsoring poor children in developing countries. Other mobile apps focus on community building: an "I" to "we" shift in which individuals are encouraged to prioritize living in a community and doing volunteer work to help others (Mossbridge 2015). For example, the app Charity Miles gives donations for running, walking, or biking a certain distance.

Although research on the effect of these positive psychology and cognitive-restructuring apps is limited, several studies have reported that they can improve general well-being (Runyan and Steinke 2015). An RCT (N=102) on the effect of directing the user's attention to gratitude and thankful events showed that keeping a diary of gratitude and thankful events led to significantly fewer depressive symptoms and reduced stress levels (Cheng et al. 2015). The stress reduction lasted for 3 months, and the depressive symptoms continued to decrease during the 3-month posttreatment follow-up. In another RCT (N=81), Runyan et al. (2013) reported that individuals who received four daily gratitude reminders had better short-term positive mood compared with control participants who received one message a day or no messaging. However, the effects were not significant after 1 month. A small pilot study (N=90) found that individuals who received basic empathy-related text messages donated more time to helping others and had more prosocial motivations than did the control group receiving no treatment (Konrath et al. 2015).

Unanswered Questions

Despite the demand, several shortcomings in the broad class of meditation apps limit their efficacy as stand-alone interventions. First, people typically do not use unguided apps for more than a few weeks, reflecting a high rate of attrition (Eysenbach 2005), and developers of most products do not release findings on all their users but rather only on those who are highly motivated and compliant. For example, Happify, a cognitive-reframing app, claims that a large percentage of people who use the app "regularly" report being happier. A similar result was released by Live Happy, an app that offers eight happiness-building activities (e.g., gratitude, remembering happy times, present moment attention) based on a naturalistic single-group study, which asserted that those who used the app more often reported greater increases in subjective happiness (Parks et al. 2012). Similarly, results from dose-response studies may be influenced by other confounds such as motivation (Glück and Maercker 2011). One weakness of all of these reports is that without knowing the total number of people who try the app, there is no way to know the percentage who continue to use it. Thus, the subject sample is biased by including only people who like the app well enough to continue using it.

Furthermore, many apps use features that may be at odds with the practice of meditation. For example, approximately 28% of smartphone apps use social media to "show" people how much they have meditated (Mani et al. 2015). Others have dashboards to assess "progress" and other features associated with judgment and striving. Approximately 37% of these apps contain reports or statistics, through either graphs or texts (Plaza et al. 2013). Also, because these apps have so many components and features, sometimes it is hard to dismantle the effects or understand the mechanisms of action. Multiple features may improve user satisfaction but make it very difficult to isolate the mechanisms of action. In addition, many apps claim that they foster mindfulness or meditation when they are merely cognitive-reframing apps or timers (Mani et al. 2015). Although there is little argument against technology being used for mantra meditation (to help with focusing on a single object or sound) or for breath retraining with a pacer, many forms of meditative practice cannot be "technologized" by current approaches. If one's goal is present moment nonstriving and nonjudgmental focus, how would an app that fosters attention to immediately measurable results facilitate the desired mental state?

Certain apps, such as Pause and Personal Zen, target present moment nonjudgmental focus with a few additional features. Each of these apps guides the user to focus on a target and engage with the target nonjudgmentally. Buddha Board apps are available to foster present moment focus while letting go of tangible outcomes by drawing something that disappears after a few moments. Although the effectiveness of these apps is unclear, they are within the framework of the operational definition of mindfulness. Some apps (e.g., Headspace) require monthly fees, but most are inexpensive, and free guided meditations are available for users to test, such as those offered by the UCLA Mindful Awareness Research Center.

Virtual Reality

Virtual reality therapies are emerging as viable technology-based treatments for mental health disorders. Reviews indicate that virtual reality is an empirically supported means to treat phobias, assess cue reactivity for substances, and develop new meditation-focused treatments, although empirical literature on the latter is limited (Gonçalves et al. 2012; Gromala et al. 2015; Kosunen et al. 2016). Products such as DEEP, Guided Meditation VR, and Eden River are being sold directly to consumers for use via virtual reality technologies, including Google Cardboard and Oculus Rift. These technologies create immersive environments where individuals have a closer connection to the target goal (e.g., nature) through interactive avatars, augmented reality paradigms, adaptive virtual worlds, and virtual diagnostic and intervention tools. Although still in their infancy, virtual reality therapies will receive considerably more attention in the near future.

Technology-Guided Breath Awareness and Retraining

Breath awareness and retraining practices, embedded in nearly every form of meditation, mindfulness, yoga, and other practices, are also used in digital tools. As highlighted by Brown et al. (2013), breath retraining is one of the most often developed technology-based meditation tools. It is delivered in a variety of ways, such as guided audio or video tutorials, Web-based and mobile customizable breathing pacers, and computer-based and mobile physiological monitoring and feedback systems. Breathing pacers using sound or visual cues are employed in numerous apps to assist users in learning the proper rate of breathing for a specific goal. However, unlike a live instructor, apps are limited in that they cannot observe and correct a user's improper breathing techniques.

A more fundamental limitation is that many people are unfamiliar with the state of mind they need to achieve. One role of the clinician is to help the patient recognize when he or she has attained the desired state and learn how to maintain it. The use of auditory signals to trigger inspiration and expiration is a simple, easy-to-use tool (Grossman and Taylor 2007). Pacers guide specific breathing rates (e.g., 3.5–5 breaths/minute for arousal reduction and 6 breaths/minute for mental focus). The hundreds, possibly thousands, of breathing pacing apps include those that target specific symptoms or conditions and those built within a meditation app with multiple features. For example, the Do As One app, a simple breath pacer, encourages users to synchronize their breathing with others who are using the same app at the same time to create a feeling of shared experience. Overall, these apps simply guide a user's breathing to a specified pattern. The clinician may help the patient find the apps that are most appropriate and appealing.

In several studies, breathing pacers have been shown to be effective in changing physiological parameters such as heart rate variability (Brown et al. 2013), and in one study they were as good as biofeedback training (Wells et al. 2012). However, in these studies, participants were initially trained by a practitioner on proper breathing and then were taught to use the technology outside of therapy sessions. Proper training is typically not included in most breathing pacers. Because many individuals have trouble learning optimal breathing techniques on their own, it is questionable to generalize the findings of these studies to remote (not guided by a clinician) app practice only. Despite this limitation, breathing pacer apps can be useful in guiding the breathing pace and especially useful when used in combination with biofeedback.

Breath-Based Biofeedback Devices

Office-based biofeedback, one of the oldest forms of technology integrated into mind-body treatments, has expanded into the portable and wearable direct-to-consumer markets. The original home training device introduced in the 1970s was the GSR2, which measured sympathetic arousal via finger skin conductance. Later, computer-based programs appeared (e.g., Journey to Wild Divine), followed by portable devices with computer interfaces (e.g., emWave, StressEraser, NeuroSky, Muse). The current wave offers wearable sensors.

Self-guided ambulatory breath-retraining biofeedback devices have the largest empirical literature base, followed by neurofeedback devices. Reviews of technology-based breath retraining for mental health treatment include numerous studies of depression, anxiety disorders, insomnia, stress, and other disorders (Brown et al. 2013; Wheat and Larkin 2010). Breath-retraining biofeedback systems offer individualized feedback based on targeted physiological parameters, such as respiration rate and heart rate variability (HRV), which are either directly related to respiration or highly correlated with changes in respiration. Respiratory strain gauge systems (e.g., RESPeRATE) can be used to provide direct assessment of respiratory rate. Research on ambulatory strain gauge devices highlights their efficacy in helping individuals breathe properly, reduce blood pressure, and reduce overall arousal (Gavish 2010). However, these devices require the individual to wear a burdensome chest or abdomen strap, which reduces long-term use. Newer consumer devices, such as Spire, measure respiration during activity using a motion sensor worn on the belt or pants, but no research on their efficacy has been published.

Another class of breath-retraining biofeedback is through HRV training. HRV biofeedback is typically performed by sampling real-time heart rates and displaying the natural increases during inspiration and decreases during expiration—a phenomenon called *respiratory sinus arrhythmia*—on the screen alone or with a Fourier transformation of the HRV data into frequency spectra. The goal of HRV biofeedback is to reduce breathing frequency to a rate unique to the individual such that real-time heart rate and respiration covary in a perfect phase relationship (Lehrer et al. 2000; Vaschillo et al. 2004). Ambulatory and office-based HRV biofeedback studies have yielded positive results for anxiety, depression, general stress, performance enhancement, hypertension, and cognitive performance (Gevirtz 2013).

Several HRV biofeedback devices on the market (e.g., emWave/Inner Balance, Sona, and StressEraser) and office-based products are available to practitioners interested in helping clients learn self-regulation through breath-retraining biofeedback and present moment positive emotions. With the advent of heart rate wearables, app designers are trying to integrate HRV assessment into their schema, including mobile apps that use the flashlight to attempt to generate an HRV signal. Because HRV needs a very high sampling rate and accurate sensors compared with simple heart rate measurement, devices that use the smartphone camera to detect a fingertip pulse should be used with caution until they are validated. Newer tools that measure HRV passively to assess autonomic function via video and wearables will soon be available, enabling ongoing passive assessment without the burden of a specific breathing-based device.

Other biofeedback devices do not focus on breath retraining but rather target a change in biological state. Tools that measure and provide feedback on sympathetic arousal via skin conductance and peripheral skin temperature also assess physiological stress. They guide users to alter their physiology with a range of self- and clinician-guided techniques that manipulate the physiological target indirectly. For example, both mindfulness meditation and slowing one's breath may reduce sympathetic arousal as measured through skin conductance. Unlike HRV biofeedback, which requires a specific pace of breathing to manipulate signals, these methods of biofeedback allow more flexibility in the type of practice used to achieve a desired state.

Electroencephalogram (EEG) biofeedback or neurofeedback uses feedback on EEG signals to modify the brain's electrical activity patterns to achieve a desired state. See Chapter 3 ("Complementary and Integrative Medicine in Child and Adolescent Psychiatric Disorders") and Chapter 26 for reviews of clinician-administered neurofeedback therapies. Commercial neurofeedback devices directly available to consumers, such as NeuroSky or Muse, use minimal sensors to obtain basic delta-beta frequencies that help users chart and alter their EEG activity. However, little research is available on the validity of the data collected in real-world settings, user attrition, and long-term outcomes when these devices are used without clinician guidance.

Nearly all forms of biofeedback have a strong empirical base, and consumers enjoy the biofeedback process because it engages them in new awareness and knowledge of their bodies. However, it is unclear whether similar results could be achieved with meditation alone or how the awareness of changes in physiological and neurological activity may serve as a distinct mechanism of action. Biofeedback can be a tool to enhance understanding of the mind-body connection in different contexts and states, thereby providing guidance toward specific goals.

Entrainment

Entrainment entails coupling an exogenous rhythm with an endogenous rhythm to achieve some desired state. Although there are *active* forms of entrainment (e.g., musically based breathing pacers) (Grossman and Taylor 2007), we refer to *passive* entrainment, in which the user is not actively involved in the process but rather passively allows external stimulation to change a physiological parameter, such as brain wave frequencies or heart rate. Several categories of entrainment exist, including music (e.g., binaural beats), brain-based electrical stimulation, and direct nerve stimulation. When presented with two different sound waves at frequencies below 1,500 Hz, the listener will perceive a third tone (an auditory illusion)—a binaural beat—whose frequency equals the difference between the two waves. For example, for waves of 560 Hz and 550 Hz, the binaural beat would be 10 Hz. Numerous binaural beat mobile apps are available for Android and iOS phones. Overall, the literature on binaural beats is limited and mixed, with some studies showing no effects on EEG frequencies (Vernon et al. 2014) and others showing entrainment (da Silva et al. 2015). Some authors suggest that a subset of people respond to binaural beats, although a mechanism that might differentiate responders from nonresponders is unknown.

Transcranial direct current stimulation (tDCS) uses constant and low current to deliver neurostimulation to the brain via scalp electrodes. Used to treat brain injuries and depression, tDCS alters spontaneous cortical activity, thereby altering cognitive processing (Kuo and Nitsche 2012; Meron et al. 2015). The literature on tDCS is fairly robust, with meta-analyses indicating small to moderate effects for depression (Meron et al. 2015). Also, tDCS also appears to benefit working memory in healthy adults and psychiatric populations (Hill et al. 2016). For a review of portable commercial tDCS devices, see Chapter 27, "Cranial Electrotherapy Stimulation in the Psychiatric Setting." Other techniques, such as vagus nerve stimulation, are shifting from surgically implanted devices to direct-to-consumer external stimulation (e.g., NEMOS, a transcutaneous vagal nerve stimulator that consists of a stimulation unit and ear electrode). Overall, research indicates that electrical stimulation entrainment is a promising means to target mechanisms associated with improved mental health and well-being in clinical samples. Clinicians are advised to learn more about new entrainment products as they come onto the market to ensure that they are validated and proven safe and efficacious.

Technology to Enhance Practice

The tools reviewed in this chapter can be used as adjuncts to a clinician's existing practices or as self-help tools. Beyond their function as platforms for disseminating more personalized care, they constitute a therapeutic resource that most health care practitioners cannot provide: objective real-time guidance when the health care provider is not present. Technology-based assessment interventions enhance service delivery by 1) offering new types of services such as biofeedback; 2) extending practice beyond the clinic using practice tools; 3) increasing therapeutic salience of treatment goals and practices through reminders and app-based push alerts; 4) providing ongoing monitoring by objective recording of practice adherence; 5) providing ongoing assessment through real-time data (e.g., wearables) or self-report; 6) employing just-in-time interventions when individuals need them most, on the basis of physiological feedback; and 7) providing social connections through audio, video, and other means to encourage isolated individuals to practice. These tools can be viewed as sequential care guidance on the journey toward self-integration and resilience. Such benefits are driving the wave of new products and services, but we are still in the very early stages of development and understanding regarding their pitfalls and mechanisms of action.

Understanding Limitations of Technologies

Integrating technology into psychiatric care can be as simple as recommending a device, app, or Web site to patients. For some technologies, a basic level of knowledge is sufficient, whereas for others, some advanced training is needed. Practitioners can decide how much technology to integrate into care, depending on their level of comfort and understanding. Before recommending a technology, clinicians are advised to try the technology for themselves for at least 2 weeks to better understand the nuances of the app as well as the burden and effort needed to comply with tasks. For access to more sophisticated biofeedback or virtual reality software, clinicians need to obtain training and oversight or refer the patient to a qualified provider.

Data Security and Privacy

Integrating technology into treatment may pose challenges related to data privacy and confidentiality. Understanding where and how the data are being entered, transmitted, and stored and what type of data are being collected (e.g., personal health care information vs. appointment reminders) requires careful consideration. Because meditation apps and devices usually do not target a specific disease state or diagnosis, there is less concern about the type of data being collected. Regardless, practitioners should be aware of regulations and privacy rules, especially when interacting with patients via technology. For example, social media–based support groups are emerging as a medium for interactive support, but participants need to be informed that social media sites such as Facebook obtain information about their support group activity and participation. Similarly, sending a text message is perhaps the least secure form of communication because texts are stored in multiple databases.

Consent

The consent process must be transparent in presenting the types of data storage and transmission breach risks a participant might be vulnerable to, as well as which organizations might have access to the participant's data. DHT consent forms likely will need to include information such as the scope of digital communication, what information will be communicated and how, inherent privacy risks of communication, security and storage of communication, the use of outside vendors who have access to the communications, security of external vendor apps, procedures for lost provider devices, training on how to secure communication devices, lack of control over timing of digital communication, likelihood of missed communication interaction, the inappropriateness of digital communication as an emergency platform, recorded digital communication as part of the patient's health record, risk of misinterpretation in text-based communication (e.g., cryptic tone or context), possible charges incurred by the patient, protection of agency and agency staff devices, and opt-out and help options (Muench 2014). Understanding each of these components takes careful consideration.

Addressing Patient Concerns

Despite most patients' enthusiasm for DHTs, they have concerns that need to be addressed. First is the Orwellian nature of real-world monitoring when adherence tracking or other passive sensing is used. Patients may not feel comfortable being continuously monitored outside the treatment setting, and some will consider it an intrusion on their privacy. Exploring these feelings and deciding on the appropriate level of monitoring on the basis of patient preferences are often warranted. Second, patients need to be trained in the use of these systems because evidence shows that comfort with technology is a driver of patient use (Ranney et al. 2012). Training should cover how to deal with privacy, communication expectations, emergencies, and service outages. Unfortunately, the cost of the more expensive biofeedback devices and smartphones is beyond what many patients can afford, and clinicians should be sensitive to these economic barriers before recommending specific devices. These factors may limit DHT integration into practice. It is, therefore, imperative to any digital integration effort that treatment providers take into account their population's needs and constraints.

Validation and Targets

One of the greatest concerns associated with devices that measure a physiological parameter or behavioral target (e.g., the steps taken while walking) is obtaining valid real-world data. Many products have not been validated against standard equipment, and many do not have U.S. Food and Drug Administration approval or 510(k) exempt status. Clinicians should be aware of the evidence base for these products and their efficacy. Although a simple customizable breathing pacer needs only face validity, newer entrainment devices should be researched thoroughly. In addition to validation, we need clearer operational definitions of the practices. Trying to provide feedback on an ambiguous target is difficult. What does it mean to increase alpha EEG frequency or stimulate the vagus nerve? Does it constitute meditation, a derivative, or something completely different? What are the ancillary benefits of these practices? How does targeting a specific parameter help or hinder long-standing meditative practices? Such questions need to be addressed as technologies become an integrated part of clinical practice.

Human Support

Technology can drive us more inward, away from meaningful connections and closeness with others (Przybylski and Weinstein 2013). However, technology also can be used to bring us closer together by connecting remotely to loved ones and sharing positive experiences. Use of technologies to connect people who feel isolated to a video chat group peer meditation or a provider-led session is a simple but meaningful advance. Nevertheless, self-guided and peer-based connections for health via technology often have high attrition rates. Mohr et al. (2011) stressed the importance of human accountability in technology-based interventions, particularly because of the demotivating nature of automated human-computer interaction over the long term and ethical concerns about the effects of automated systems on severely ill populations. Overall, technologies are best considered as adjuncts and enhancements to care rather than as substitutes for human contact and guidance.

KEY POINTS

- Stand-alone and adjunctive technologies extend care outside the office or clinic, increase compliance, and provide new tools for patient care.

- Most mobile apps are digitized methods for conventional practices (similar to an audio compact disc or breathing pacer).

- Technology-based apps may benefit patients who have difficulty learning specific techniques or adhering to unstructured practices.

- The evidence base for biofeedback and neurofeedback is robust but is limited for newer mobile apps.

- Before recommending technology-based apps, clinicians are advised to read the literature, consult with experienced colleagues, and try the products themselves.

References

Albertson ER, Neff KD, Dill-Shackleford KE: Self-compassion and body dissatisfaction in women: a randomized controlled trial of a brief meditation intervention. Mindfulness 6(3):444–454, 2015

Brown RP, Gerbarg PL, Muench F: Breathing practices for treatment of psychiatric and stress-related medical conditions. Psychiatr Clin North Am 36(1):121–140, 2013 23538082

Carissoli C, Villani D, Riva G: Does a meditation protocol supported by a mobile application help people reduce stress? Suggestions from a controlled pragmatic trial. Cyberpsychol Behav Soc Netw 18(1):46–53, 2015 25584730

Cavanagh K, Strauss C, Cicconi F, et al: A randomised controlled trial of a brief online mindfulness-based intervention. Behav Res Ther 51(9):573–578, 2013 23872699

Cheng ST, Tsui PK, Lam JH: Improving mental health in health care practitioners: randomized controlled trial of a gratitude intervention. J Consult Clin Psychol 83(1):177–186, 2015 25222798

Chittaro L, Vianello A: Computer-supported mindfulness: evaluation of a mobile thought distancing application on naive meditators. Int J Hum Comput Stud 72(3):337–348, 2014

Crane C, Crane RS, Eames C, et al: The effects of amount of home meditation practice in mindfulness based cognitive therapy on hazard of relapse to depression in the Staying Well After Depression Trial. Behav Res Ther 63:17–24, 2014 25261599

da Silva VF, Ribeiro AP, Dos Santos VA, et al: Stimulation by light and sound: therapeutics effects in humans: systematic review. Clin Pract Epidemol Ment Health 11:150–154, 2015 26161130

Eysenbach G: The law of attrition. J Med Internet Res 7(1):e11, 2005 15829473

Gavish B: Device-guided breathing in the home setting: technology, performance and clinical outcomes. Biol Psychol 84(1):150–156, 2010 20193729

Gevirtz R: The promise of heart rate variability biofeedback: evidence-based applications. Biofeedback 41(3):110–120, 2013

Glück TM, Maercker A: A randomized controlled pilot study of a brief web-based mindfulness training. BMC Psychiatry 11:175, 2011 22067058

Gonçalves R, Pedrozo AL, Coutinho ESF, et al: Efficacy of virtual reality exposure therapy in the treatment of PTSD: a systematic review. PLoS One 7(12):e48469, 2012 23300515

Gromala D, Tong X, Choo A, et al: The virtual meditative walk: virtual reality therapy for chronic pain management. Paper presented at the 33rd Annual ACM Conference on Human Factors in Computing Systems, Seoul, Republic of Korea, 2015

Grossman P, Taylor EW: Toward understanding respiratory sinus arrhythmia: relations to cardiac vagal tone, evolution and biobehavioral functions. Biol Psychol 74(2):263–285, 2007 17081672

Hill AT, Fitzgerald PB, Hoy KE: Effects of anodal transcranial direct current stimulation on working memory: a systematic review and meta-analysis of findings from healthy and neuropsychiatric populations. Brain Stimul 9(2):197–208, 2016 26597929

Howells A, Ivtzan I, Eiroa-Orosa FJ: Putting the 'app' in happiness: a randomised controlled trial of a smartphone-based mindfulness intervention to enhance wellbeing. J Happiness Stud 17(1):163–185, 2014

Hughes JJ: How conscience apps and caring computers will illuminate and strengthen human morality, in Intelligence Unbound: Future of Uploaded and Machine Minds. Edited by Blackford R, Broderick D. Chichester, UK, Wiley, 2014, pp 26–34

Konrath S, Falk E, Fuhrel-Forbis A, et al: Can text messages increase empathy and prosocial behavior? The development and initial validation of text to connect. PLoS One 10(9):e0137585, 2015 26356504

Kosunen I, Salminen M, Järvelä S, et al: Neuroadaptive and immersive virtual reality meditation system. Paper presented at the 21st International Conference on Intelligent User Interfaces, Sonoma, CA, March 2016

Kuo MF, Nitsche MA: Effects of transcranial electrical stimulation on cognition. Clin EEG Neurosci 43(3):192–199, 2012 22956647

Lehrer PM, Vaschillo E, Vaschillo B: Resonant frequency biofeedback training to increase cardiac variability: rationale and manual for training. Appl Psychophysiol Biofeedback 25(3):177–191, 2000 10999236

Ly KH, Trüschel A, Jarl L, et al: Behavioural activation versus mindfulness-based guided self-help treatment administered through a smartphone application: a randomised controlled trial. BMJ Open 4(1):e003440, 2014 24413342

Mani M, Kavanagh DJ, Hides L, et al: Review and evaluation of mindfulness-based iPhone apps. JMIR Mhealth Uhealth 3(3):e82, 2015 26290327

Meron D, Hedger N, Garner M, et al: Transcranial direct current stimulation (tDCS) in the treatment of depression: systematic review and meta-analysis of efficacy and tolerability. Neurosci Biobehav Rev 57:46–62, 2015 26232699

Mohr DC, Cuijpers P, Lehman K: Supportive accountability: a model for providing human support to enhance adherence to eHealth interventions. J Med Internet Res 13(1):e30, 2011 21393123

Mossbridge J: Designing transcendence technology, in Psychology's New Design Science and the Reflective Practitioner. Edited by Imholz SC, Sachter J. New York, Oxford University Press, 2015

Muench F: The promises and pitfalls of digital technology in its application to alcohol treatment. Alcohol Res 36(1):131–142, 2014 26259008

Parks AC, Della Porta MD, Pierce RS, et al: Pursuing happiness in everyday life: the characteristics and behaviors of online happiness seekers. Emotion 12(6):1222–1234, 2012 22642345

Plaza I, Demarzo MMP, Herrera-Mercadal P, et al: Mindfulness-based mobile applications: literature review and analysis of current features. JMIR Mhealth Uhealth 1(2):e24, 2013 25099314

Przybylski AK, Weinstein N: Can you connect with me now? How the presence of mobile communication technology influences face-to-face conversation quality. J Soc Pers Relat 30(3):237–246, 2013

Ranney ML, Choo EK, Wang Y, et al: Emergency department patients' preferences for technology-based behavioral interventions. Ann Emerg Med 60(2):218–27.e48, 2012 22542311

Riva G, Baños RM, Botella C, et al: Positive technology: using interactive technologies to promote positive functioning. Cyberpsychol Behav Soc Netw 15(2):69–77, 2012 22149077

Runyan JD, Steinke EG: Virtues, ecological momentary assessment/intervention and smartphone technology. Front Psychol 6:481, 2015 25999869

Runyan JD, Steenbergh TA, Bainbridge C, et al: A smartphone ecological momentary assessment/intervention "app" for collecting real-time data and promoting self-awareness. PLoS One 8(8):e71325, 2013 23977016

Vaschillo E, Vaschillo B, Lehrer P: Heartbeat synchronizes with respiratory rhythm only under specific circumstances. Chest 126(4):1385–1386, author reply 1386–1387, 2004 15486413

Vernon D, Peryer G, Louch J, et al: Tracking EEG changes in response to alpha and beta binaural beats. Int J Psychophysiol 93(1):134–139, 2014 23085086

Villani D, Riva G: Does interactive media enhance the management of stress? Suggestions from a controlled study. Cyberpsychol Behav Soc Netw 15(1):24–30, 2012 22032797

Wells R, Outhred T, Heathers JA, et al: Matter over mind: a randomised-controlled trial of single-session biofeedback training on performance anxiety and heart rate variability in musicians. PLoS One 7(10):e46597, 2012 23056361

Wheat AL, Larkin KT: Biofeedback of heart rate variability and related physiology: a critical review. Appl Psychophysiol Biofeedback 35(3):229–242, 2010 20443135

Index

*Page numbers printed in **boldface** type refer to tables or figures.*

367